Leong's Manual of Diagnostic Antibodies for Immunohistology

Third Edition

Leong's Manual of Diagnostic Antibodies for Immunohistology

Third Edition

Edited by

Runjan Chetty
The Laboratory Medicine Program, University Health Network,
Toronto, Ontario, Canada

Kumarasen Cooper
University of Pennsylvania Hospital,
Philadelphia, PA, USA

Allen M. Gown
PhenoPath Laboratories, Seattle, WA, and
University of British Columbia, Vancouver, BC, Canada

CAMBRIDGE UNIVERSITY PRESS

CAMBRIDGE
UNIVERSITY PRESS

University Printing House, Cambridge CB2 8BS, United Kingdom

Cambridge University Press is part of the University of Cambridge.

It furthers the University's mission by disseminating knowledge in the pursuit of education, learning and research at the highest international levels of excellence.

www.cambridge.org
Information on this title: www.cambridge.org/9781107077782

© Cambridge University Press, 2016

This publication is in copyright. Subject to statutory exception
and to the provisions of relevant collective licensing agreements,
no reproduction of any part may take place without the written
permission of Cambridge University Press.

First edition published by Greenwich Medical Media Limited, 1999
Second edition by Greenwich Medical Media Limited, 2002
Third edition 2016

Printed in the United Kingdom by Clays, St Ives plc

A catalog record for this publication is available from the British Library

Library of Congress Cataloging in Publication data
Names: Chetty, Runjan, editor. | Cooper, Kumarasen, editor. | Gown, Allen M., editor.
Title: Leong's manual of diagnostic antibodies for immunohistology / edited by Runjan Chetty, The Laboratory Medicine Program, University Health Network, Toronto, Ontario, Canada, Kumarasen Cooper, University of Pennsylvania Hospital, Philadelphia, PA, USA, Allen Gown, PhenoPath Laboratories, Seattle, WA, and University of British Columbia, Vancouver, BC, Canada.
Description: Third edition. | Cambridge, United Kingdom : Cambridge University Press, 2016. | Includes bibliographical references and index.
Identifiers: LCCN 2016026408 | ISBN 9781107077782 (hardback)
Subjects: LCSH: Immunoglobulins – Handbooks, manuals, etc.
Classification: LCC QR186.7 .L46 2016 | DDC 616.07/98 – dc23 LC record available at https://lccn.loc.gov/2016026408

ISBN 978-1-107-07778-2 Hardback

Cambridge University Press has no responsibility for the persistence or accuracy of URLs for external or third-party internet websites referred to in this publication, and does not guarantee that any content on such websites is, or will remain, accurate or appropriate.

....

Every effort has been made in preparing this book to provide accurate and up-to-date information which is in accord with accepted standards and practice at the time of publication. Although case histories are drawn from actual cases, every effort has been made to disguise the identities of the individuals involved. Nevertheless, the authors, editors and publishers can make no warranties that the information contained herein is totally free from error, not least because clinical standards are constantly changing through research and regulation. The authors, editors and publishers therefore disclaim all liability for direct or consequential damages resulting from the use of material contained in this book. Readers are strongly advised to pay careful attention to information provided by the manufacturer of any drugs or equipment that they plan to use.

It is with much nostalgia that we dedicate the third edition of this book to Professor Anthony S.-Y. Leong, BBS, MD, FRCPA who passed away in 2011. In honor of Professor Leong's memory we have decided to entitle the book *Leong's Manual of Diagnostic Antibodies for Immunohistology*. This is a befitting tribute to Tony's brainchild, which was first published in 1999. More importantly, we are deeply indebted to his wife Wendy and children Joel and Trishe for their unconditional support to publish this third edition.

Contents

List of contributors	page xi
Preface to the first edition	xiii
Preface to the second edition	xv
Preface to the third edition	xvii
Note	xviii
Introduction	xix

Section 1: Antibodies

α-Fetoprotein (AFP)	3
α-Smooth muscle actin (α-SMA)	5
AMACR	7
Amyloid	11
Anaplastic lymphoma kinase (ALK)	13
Androgen receptor	15
Anti-apoptosis	17
Arginase-1	21
Bcl-2	23
Bcl-6	25
Ber-EP4	27
β-hCG (human chorionic gonadotropin)	29
BOB-1	31
Brachyury	33
CA125	35
N/97-Cadherin/E-Cadherin	37
CAIX	39
Calcitonin	41
h-Caldesmon	43
Calponin	45
Calreticulin	47
Calretinin	49
Candida albicans	51
Carcinoembryonic antigen (CEA)	53
Catenins α, β, γ	55
CD1	57
CD2	59
CD3	61
CD4	63
CD5	65
CD7	67
CD8	69
CD9	71
CD10 (CALLA)	73
CD11	75
CD15	77
CD19	79
CD20	81
CD21	83
CD23	85
CD24	87
CD25	89
CD30 (Ki-1)	91
CD31	95
CD33	97
CD34	99
CD35	101
CD38	103
CD40	105
CD43	107
CD44	109
CD45 (leukocyte common antigen)	111
CD54 (ICAM-1)	115
CD56 (neural cell adhesion molecule)	117
CD57	119
CD68	123
CD71	125
CD74 (LN-2)	127
CDw75 (LN-1)	129
CD79a	131
CD99 (p30/32^{MIC2})	133
CD103	135
CD117 (KIT)	137
CD123	139
CD138	141
CD163	143
CDK4	145

CDX2 (caudal type homeobox 2)	147	*Helicobacter pylori*	253
c-*erb*B-2 (*HER2, neu*)	149	Hep Par 1 (hepatocyte marker)	255
Chlamydia	153	Hepatitis B core antigen (HBcAg)	257
Chromogranin	155	Hepatitis B surface antigen (HBsAg)	259
c-Myc	157	Herpes simplex virus I and II (HSV I and II)	261
Collagen type IV	159	HHV-8 LANA-1	263
CXCL13	161	HLA-DR	265
Cyclin D1 (Bcl-1)	163	HMB-45 (melanoma marker)	267
Cytokeratins	165	hMLH1 and hMSH2 (mismatch repair proteins)	271
Cytokeratin 5/6 (CK5/6)	169	Human immunodeficiency virus (HIV)	273
Cytokeratin 7 (CK7)	171	Human papillomavirus (HPV)	275
Cytokeratin 19 (CK19)	173	Human parvovirus B19	277
Cytokeratin 20 (CK20)	175	Human placental lactogen (hPL)	279
Cytokeratins: AE1/AE3	177	Immunoglobulins: Igκ, Igλ, IgA, IgD, IgE, IgG, IgM	281
Cytokeratins: 34βE12	179	IgG4	285
Cytokeratins: CAM 5.2	181	Inhibin	287
Cytokeratins: MAK-6	183	Islet1	289
Cytokeratins: MNF116	185	Ki-67 (MIB1, Ki-S5)	291
Other pan-cytokeratin cocktails	187	Laminin	293
Cytomegalovirus (CMV)	189	Mammaglobin	295
Cytotoxic molecules (TIA-1, granzyme B, perforin)	191	MART-1/Melan-A	297
D2-40	193	MDM-2 protein	299
DBA.44 (hairy cell leukemia)	195	Measles	301
Desmin	197	Mel-CAM (CD146)	303
Desmoplakins	199	Mesothelin	305
DOG1	201	Metallothioneins	307
DPC4/SMAD4	203	Microphthalmia transcription factor (MiTF)	309
EMA (epithelial membrane antigen)	205	Mitochondria	311
Epidermal growth factors: EGFR	207	MOC-31	313
Epidermal growth factors: TGF-α	209	MSA (muscle-specific actin)	315
Epstein–Barr virus, LMP	211	MUM1	317
ERG	213	Mutated BRAF V600E	319
Erythropoietin	215	Mutated IDH-1 (mIDH1-R132H, R132S, R132G)	321
Factor VIII RA (von Willebrand factor)	217	Mycobacterial antigen	323
Factor XIIIa	219	Myeloperoxidase	325
Fas (CD95) and Fas-ligand (CD95L)	221	MyoD1	327
Fascin	223	Myogenin	329
Ferritin	225	Myoglobin	331
Fibrin	227	Napsin-A	333
Fibrinogen	229	Neurofilaments	335
Fibronectin	231	Neutrophil elastase	337
Fli-1	233	nm23/*NME1*	339
FMC-7	235	NUT	341
Forkhead box L2 (FOXL2)	237	OCT2	343
GATA binding protein 3 (GATA3)	239	OCT4	345
Glial fibrillary acidic protein (GFAP)	243	OLIG2 (oligodendrocyte transcription factor 2)	347
Glut-1	245	Osteopontin	349
Glypican-3	247	p16	351
Gross cystic disease fluid protein 15 (GCDFP-15, BRST-2)	249	p27^{kip1}	353
		p40	355
HBME-1 (mesothelial cell)	251	p53	357

p63	359
Pancreatic hormones: insulin, somatostatin, vasoactive intestinal polypeptide, gastrin, glucagon, pancreatic polypeptide	361
Parafibromin (CDC73)	365
Parathyroid hormone	367
Parathyroid hormone-related protein (PTHrP)	369
PAX-2 (paired box gene 2)	371
PAX-5	373
PAX-8	375
PD-1	377
P-glycoprotein (P-170), multidrug resistance (MDR)	379
Phosphohistone H3 (pHH3)	381
PIT1 (*POU1F1*)	383
Pituitary hormones: ACTH, FSH, hGH, LH, PRL, TSH	385
PLAP (placental alkaline phosphatase)	389
PMS2	391
Pneumocystis jirovecii	393
Pregnancy-specific β-1-glycoprotein (SP1)	395
Progesterone receptor (PR)	397
Protein gene product 9.5 (PGP 9.5)	399
Proto-oncogene tyrosine-protein kinase 1 (ROS1)	401
pS2	403
PSA (prostate-specific antigen)	405
PSAP (prostate-specific acid phosphatase)	407
PTEN (phosphatase and tensin homolog deleted on chromosome 10)	409
Rabies	411
Retinoblastoma gene protein (P110^{RB}, Rb protein)	413
S100	415
SALL4	417
SDHB (succinate dehydrogenase complex, subunit B)	421
Serotonin	423
Simian virus 40 (SV40 T antigen)	425
SMARCB1	427
Smooth muscle myosin heavy chain	429
SOX9	431
SOX10	433
Spectrin/fodrin	435
Surfactant apoprotein A	437
Synaptophysin	439
Tau	441
T-cell receptor	443
Tenascin	445
Terminal deoxynucleotidyl transferase (TdT)	447
TFE3	449
Thrombomodulin	451
Thyroglobulin	453
TLE1	455
Topoisomerase IIα	457
Transthyretin (prealbumin, TTR)	459
Tyrosinase	461
Tyrosine hydroxylase	463
Ubiquitin	465
Ulex europaeus agglutinin 1 lectin (UEA-1)	467
VEGF (vascular endothelial growth factor)	469
Villin	471
Vimentin	473
VS38	475
WT1	477

Section 2: Appendices

Appendix 1 Selected antibody panels for specific diagnostic situations — 481

1.1	Bone/soft tissue – chondroid-like tumors	481
1.2	Brain – metastatic carcinoma vs. glioblastoma vs. meningioma	481
1.3	Childhood round cell tumors	481
1.4	Gastrointestinal and aerodigestive tract mucosa – basaloid squamous vs. adenoid cystic vs. neuroendocrine carcinoma	482
1.5	Gonads – germ cell tumors vs. somatic adenocarcinoma	482
1.6	Granulocytic sarcoma vs. lymphoma vs. carcinoma vs. plasmacytoma	482
1.7	Intracranial tumors	482
1.8	Liver – hepatocellular carcinoma vs. metastatic carcinoma vs. cholangiocarcinoma	483
1.9	Lung – clear cell tumors	483
1.10	Lymph node – round cell tumors in adults	483
1.11	Undifferentiated round cell tumors	483
1.12	Mediastinal tumors	484
1.13	Nasal tumors	484
1.14	Pelvis – metastatic colonic adenocarcinoma vs. ovarian endometrioid carcinoma	484
1.15	Perineum – prostatic vs. bladder vs. rectal carcinoma	484
1.16	Peritoneum – myxoid tumors	484
1.17	Pleura – mesothelioma vs. carcinoma	485
1.18	Retroperitoneum – renal cell carcinoma vs. adrenocortical carcinoma vs. pheochromocytoma	485
1.19	Retroperitoneum – vacuolated/clear cell tumor	485
1.20	Skin – adnexal tumors	485
1.21	Skin – basal cell carcinoma vs. squamous carcinoma vs. adnexal carcinoma	485
1.22	Skin – pagetoid tumors	486
1.23	Skin – spindle cell tumors	486
1.24	Soft tissue – epithelioid tumors	486
1.25	Soft tissue – spindle cell, fasciculated	486

1.26	Soft tissue – myxoid tumors	487
1.27	Soft tissue – pleomorphic tumors	487
1.28	Extraskeletal myxoid/chondroid tumors	487
1.29	Stomach – undifferentiated spindle cell tumors	487
1.30	Thyroid carcinomas	488
1.31	Urinary tract – spindle cell proliferations	488
1.32	Uterine cervix – endometrial vs. endocervical carcinoma	488
1.33	Uterus – trophoblastic cells	488
1.34	Uterus – immunophenotyping of syncytiotrophoblasts in trophoblastic proliferations	489
1.35	Brain intraventricular tumors	489
1.36	CNS small-cell tumors	490
1.37	Tissue-associated antigens in "treatable tumors"	490
1.38	Epithelial tumors which may co-express vimentin intermediate filaments	490
1.39	Mesenchymal tumors which may co-express cytokeratin	491
1.40	Tumors which may co-express three or more intermediate filaments	491

Appendix 2 Antibody panels for lymphoid neoplasms   493

2.1	Useful markers in B-cell neoplasms	493
2.2	Useful markers of T-cell neoplasms	494
2.3	Markers of Reed–Sternberg cells	494
2.4	Useful markers of monocytes/macrophages	495
2.5	Markers of myeloid cells	495
2.6	Useful markers of natural killer (NK) cells	495
2.7	Markers of follicular dendritic cells	495
2.8	Panel for small-cell lymphomas	496

Appendix 3 Antibody applications   497

Contributors

Sandra D. Bohling, MD
Pathologist and Associate Director of Hematopathology and Clinical PCR Services, PhenoPath Laboratories, Seattle, WA, USA

Runjan Chetty, MBBCh, FFPath, FRCPA, FRCPath, FRCPC, DPhil,
Interim Medical Director, Laboratory Medicine Program, University Health Network, Professor, University of Toronto, Toronto, Canada

Carol Cheung, MD, PhD, JD, FRCPC
Medical Director, Immunopathology Laboratory, Laboratory Medicine Program, University Health Network, Assistant Professor, University of Toronto, Toronto, Canada

Kumarasen Cooper, MBChB, FFPath, FRCPath, DPhil
Professor, University of Pennsylvania Hospital, Philadelphia, PA, USA

Kossivi E. Dantey, MD
Bone and Soft Tissue Pathology Fellow, Department of Pathology, University of Pittsburgh Medical Center, Pittsburgh, PA, USA

Charuhas Deshpande, MD
Associate Professor at the Pennsylvania Hospital, Department of Pathology and Laboratory Medicine, University of Pennsylvania Health System, Philadelphia, PA, USA

Allen M. Gown, MD
Director, PhenoPath Laboratories, Seattle, Washington, USA; and University of British Columbia, Vancouver, BC, Canada

Jui-Han Huang, MD, PhD
Assistant Professor at the Pennsylvania Hospital, Department of Pathology and Laboratory Medicine, University of Pennsylvania Health System, Philadelphia, PA, USA

Harry Hwang, MD
Director, Molecular Pathology, PhenoPath Laboratories, Seattle, WA, USA

Steven J. Kussick, MD, PhD
Associate Medical Director and Director, Hematopathology and Flow Cytometry, PhenoPath Laboratories, Seattle, WA, USA

Priti Lal, MD, FCAP
Associate Professor, Pathology, Perelman School of Medicine, and Director of the GU subdivision at the Department of Pathology, University of Pennsylvania Hospital, Philadelphia, PA, USA

Maria Martinez-Lage, MD
Assistant Professor in Neuropathology and Surgical Pathology, Department of Pathology and Laboratory Medicine, Perelman School of Medicine, University of Pennsylvania, Philadelphia, PA, USA

David Ng, MD
Hematopathologist, PhenoPath Laboratories, Seattle, WA, USA

M. Carolina Reyes MD
Assistant Professor, Department of Pathology, University of Pennsylvania Hospital, Philadelphia, PA, USA

Stefano Serra, MD
University Health Network, Assistant Professor of Pathology, University of Toronto, Toronto, Canada

Stuti G. Shroff, MD, PhD
Assistant Professor of Anatomic Pathology, Department of Pathology and Laboratory Medicine, University of Pennsylvania Hospital, Philadelphia, PA, USA

Kristen M. Stashek, MD
Assistant Professor of Clinical Pathology and Laboratory Medicine, Perelman School of Medicine, University of Pennsylvania, Philadelphia, PA, USA

Preface to the first edition

The rapid acceptance and entrenchment of immunohistochemistry as an important and, in some cases, indispensable adjunct to morphological examination and diagnosis has imposed the necessity for anatomical pathology laboratories to be proficient in immunostaining procedures. However, for immunohistochemical stains to be meaningful, technical competence must be accompanied by a familiarity with the characteristics and specificities of the reagents employed. In particular, the medical technologist and pathologist must have knowledge of the sensitivity and specificity of the primary antibody employed, the nature of the epitope demonstrated by each antibody and its sensitivity to common fixatives. They should be equally conversant with protocols for tissue processing as well as the various methods of antigen/epitope retrieval which are appropriate for the demonstration of the specific protein sought for in the tissue section or cell preparation.

The versatility and contributions of immunohistochemistry to diagnostic pathology, particularly in the areas of tumor diagnosis, lineage identification, prognostication and therapy are largely dependent on the ever-increasing range of antisera and monoclonal antibodies that are commercially available. However, this latter feature is a two-edged sword. While the extensive spectrum of antibodies allows the identification of a wider and wider range of cellular antigens, the user must also be familiar with the properties and characteristics of each of these many antibodies.

This book provides a comprehensive list of antisera and monoclonal antibodies that have useful diagnostic applications in tissue sections and cell preparations. Various clones, which are commercially available to detect the same antigen, are listed and the sensitivities and specificities of the antibodies are discussed. Importantly, our own experience with these reagents is provided together with pertinent references. While as many available sources of antibodies are provided, it is acknowledged that the listing cannot be exhaustive and only major sources are covered. A brief coverage of the diagnostic approach to the general categories of the poorly differentiated round cell and spindle cell tumors in various anatomical sites using panels of selected antibodies is provided in the form of tables. Staining protocols and antigen/epitope retrieval procedures including those employing enzymes, microwaves and heat are also given in detail.

It is hoped that this compendium will provide a source of useful and practical information to both the diagnostic as well as research laboratory.

Anthony S.-Y. Leong
Kumarasen Cooper
F. Joel W.-M. Leong

Preface to the second edition

Since the publication of the 1st edition of this book in 1999, the role of immunohistology in diagnostic pathology has consolidated further and continued to expand. Immunohistology has rapidly become an integral part of microscopic examination and diagnosis, occupying a position of importance only next to the hematoxylin and eosin section and usurping many of the diagnostic roles of histochemical stains and electron microscopy. There is widespread use of immunohistology in diagnostic services throughout the world and in the field of oncologic pathology and as many as 25% of tumors require immunostaining for accurate diagnosis. The percentage is considerably higher in the case of anaplastic and pleomorphic tumors where morphologic features to allow accurate typing of the tumor are absent. With the introduction of Herceptin as the first antibody treatment for cancer, immunolabeling for the Herceptin or c-*erb*B-2 antigen has empowered immunostaining even further. The detection of other antigens such as CD117 (c-*kit*) provides equally important information that predicts response to the specific therapeutic agent SYT-571. Immunostaining is a requirement for the examination of sentinel node biopsies in most treatment protocols. The role of immunostaining in cancer pathology continues to increase so that it now is employed not only for diagnosis but also for other parameters including prognosis, microscopic tumor staging, prediction of response to therapy, and for the selection of specific therapeutic agents. Immunostaining also provides invaluable information for the understanding of tumorigenesis and the identification of carrier states through the identification of gene products.

Automation in immunohistology is well established with a variety of machines employing a number of different patented techniques for antibody incubation. Such instruments have the main advantage of consistency over manual techniques rather than cost or labor savings. Many autoimmunostainers suffer from the disadvantage of rigid incubation times so that overnight incubation of primary antibodies at room temperature or at 4 °C is impossible or difficult to perform as an automated procedure. Optimal conditions for antigen detection have thus given way to expediency.

The threshold of antigen detection continues to be lowered as more sensitive detection methods are developed, the tyramide signal amplification or catalyzed reporter deposition system being a notable example. Modifications of amplification systems that employ multiple antibody layers such as the mirror image complementary antibody (MICA) detection system also continue to be introduced. Such systems increase the cost of the procedure, making it prohibitive to use routinely or in high volumes. Furthermore, they sometimes produce undesirable background staining if not optimally employed.

Undoubtedly, a major milestone in immunohistology was the introduction of heat-induced antigen retrieval, which lowered antigen detection thresholds sufficiently that most proteins of diagnostic interest could be demonstrated with standard detection systems. A variety of methods to generate heat for retrieval have been introduced with minor differences in efficacy so that the method of choice has been very much influenced by familiarity or convenience of use. This was so until the recent demonstration that superheating to 120 °C, attained under pressure, appeared to lower detection thresholds further than conventional methods. This is in keeping with the concept that both time and temperature are major influences in heat-induced antigen retrieval. The pH of the retrieval solution is another major factor, and it has been demonstrated that the majority of antigens are better enhanced following retrieval at alkaline pH. The breaking of protein cross-linkages induced by aldehyde fixatives is the prevalent concept in heat-induced antigen retrieval. However, the true mechanism of antigen retrieval continues to elude us, particularly as it has been shown that ultrasound, which generates negligible heat, can be an effective form of antigen retrieval. Furthermore, microwave heating also enhances immunostaining of tissues fixed in a non-cross-linking fixative such as ethanol, suggesting that heating may unmask epitopes by mechanisms other than through the breakage of cross-linkages.

While the great majority of diagnostic antibodies are highly sensitive, highly specific antibodies are few and far between. Other than those raised to specific gene products most antibodies, at best, are only tissue-selective and their effective usage is to some extent dependent on knowledge of the range of tissues that the reagent may label, specific or otherwise. As often is the case, with the progression of time and usage, newly developed antibodies are found to stain an increasing range of cells besides what they were intended for. Much of this 2nd edition is devoted to this aspect of antibody properties as well as to newer applications. Pertinent references are updated and new diagnostic panels are provided. Also, newly produced antibodies are discussed, particularly as there are now a number of antibodies available that have been raised against specific gene or fusion gene products that are of diagnostic importance.

Anthony S.-Y. Leong
Kumarasen Cooper
F. Joel W.-M. Leong
October 2002

Preface to the third edition

Much of what was written in the prefaces of the first two editions is still pertinent to the practice of immunohistology today, albeit 16 years later, and will not be repeated. Runjan Chetty and Allen Gown are welcome and refreshing additions to the editorship, each bringing his own brand of expertise to this compilation, alongside contributions from many new authors. The format of the first two editions has been retained, with an alphabetic listing of antibodies enabling quick and easy reference, followed by updated tables covering common neoplasms and targeted differential diagnoses. With the burgeoning expansion of available commercial antibodies for immunohistology, this new edition has been enhanced by the addition of several new antibodies, and we are very grateful to the numerous contributors for their valued efforts. In order to maintain the size and weight of this tome, while retaining its usefulness as a manual, the number of quoted references has been restricted to a select few.

Recent years have seen an exponential growth in molecular technology, along with the development of an expanded range of targeted therapies, establishing an enhanced level of standard of care. Key to this molecular evolution, an accurate and complete surgical pathology reporting of neoplasms, supported by equally proficient and excellent immunohistology, remains the diagnostic mainstay leading to efficacious state-of-the-art clinical management of patients. The role of immunohistology as a diagnostic, prognostic, and predictive tool, and, more recently, in the identification of gene products, is still critical for patient care since this technology evolved in the 1970s.

We trust that this compendium of antibodies for the detection of tissue and cellular antigens will be practical and useful for trainees, as well as for both recently initiated and experienced pathologists.

Kumarasen Cooper
Runjan Chetty
Allen M. Gown

Note

Sources/clones lists are not exhaustive. They all refer to antibodies reactive against human epitopes; the search was performed at www.biocompare.com and www.antibodyresource.com, last accessed on November 14, 2014, from Philadelphia, USA.

Introduction

This book discusses diagnostic antibodies and antisera in alphabetical order and provides the background, applications, and diagnostic pitfalls of each reagent, together with pertinent references. Common clones of diagnostic relevance and some sources are listed, but this is not intended to be exhaustive; furthermore, it is mainly antibodies shown to be immunoreactive in fixed paraffin-embedded tissue sections that are discussed, as paraffin sections remain the mainstay of diagnostic histopathology.

Diagnostic approach

Diagnostic antibodies should not be employed in isolation, but always as part of a panel of antibodies directed to the entities considered in differential diagnosis. As the latter is derived from the cytomorphologic appearances of the tumor, it is evident that immunohistochemical diagnosis is morphology-based. For this reason we favor "immunohistology" over the more established term "immunohistochemistry," as it emphasizes the relationship of immunostaining to morphology and that immunostaining is not a test procedure but an integral component of microscopic diagnosis. To assist with the diagnostic process, both antibodies to markers recognized as being expressed by the tumor in question and those associated with entities considered in differential diagnoses should make up the panel. As markers are almost never tissue-specific, the application of a panel of antibodies will generate an immunophenotypic profile comprising both positive and negative findings which, in combination, produce the most accurate results. By defining the immunophenotype of the tissue tested, the errors of false-positive and false-negative staining will be reduced and the highest diagnostic yield obtained. For example, anaplastic large-cell lymphoma has carcinoma and melanoma as morphologic mimics. Anaplastic large-cell lymphoma may express epithelial membrane antigen (EMA) in about 45% of cases, and may fail to stain for CD45 (leukocyte common antigen) in as many cases. These findings, taken in isolation, may be mistaken for those of a carcinoma. However, if antibodies to vimentin, broad-spectrum cytokeratin, S100, and HMB-45 (melanoma-associated antigen) are also employed, the error will be averted as the profile of EMA+, CD45−, VIM+, CK−, S100−, HMB-45− fits best with that of anaplastic large-cell lymphoma, in the context of the differential diagnoses. In some situations it may be necessary to perform the immunostaining in two stages. A primary panel of antibodies provides the major categorization of the tumor, and a secondary panel allows further subtyping. For example, positivity for CD30 will be useful for the confirmation of the diagnosis of anaplastic large-cell lymphoma and lineage typing can be further performed.

As an alternative, the algorithmic approach may be adopted, but whichever approach is favored, it is important that antibodies directed to all entities considered in differential diagnosis be employed. Of course, exceptions to this rule include the application of immunostaining for prognostic markers and the identification of infectious agents in tissue sections.

Standardization and optimization of immunostaining

Much has been discussed about standardization in immunohistology, but this goal is difficult or impossible to achieve simply because fixatives, durations of fixation, and methods of tissue processing employed by laboratories are different. The ability to demonstrate various tissue antigens is very much dependent on their preservation and therefore on the method of fixation and processing employed. With the vastly different practices in laboratories throughout the world, it is clear that standardization as a goal may be impossible to achieve.

It would be more appropriate to aim for optimization of immunostaining within the individual laboratory. This means consistency, reproducibility, and the ability to obtain the optimal results with the method of fixation and processing employed. To this end, it is necessary for each laboratory to adopt a method of fixation and tissue processing which will allow the optimal antigen preservation and yet not compromise cytomorphological preservation. It may be appropriate to examine each fixation and processing step and adjust for optimization, remembering that antigen preservation may also be influenced by the surgeon or physician who has responsibility for placing the excised specimen into the fixative, to avoid the effects of cold ischemic time on immunohistochemistry.

Antigen retrieval

It is imperative to test every new antibody on tissue blocks processed in your own laboratory. While reagent dilutions and tissue preparation instructions provided by the manufacturers are useful guides, they are universal recommendations and not individualized. It is necessary to evaluate various methods of antigen retrieval and to determine, by titration, antibody concentrations that are optimal for tissue processed in your laboratory. The introduction of the heat-induced epitope retrieval (HIER) procedure has contributed significantly to our ability to optimize immunostaining procedures, and HIER must be evaluated for each new antibody used. With very rare exceptions, we have not found HIER to be deleterious to the majority of diagnostic antigens and recommend that it be applied as a routine before any immunostaining is performed. The combination of HIER with enzymatic digestion should also be explored for some antigens. A variety of methods for HIER have become popular, including the use of microwave irradiation, pressure cooker heating, steaming, wet autoclaving, and simple boiling. While there continues to be debate on the actual mechanism of antigen retrieval induced by heating of deparaffinized tissue sections and the role of microwave irradiation, there is general agreement that the threshold of antigen staining is largely dependent on both temperature and the duration of heating. Superheating to 120 °C, attained under pressure, produces the most effective antigen retrieval.

Controls

Diagnostic interpretation in immunohistology includes the assessment of internal positive control cells or tissues. Many test sections contain normal tissue that expresses the antigen being tested. Positive controls should also be used routinely in each antibody staining run, remembering that it is more appropriate to employ neoplastic tissues known to express equivalent amounts of the antigen tested rather than non-lesional tissues that may express much higher levels of antigen. A negative control of tissues known not to express the antigen should also be employed. In addition, a nonspecific negative reagent control should be employed in place of the primary antibody to evaluate nonspecific staining. Ideally, a negative reagent control contains the same isotype as the primary antibody but exhibits no specific reactivity with human tissues in the same matrix or solutions as the primary antibody. All control tissues should be fixed, processed, and embedded in a manner identical to the test sample.

In addition to these technical aspects, consideration should also be given to the nature of the diagnostic specificity of the antibodies used and the properties of the target antigen. Much of this information is theoretical and beyond the control of the diagnostic laboratory. Nonetheless, you should have some familiarity with this aspect of the reagents. The information is often available in the literature, and it may be found in the product profiles provided by the manufacturer.

It is clear from the foregoing that immunohistology is not a simple matter of a positive or negative stain. While it is a powerful diagnostic tool, immunostaining is only an adjunct to histologic examination and requires careful optimization if it is to produce the highest diagnostic yield.

This book contains antibodies and antisera which we consider to be of diagnostic relevance. With the exception of a small number, such as the cytokeratins and the pituitary and pancreatic hormones, the antibodies are discussed separately and listed in alphabetical order for easy reference. The antibodies are listed under their main and alternate names, but specific clone numbers are not indexed.

Selected references

Gown AM, de Wever HT, Battifora H. Microwave-based antigenic unmasking: a revolutionary new technique for routine immunohistochemistry. *Applied Immunohistochemistry* 1993; 1: 256–66.

Gown AM, Leong AS-Y. Immunohistochemistry of "solid" tumors: poorly differentiated round cell and spindle cell tumors II. In Leong AS-Y, ed. *Applied Immunohistochemistry for the Surgical Pathologist*. London: Edward Arnold, 1993, pp. 73–108.

Leong AS-Y. Diagnostic immunohistochemistry: problems and solutions. *Pathology* 1992; 24: 1–4.

Leong AS-Y, Gown AM. Immunohistochemistry of "solid" tumors: poorly differentiated round cell and spindle cell tumors I. In Leong AS-Y, ed. *Applied Immunohistochemistry for the Surgical Pathologist*. London: Edward Arnold, 1993, pp. 23–72.

Leong AS-Y, Haffajee Z, Lee ES, Kear M, Pepperral D. Superheating antigen retrieval. *Applied Immunohistochemistry and Molecular Morphology* 2002; 10: 263–8.

Leong AS-Y, Milios J. An assessment of the efficacy of the microwave antigen-retrieval procedure on a range of tissue antigens. *Applied Immunohistochemistry* 1993; 1: 267–74.

Leong AS-Y, Wick MR, Swanson PE. Immunohistology and ultrastructural features in site-specific epithelial neoplasm–an algorithmic approach. In *Immunohistology and Electron Microscopy of Anaplastic and Pleomorphic Tumors*. Cambridge: Cambridge University Press, 1997, pp. 20–40.

Li X, Deavers MT, Guo M, *et al.* The effect of prolonged cold ischemic time on estrogen receptor immunohistochemistry in breast cancer. *Modern Pathology* 2013; 26: 71–8.

Lin F, Chen Z. Standardization of diagnostic immunohistochemistry: literature review and Geisinger experience. *Archives of Pathology and Laboratory Medicine* 2014; 138: 1564–77.

Shi SR, Key ME, Kalra KL. Antigen retrieval in formalin-fixed, paraffin-embedded tissues: an enhancement method for immunohistochemical staining based on microwave oven heating of tissue sections. *Journal of Histochemistry and Cytochemistry* 1991; 39: 741–8.

Taylor CR. An exaltation of experts: concerted efforts in the standardization of immunohistochemistry. *Applied Immunohistochemistry* 1993; 1: 232–43.

Yildiz-Aktas IZ, Dabbs DJ, Bhargava R. The effect of cold ischemic time on the immunohistochemical evaluation of estrogen receptor, progesterone receptor and HER2 expression in invasive breast carcinoma. *Modern Pathology* 2012; 25: 1098–105.

SECTION 1
Antibodies

α-Fetoprotein (AFP)

Sources/clones

Accurate, Biodesign (polyclonal), Biogenesis (219-2, BIOAFP003, polyclonal), Biogenex (A-013-01), Bioprobe (F2, C3), Cymbus Bioscience (946.11), Dako (polyclonal), Immunotech (IC5, C3), Pierce (ZGAFP1), Sigma (C3), Zymed (ZSA06, ZMAF2, polyclonal).

Fixation/preparation

The antibody is immunoreactive in routinely prepared sections. HIER enhances staining.

Background

α-Fetoprotein (AFP) is a glycoprotein composed of 590 amino acid residues. Cells of the embryonic yolk sac, fetal liver, and intestinal tract synthesize this glycoprotein. By immunostaining, the antigen is detectable in hepatocellular carcinoma, and gonadal and extragonadal germ cell tumors including yolk sac tumors. It is otherwise not present in adult tissues.

Applications

Staining for AFP is largely used for the identification of the glycoprotein in germ cell tumors and in the separation of hepatocellular carcinoma (HCC) from its mimics such as cholangiocarcinoma and metastatic carcinoma in the liver (Appendix 1.8). Unfortunately, although specific, AFP is of low sensitivity and estimated to be present in no more than 44% of hepatocellular carcinomas. Other antibodies employed in a panel may be useful in this context. They include anti-albumin (specific to HCC but not a sensitive marker), cytokeratin 19 (expressed by bile duct epithelium and cholangiocarcinoma), cytokeratin 20 (expressed by both cholangiocarcinoma and gastrointestinal tract tumors), polyclonal CEA (highlights bile canaliculi in HCC but stains the cytoplasm of cholangiocarcinoma and metastatic adenocarcinoma diffusely), α-1-antitrypsin (found in HCC but is of low specificity, being expressed in various carcinomas), sialoglycoproteins such as B72.3 and Leu-M1 (found in some metastatic adenocarcinomas). Other mimics of HCC are hepatoid tumors that have immunophenotypic characteristics similar to that of HCC including staining for AFP, canalicular staining for CEA and α-1-antitrypsin. Such tumors have been seen in ovary, testis, urinary bladder, breast, lung, thymus, stomach, colon, gallbladder, and pancreas, and focally in germ cell tumors, and represent areas of true hepatocellular differentiation.

Comments

A-013-01 is used routinely following HIER.

Selected references

Chedid A, Chejfec G, Eichorst M, et al. Antigenic markers for hepatocellular carcinoma. *Cancer* 1990; 65: 84–7.

Fucich LF, Cheles MK, Thung SN, et al. Primary versus metastatic hepatic carcinoma. An immunohistochemical study of 34 cases. *Archives of Pathology and Laboratory Medicine* 1994; 118: 927–30.

Guindi M. Yazdi HM, Gilliatt MA. Fine needle aspiration biopsy of hepatocellular carcinoma. Value of immunocytochemical and ultrastructural studies. *Acta Cytologica* 1994; 38: 385–91.

Leong AS-Y, Sormunen RT, Tsui WM-S, Liew CT. Immunostaining for liver cancers. *Histopathology* 1998; 33: 318–24.

NOTES

α-Smooth muscle actin (α-SMA)

Sources/clones

Accurate (1A4), Biodesign (asm-1, A4), Biogenex (1A4), Cymbus Bioscience (asm-1), Dako (1A4), Enzo (CGA7), ICN (1A4), Immunotech (1A4), Medac (TCS), Novocastra (asml), RDI (asm-1), Sigma (1A4) and Zymed (Z060).

Fixation/preparation

Several of the antibody clones to α-smooth muscle actin (α-SMA) are immunoreactive in fixed paraffin-embedded sections. HIER at 120 °C enhances immunolabeling.

Background

Cytoplasmic actins vary in amino acid sequences and can be separated by electrophoresis into six different isotopes, all having the same molecular weight of 42 kDa. α-Actins are found in muscle cells, beta- and gamma-actins may be present in muscle cells as well as most other cell types in the body including non-muscle cells. Striated and smooth muscle fibers differ in their expression of actin isotypes, and this has formed the basis for the generation of antibodies directed at muscle-specific actin subtypes. HHF35 (muscle-specific actin) identifies all four actin isoforms present in smooth muscle as well as skeletal muscle cells, pericytes, myoepithelial cells, and myofibroblasts. In contrast, antibodies to α-SMA specifically identify the single α-isoform characteristic of smooth muscle cells and those cells with myofibroblastic differentiation.

Applications

Antibodies to α-SMA are used in several diagnostic situations. These include the identification of myoepithelial cells, which are admixed with epithelial cells in benign proliferative lesions of the breast, salivary, and sweat glands, allowing their distinction from neoplastic proliferations. Myoepithelial cells also line benign ductules of the breast, compared to their absence in neoplastic tubules. α-SMA is also a useful marker to identify myofibroblastic differentiation and has been used in studies of idiopathic pulmonary fibrosis and of the fibrogenic Ito cells in the liver. In diagnostic pathology, α-SMA is used mostly as a discriminator of smooth muscle tumors in the identification of spindled and pleomorphic tumors. It is important to emphasize that this marker should not be used in isolation. Because myogenic determinants are not always synthesized by normal and neoplastic cells simultaneously, the highest diagnostic yield is obtained with a panel of antibodies that include α-SMA, desmin, and muscle-specific actin (Appendix 1.23, 1.24). In the diagnostic context of the morphologically indeterminate spindle cell tumor, it should also be remembered that myofibroblasts might express these myogenic markers. However, expression of desmin tends to be focal and within scattered cells in myofibroblastic proliferations, and these cell types show a thin and fragmented basal lamina compared to the thick, irregular, and long runs of basal lamina around smooth muscle tumors. Myofibroblastic proliferations may display a characteristic "tram-track" pattern of distribution of muscle actins distributed in a subplasmalemmal location. Furthermore, smooth muscle cells may express low-molecular-weight cytokeratin. α-SMA positivity is also observed in adult and juvenile granulosa cell tumors, and in the theca externa and focally in the cortex-medulla of the ovary. Myofibroblastic differentiation is not uncommon in malignant fibrous histiocytoma, so "pleomorphic myofibrosarcoma" has been suggested as an alternative name for this tumor. α-SMA is a useful marker to identify myoepithelial cells and has been used to show the presence of myoepitheliomas in several extrasalivary sites such as the breast, larynx, retroperitoneum, and, more recently, the skin.

Some melanomas may exhibit an aberrant immunophenotype that includes contractile proteins α-SMA and desmin. SMA-positive cells have been suggested to play a role in the pathogenesis of tubulointerstitial damage in the kidney. The significance of muscle actin expression observed in mesotheliomas is presently unknown. α-SMA expression and staining has recently been demonstrated in articular chondrocytes.

Comments

Clone 1A4 produces the best results in our hands. Immunoreactivity appears not to be enhanced by boiling or proteolytic digestion and is best demonstrated following retrieval at 120 °C in citrate buffer at pH 6.0.

Selected references

Banerjee SS, Harris M. Morphological and immunophenotypic variations in malignant melanoma. *Histopathology* 2000; 36: 387–402.

Kinner B, Spector M. Smooth muscle actin expression by human articular chondrocytes and their contraction of a collagen–glycoasaminoglycan matrix in vitro. *Journal of Orthopedic Research* 2001; 19: 233–41.

Kung IT, Thallas V, Spencer EJ, Wilson SM. Expression of muscle actins in diffuse mesothelioma. *Human Pathology* 1995; 26: 565–70.

Kutzner H, Mentzel T, Kaddu S, *et al.* Cutaneous myoepithelioma: an under-recognised cutaneous neoplasm composed of myoepithelial cells. *American Journal of Surgical Pathology* 2001; 25: 348–55.

Leong AS-Y, Milios J, Leong FJ. Patterns of basal lamina immunostaining in soft-tissue and bony tumors. *Applied Immunohistochemistry* 1997; 5: 1–7.

Ohta K, Mortenson RL, Clark RA, *et al.* Immunohistochemical identification and characterization of smooth muscle-like cells in idiopathic pulmonary fibrosis. *American Journal of Respiratory & Critical Care Medicine* 1995; 152: 1659–65.

Raymond WA, Leong AS-Y. Assessment of invasion in breast lesions using antibodies to basement membrane component and myoepithelial cells. *Pathology* 1991; 23: 291–7.

Santini D, Ceccarelli C, Leone O, *et al.* Smooth muscle differentiation in normal human ovaries, ovarian stromal hyperplasia and ovarian granulosa-stromal cell tumors. *Modern Pathology* 1995; 8: 25–30.

AMACR

Sources/clones

Clone 13H4: Biocare Medical, Walnut Creek, CA; Corixa Corporation, Seattle, WA; Zeta, DAKO, Carpinteria, CA, USA

Clone P504S: Abgenix Biopharma Inc., Vancouver, BC, Canada; Zeta Corp, Sierra Madre, CA, USA

Fixation/preparation

Standardized for formalin-fixed paraffin-embedded tissue. Cytoplasmic immunohistochemical stain.

Background

α-Methylacyl CoA racemase (AMACR), also called P504S, is a mitochondrial and peroxisomal enzyme involved in the metabolism of branched chain fatty acid and bile acid intermediates. It catalyzes the racemization of α-methyl branched carboxylic coenzyme A thioesters. Deficiency of AMACR is associated with certain adult-onset sensory motor neuropathies. The National Cancer Institute Cancer Genome Anatomy Project Expressed Sequence Tags (ESTs) and Serial Analysis of Gene Expression (SAGE) databases found variable levels of AMACR protein overexpression in a wide range of tissues and cancers including colorectal, prostate, ovarian, breast, bladder, lung, and renal cell carcinomas. Additionally AMACR is expressed in lymphoma and melanoma. AMACR is thus considered a common abnormality in human cancers and is thought to participate in the early stages of development. Prostate and colorectal carcinomas show the highest expression, at 92% and 83% respectively. In prostate carcinoma, AMACR is overexpressed in high-grade prostatic intraepithelial neoplasia (high-grade PIN), invasive adenocarcinoma, and metastatic androgen-independent prostate cancer. AMACR is extensively used as an adjunct immunohistochemical marker for diagnosis of challenging prostate biopsies.

AMACR has also emerged as a putative therapeutic target in cancer treatment. While overexpression of AMACR is seen in a high percentage of the cancers named above, it is either negative or minimally expressed in the adjacent normal tissue. This property makes it a potential candidate for targeted therapy, either as an antibody or as an enzyme inhibitor.

Applications

A. **Use of AMACR in the diagnosis of prostate carcinoma**

AMACR is a sensitive (82–100%) and relatively specific (70–100%) marker for prostate cancer. It is most specific if circumferential luminal to subluminal and diffuse cytoplasmic staining is noted. It is a commonly used tool in the diagnosis of morphologically difficult prostatic adenocarcinomas, in combination with basal cell markers including p63 and 34BE12 (CK903).

1. **AMACR for evaluation of minimal prostatic adenocarcinoma and atypical proliferations**

    Immunohistochemical assays for AMACR have become part of routine surgical pathology practice during the past few years. A cocktail stain containing racemase along with p63 and CK903 is becoming increasingly common in the workup of atypical small acinar proliferations (ASAPs) and to support the diagnosis of small foci of prostatic adenocarcinomas. Approximately 10% of cases thought to be atypical can be diagnosed as carcinoma after addition of AMACR to the basal cell marker cocktail. Approximately 45% of atypical diagnoses, rendered by experts, converted to a definitive diagnosis of carcinoma after a positive AMACR.

    AMACR staining is not uniform in prostate carcinoma. Approximately 23% of carcinomas are weakly positive, 41% moderately positive, and 35% strongly positive. Histologically benign prostate tissue can sometimes be positive (~8% of cases).

Additionally, premalignant and benign entities that are known to lose basal cell markers may also be positive for AMACR, such as atypical adenomatous hyperplasia (14% of cases), atrophy, partial atrophy, and crowded benign glands.

Conversely, approximately 18% of cases considered to be carcinoma by H&E may be negative for AMACR and basal cell markers. While initial studies suggested that AMACR was uniformly and strongly positive in 97–100% of prostate cancers, more recently only about 82% cancers on needle biopsies were found to be positive.

It is also important to note that unusual morphologic variants including foamy gland, pseudohyperplastic, and atrophic prostate cancers are less frequently positive for AMACR expression, with only 69–80% of cases staining positive. The diagnostic implications of these findings are that while AMACR is a great addition to the armamentarium of stains for the workup of ASAP, it has its limitations. Interpretations based on a positive or negative AMACR should be made with caution, keeping in mind the impression made on H&E.

A cancer diagnosis based on H&E-stained section should not be downgraded to "atypical" on the basis of a negative AMACR.

Use of triple stain (PIN4 cocktail, p63, and 34beta12) or in combination with CK5/6 and p63 is found to increase specificity for detecting prostatic adenocarcinoma in limited needle biopsy material.

2. **AMACR expression in prostatic "pseudoneoplasms"**

   Widely recognized mimics of prostatic adenocarcinoma include atypical adenomatous hyperplasia (AAH), adenosis, atrophy, post-atrophic hyperplasia, basal cell metaplasia, and seminal vesicle or ejaculatory duct epithelium. A small number of AAH cases (4/40) reveal focal staining, hence AMACR staining is helpful in distinguishing most, but not all, cases of AAH from adenocarcinoma. Foci of atrophic glands as well as post-atrophic hyperplasia have been shown to be positive for AMACR in 0–36% of cases.

3. **AMACR staining in post-treatment prostate carcinoma**

   Radiation therapy has no effect on the staining of prostatic adenocarcinoma in needle biopsies, TURP (transurethral resection of prostate) chips, or salvage radical prostatectomies. On the other hand, benign glands with radiation atypia are found to be negative. A significant decrease in the intensity of AMACR staining is noted in hormone-refractory prostatic adenocarcinoma when compared to clinically localized cancer. To assess residual post-treatment prostatic adenocarcinoma, a panel of stains containing AMACR is useful.

B. **AMACR in renal tumors**

   Contemporary classification of renal tumors is based on clinical, morphological, and molecular genetic characteristics. With the emergence of numerous distinct genetic subtypes, often with overlapping histological features, immunohistochemical stains have come to play an increasingly important role in their accurate classification. AMACR has been found to be strongly expressed in papillary renal cell carcinomas, mucinous tubular and spindle cell carcinoma, and acquired cystic disease-associated renal cell carcinoma (RCC).

   In a poorly differentiated RCC, or in cases with overlapping histological appearances, AMACR forms a useful adjunct.

   Renal tumors with clear and papillary features are often encountered in our daily practice. In this setting the differential diagnoses will include CCRCC (clear cell renal cell carcinoma), PRCC (papillary renal cell carcinoma) with clear cell changes, CCPRCC (clear cell papillary renal cell carcinoma), and Xp11 translocation RCC. While the majority of CCRCCs present with sheet-like growth patterns, rarely, true papillae can be seen. PRCCs can have clear cells, and Xp11.2 translocation RCCs can have clear cells growing as solid sheets and/or lining true papillae. Given the overlapping histological features of these genetically and prognostically distinct entities, immunohistochemical stains for accurate classification become essential.

   A panel of stains that includes CAIX, CK7, AMACR, TFE3, and cathepsin K can be used as follows:
   - CCRCC is positive for CAIX, while being negative for CK7 and AMACR. Rare cases may show some focal weak staining with AMACR.
   - PRCC with clear cell features is strongly positive for CK7 and AMACR. Focal CAIX staining may be seen.
   - CCPRCC is positive for CK7 and CAIX, while being negative for AMACR.
   - Xp11 translocation RCC is positive for AMACR, TFE3, and cathepsin K. The majority are negative for CK7, but focal positivity for CK7 may be seen. CAIX may be focally positive as well.

C. **Positive AMACR staining in other sites**
   1. In the gastrointestinal tract:
      a. Colon adenomas with high-grade dysplasia stain positive for AMACR.
      b. Barrett-related dysplasia is found to be positive: 93% of cases with high-grade dysplasia and 44% of

cases with low-grade dysplasia have been reported positive.
   c. Stomach adenocarcinoma may also show positivity for AMACR in approximately 25% of cases.
2. Extramammary Paget's disease: 71% of cases are reportedly positive.

Selected references

Dabir PD, Ottosen P, Hoyer S, Hamilton-Dutoit S. Comparative analysis of three- and two-antibody cocktails to AMACR and basal cell markers for the immunohistochemical diagnosis of prostate carcinoma. *Diagnostic Pathology* 2012; 7: 81.

Hameed O, Humphrey PA. p63/AMACR antibody cocktail restaining of prostate needle biopsy tissues after transfer to charged slides: a viable approach in the diagnosis of small atypical foci that are lost on block sectioning. *American Journal of Clinical Pathology* 2005; 124: 708–15.

Jiang Z, Woda BA, Rock KL, *et al.* P504S: a new molecular marker for the detection of prostate carcinoma. *American Journal of Surgical Pathology* 2001; 25: 1397–404.

Rubin MA, Zhou M, Dhanasekaran SM, *et al.* alpha-Methylacyl coenzyme A racemase as a tissue biomarker for prostate cancer. *JAMA* 2002; 287: 1662–70.

Shi XY, Bhagwandeen B, Leong AS. p16, cyclin D1, Ki-67, and AMACR as markers for dysplasia in Barrett esophagus. *Applied Immunohistochemistry and Molecular Morphology* 2008; 16: 447–52.

Zhou M, Aydin H, Kanane H, Epstein JI. How often does alpha-methylacyl-CoA-racemase contribute to resolving an atypical diagnosis on prostate needle biopsy beyond that provided by basal cell markers? *American Journal of Surgical Pathology* 2004; 28: 239–43.

Zhou M, Chinnaiyan AM, Kleer CG, Lucas PC, Rubin MA. Alpha-Methylacyl-CoA racemase: a novel tumor marker over-expressed in several human cancers and their precursor lesions. *American Journal of Surgical Pathology* 2002; 26: 926–31.

NOTES

Amyloid

Sources/clones

Amyloid-A (AA)

American Research Products (REU86.2), Axcel/Accurate (mcl), Biogenesis (polyclonal), Biosource (5G6), Calbiochem/Novocastra (polyclonal), Dako (monoclonal, polyclonal anti-AA), Sanbio/Monosan/Accurate (REU86.2).

Transthyretin (ATTR/pre-albumin)

Axcel/Accurate (polyclonal), Biodesign (polyclonal), Biogenesis (polyclonal), Dako (polyclonal).

β2-microglobulin (Aβ2M)

Accurate (FMC16, polyclonal), Accurate/Sigma Chemical (BM63), Advanced Immunochemical (1F10, 2G3, 6G12), American Research Products (1672–18), Biodesign (GJ14, polyclonal), Biogenesis (B2M01), Biosource (MIG-85), Cymbus Bioscience (GJ14, polyclonal), Pharmingen (TU99), Sanbio/Monsan (B2M01), Zymed (Z022).

Amyloid-β precursor protein (βAPP)

Boehringer Mannheim (polyclonal), Dako (6F/3D), Zymed (LN27).

Fixation/preparation

These antibodies are applicable to formalin-fixed paraffin-embedded tissue sections.

Background

The amyloidoses are characterized by local, organ-limited, or generalized proteinaceous deposits of autologous origin. The pattern of distribution, progress of disease, and complications are dependent on the fibril protein. Amyloid is characterized by the following: (1) a typical green birefringence with polarized light after Congo red staining, (2) non-branching linear fibrils with a diameter of 10–12 nm, and (3) an x-ray diffraction pattern which is consistent with Pauling's model of a cross-β fibril. The diagnosis and classification of amyloidosis requires both histological proof and detection of the amyloid fibril: histochemical confirmation of amyloid deposits using Congo red evaluation in polarized light followed by identification of the fibril protein by immunostaining, thereby revealing the probable underlying disease. Apart from the rare familial syndromes, localized forms of amyloid affect certain organs or lesions (Aβ in brain, calcitonin in medullary carcinoma, islet amyloid polypeptide in insulinomas or islets of Langerhans). The five major different fibril proteins are usually associated with the most common generalized amyloid syndromes: amyloid A (AA), amyloid of λ- (Aλ) and κ- (Aκ) light chains, of transthyretin (ATTR) and β2-microglobulin origin. These fibril proteins may be deposited in a wide variety of tissues and organs. They therefore have to be considered in the investigation of any biopsy considered to be amyloidogenic.

Applications

In most instances good correlation is achieved between the immunohistochemical classification of amyloid and the underlying diseases. AA-amyloidosis is commonly associated with chronic inflammatory disorders. AL-amyloidosis (either λ- or κ- light chain origin) is linked mainly to plasma cell dyscrasias or is interpreted as being idiopathic. ATTR-amyloidosis is found in cases with familial amyloidosis. AβM-amyloidosis is associated with long-term hemodialysis.

However, a critical issue in the clinicopathological typing of amyloidosis is the interpretation of the immunostaining. Occasionally, more than one antibody may show immunostaining of amyloid deposits. Immunohistochemistry detects any associated contaminating component in the amyloid deposit (amyloid P component, apolipoprotein E, and glycosaminoglycans) and not merely the currently known obligate fibril proteins. Further, the five syndromic fibril proteins originate from plasma proteins, which may themselves "contaminate" amyloid deposits. The most critical of these are the immunoglobulin light chains. Based on these aberrant staining patterns, it has been proposed that the identification of a fibril protein with a single antibody demonstrates an even and homogeneous immunostaining for the entire amyloid deposit, while staining of the contaminant protein remains uneven. Instances also arise where two immunoreactive antibodies demonstrate similar uneven staining patterns, interpreted as being due to the irregular presentation of the epitope of the fibril protein resulting in a similar staining pattern as contaminating proteins. It is strongly recommended to test an additional specimen or biopsy to determine the causative fibril protein. In addition, the correlation of immunohistopathological observations and the clinical diagnosis is also mandatory to arrive at the correct classification of the amyloid fibril.

Another problem area is the false negative detection of amyloid. This can be avoided by increasing the sensitivity of detection by using both immune- and Congo red-staining methods. The latter method of detection is also influenced by the sample quality. It has long been recognized that the diagnostic yield of gastrointestinal biopsies (especially rectal) is extremely high, but these should contain submucosa. Other recommended sites include subcutaneous fat, sural nerve, heart, kidney, and bone marrow. While AA-amyloidosis is commonly detected in rectal biopsies, any involved organ or tissue is suitable for identification/classification of AL-amyloidosis. Interestingly, it has been shown that long-term hemodialysis-associated β2-microglobulin amyloid may also involve the gastrointestinal and reproductive systems in addition to the usual osteoarticular involvement.

The distinction and classification of amyloidosis has major therapeutic implications, as studies have recommended that AL-amyloidosis be treated with cytotoxic drugs (melphalan and prednisolone), while AA-amyloidosis responds better to colchicine and dimethylsulphoxide.

The role of antibodies against amyloid-β precursor protein has assisted in the diagnosis of Alzheimer's disease and early detection of axonal injury in the brain. Antibodies to transthyretin amyloid protein are useful in the diagnosis of cardiac amyloidosis and familial amyloidotic polyneuropathy.

Selected references

Iwamoto N, Nishiyama E, Ohwada J, Arai H. Distribution of amyloid deposits in the cerebral white matter of the Alzheimer's disease brain: relationship to blood vessels. *Acta Neuropathologica (Berlin)* 1997; 93: 334–40.

Jacobson DR, Pastore RD, Yaghoubian R, *et al.* Variant-sequence transthyretin (isoleucine 122) in late-onset cardiac amyloidosis in Black Americans. *New England Journal of Medicine* 1997; 336: 466–73.

Lansbury PT. In pursuit of the molecular structure of amyloid plaque: new technology provides unexpected and critical information. *Biochemistry* 1992; 31: 6865–70.

Ravid M, Shapiro J, Lang R, *et al.* Prolonged dimethylsulphoxide treatment in 13 patients with systemic amyloidosis. *Annals of Rheumatic Diseases* 1982; 41: 587–92.

Sherriff FE, Bridges LR, Sivaloganathan S. Early detection of axonal injury after human head trauma using immunocytochemistry for beta-amyloid precursor protein. *Acta Neuropathologica (Berlin)* 1994; 87: 55–62.

Shimizu M, Manabe T, Matsumoto T, *et al.* β_2 Microglobulin haemodialysis related amyloidosis: distinctive gross features of gastrointestinal involvement. *Journal of Clinical Pathology* 1997; 50: 873–5.

Sousa MM, Cardoso I, Fernandes R, *et al.* Deposition of transthyretin in early stages of familial amyloidotic polyneuropathy: evidence for toxicity of non fibrillar aggregates. *American Journal of Pathology* 2001; 159: 1993–2000.

Anaplastic lymphoma kinase (ALK)

Sources/clones

Abnova (ALK1), Cell Signaling (D5F3, D9E4), Dako (ALK1), Gennova Scientific (SP8), Neo Markers (SP8), Novocastra (5A4), Santa Cruz Biotechnology (5A4), Thermo Scientific (5A4), Ventana (D5F3).

Fixation/preparation

- Formalin-fixed paraffin-embedded tissues are suitable.
- Deparaffinize slides using xylene or xylene alternative and graded alcohols.
- Antigen retrieval is essential.
- Suitable for automated slide staining system

Background

Anaplastic lymphoma kinase (ALK), also known as ALK tyrosine kinase receptor or CD246 (cluster of differentiation 246), is an enzyme that in humans is encoded by the *ALK* gene. The *ALK* gene is located on chromosome 2p23, and codes for a protein that is expressed in some cells of the central nervous system, but in virtually no other normal human cells. ALK plays an important role in the development of the brain and exerts its effects on specific neurons in the nervous system. ALK shows the greatest sequence similarity to LTK (leukocyte tyrosine kinase). Interest in this protein among diagnostic pathologists has been related to its utility in recognizing a subset of CD30+ anaplastic large-cell lymphomas (ALCLs), with the characteristic t(2;5)(p23;q35) translocation. This translocation results in an abnormal fusion gene involving the *ALK* gene and the nucleophosmin (*NPM*) gene (located on chromosome 5q35), which codes for a ubiquitously expressed nucleolar phosphoprotein that functions in transporting components of ribosomes between the cytoplasm and nucleolus during the final stages of ribosome assembly. Transcription of this abnormal *NPM-ALK* fusion gene results in the production of an abnormal protein (called p80) that functions as a protein tyrosine kinase. The ALK antibody recognizes this abnormal human protein.

Applications

Antibodies to ALK have diagnostic, prognostic, and predictive usefulness in different situations. These situations include CD30+ anaplastic large-cell lymphoma, where ALK positivity is associated with better prognosis; and ALK lung cancer adenocarcinomas (unlike the standard ALK antibodies, the new generation of ALK antibodies are sensitive enough to demonstrate the expression of ALK in lung adenocarcinoma), where patients have been found to respond to an ALK inhibitor (crizotinib). In diagnostic pathology, inflammatory myofibroblastic tumor, rhabdomyosarcoma, and some cases of breast cancers are known to be ALK-positive. It is worth mentioning that the neoplasms harboring the characteristic t(2;5) (p23;q35) typically show both nuclear and cytoplasmic staining with ALK antibody, whereas those with variant translocations often only show cytoplasmic staining.

Staining pattern

IHC expression in selected neoplasm	IHC staining pattern
Anaplastic large-cell lymphoma	Nuclear and cytoplasmic[a]
Inflammatory myofibroblastic tumor	Cytoplasmic and nuclear[b]
ALK-positive non-small-cell lung carcinoma	Cytoplasmic

[a] In particular tumors harboring the characteristic t(2;5)(p23;q35).
[b] In epithelioid inflammatory myofibroblastic tumor.

Selected references

Cessna MH, Zhou H, Sanger WG, *et al.* Expression of ALK-1 and p80 in inflammatory myofibroblastic tumor and its mesenchymal mimics: a study of 135 cases. *Modern Pathology* 2002; 15: 931–8.

Chan JK. Newly available antibodies with practical applications in surgical pathology. *International Journal of Surgical Pathology* 2013; 21: 553–72.

Conklin CM, Craddock KJ, Have C, *et al.* Immunohistochemistry is a reliable screening tool for identification of ALK rearrangement in non-small-cell lung carcinoma and is antibody dependent. *Journal of Thoracic Oncology* 2013; 8: 45–51.

Corao DA, Biegel JA, Coffin CM, *et al.* ALK expression in rhabdomyosarcomas: correlation with histologic subtype and fusion status. *Pediatric and Developmental Pathology* 2009; 12: 275–83.

O'Bryant CL, Wenger SD, Kim M, Thompson LA. Crizotinib: a new treatment option for ALK-positive non-small-cell lung cancer. *Annals of Pharmacotherapy* 2013; 47: 189–97.

Perez-Pinera P, Chang Y, Astudillo A, Mortimer J, Deuel TF. Anaplastic lymphoma kinase is expressed in different subtypes of human breast cancer. *Biochemical and Biophysical Research Communications* 2007; 358: 399–403.

Tennstedt P, Strobel G, Bölch C, *et al.* Patterns of ALK expression in different human cancer types. *Journal of Clinical Pathology* 2014; 67: 477–81.

Wasik MA. Expression of anaplastic lymphomas kinase in non-Hodgkin's lymphomas and other malignant neoplasms: biological, diagnostic, and clinical implications. *American Journal of Clinical Pathology* 2002; 118 (Suppl 1): S81–92.

Androgen receptor

Sources/clones

Accurate (polyclonal), Biogenex (F39.4.1), Novocastra (2F12, polyclonal), Pharmingen (G122–25.3, G122–434, G122–77.14. AN1–15), Sanbio/Monosan (F39.4.1).

Fixation/preparation

The antibodies are immunoreactive in frozen sections, cell preparations, and paraffin-embedded sections; HIER enhances the last of these.

Background

The intracellular action of androgens is mediated by the androgen receptor, which is a key element of the androgen signal transduction cascade and a target of endocrine therapy for prostatic carcinoma. Qualitative and quantitative alterations of androgen receptor expression in prostatic carcinomas and their possible implications for tumor progression and treatment are therefore of diagnostic and research interest. Findings in prostatic tumor cell lines of rat and human origin suggest that reduction of androgen receptor protein expression is accompanied by an increase in tumor aggressiveness. However, immunohistochemical analysis and binding assays have demonstrated the presence of androgen receptors in all histological types of prostatic carcinoma and in both therapy-responsive and therapy-unresponsive tumors.

Applications

Many of the immunohistochemical studies of androgen receptors have been related to prostatic carcinoma and experimental animals. The androgen receptor content of prostatic carcinoma has been inversely correlated to Gleason grade in stage D2 carcinomas, although it was unrelated to extent of disease and response to hormonal therapy at three months. It has also been found that pretreatment androgen receptor expression alone is not related to prognosis of hormonally treated prostate cancer; however, when combined with Bcl-2 expression, it acts as an independent prognostic factor for clinical progression. One explanation for the discrepancy in findings may relate to the mutations that occur in the androgen receptor, which account for the variable response to hormonal therapy. These mutations produce broadened ligand specificity so that transcriptional factor activity of the receptor can be stimulated not just by dihydrotestosterone but also by estradiol and other androgen metabolites. Such activation of mutant androgen receptors by estrogen and weak androgens could confer on prostate cancer cells an ability to survive testicular androgen ablation through the activation of the androgen receptor by adrenal androgens or exogenous estrogen. Thus, mutated androgen receptors that occur prior to therapy may characterize a more aggressive disease.

The variability of androgen receptor protein content per unit nuclear area has been shown to increase with increasing histological grade, suggesting that this variability might account for the variable response to endocrine therapy in high-grade tumors. The extent of heterogeneity of androgen receptor expression may be a useful indicator of response to hormonal therapy.

Immunostaining for androgen receptor expression has been studied in other cell types including endometrium, genital melanocytes, meningiomas, most bone marrow cells other than erythroid and lymphoid cells, and urinary bladder carcinomas. Salivary duct carcinoma, a rare aggressive tumor that bears resemblance to invasive ductal carcinoma of the breast, shows frequent staining for androgen receptor, making this a possible diagnostic discriminator. Androgen receptor immunohistochemistry has been used in other salivary gland tumors that show potential apocrine differentiation, such as pleomorphic adenomas. Androgen receptor staining has been demonstrated in 45% of adenocarcinomas and 20% of squamous carcinomas of the esophagus. Androgen receptor positivity has also been noted in spindle cell lipomas.

Comments

The receptor is intranuclear in location. A cut-off of 10% androgen receptor-positive cells has been suggested to maximize assay prognostic efficiency with 48% positivity, showing significant correlation with response, time to progression, and survival, but not with grade or stage of prostatic cancer. Clone G122-25 is immunoreactive in fixed paraffin-embedded tissue sections and does not appear to cross-react with estrogen or progesterone receptors.

Selected references

Carroll RS, Zhang J, Dashmner K, *et al.* Androgen receptor expression in meningiomas. *Journal of Neurosurgery* 1995; 82: 453–60.

Hakimi JM, Rondinelli RH, Schoenberg MP, Barrack ER. Androgen-receptor gene structure and function in prostate cancer. *World Journal of Urology* 1996; 14: 329–37.

Hoang MP, Callender DL, Sola Gallego JJ, *et al.* Molecular and biomarker analyses of salivary duct carcinomas: comparison with mammary duct carcinoma. *International Journal of Oncology* 2001; 19: 865–71.

Mertens HJ, Heineman MJ, Koudstaal J, *et al.* Androgen receptor content in human endometrium. *European Journal of Obstetrics, Gynecology and Reproductive Biology* 1996; 70: 11–13.

Moriki T, Ueta S, Takashi T, *et al.* Salivary duct carcinoma: cytologic characteristics and application of androgen receptor immunostaining for diagnosis. *Cancer* 2001; 93: 344–50.

Syed S, Martin AM, Haupt H, Podolski V, Brooks JJ. Frequent detection of androgen receptors in spindle cell lipomas: an explanation of this lesion's male predominance? *Archives of Pathology and Laboratory Medicine* 2008; 132: 81–3.

Tihan T, Harmon JW, Wan X, *et al.* Evidence of androgen receptor expression in squamous and adenocarcinoma of the esophagus. *Anticancer Research* 2001; 21: 3107–14.

Zhuang YH, Blauer M, Tammela T, Tuohimaa P. Immunodetection of androgen receptor in human urinary bladder cancer. *Histopathology* 1997; 30: 556–62.

Anti-apoptosis

Sources/clones
Dako (BM-1), Monosan (Annexin V, polyclonal), Oncor (Apop Tag), Pharmingen (APO-BRDU, Annexin V-FITC).

Fixation/preparation
Various methods of detection of apoptotic bodies are available. All methods can be used on formalin-fixed paraffin-embedded tissue sections. Some require proteolytic digestion. Acetone-fixed cryostat sections and fixed cell smears may also be used.

Background
Cell death may occur by necrosis or apoptosis. Necrosis results from direct physical or chemical damage to the plasma membrane or disturbances in the osmotic balance of a cell. With the entrance of extracellular fluid into the cell, resultant cell swelling and lysis precede a subsequent inflammatory response. Furthermore, necrosis affects groups of cells, with consequent disruption of normal tissue architecture.

In contrast to necrosis, apoptotic cell death is a highly regulated physiologic process. The balance between apoptosis and cell proliferation results in the maintenance of cell homeostasis. Apoptotic bodies are rapidly engulfed by neighboring cells or macrophages, without an inflammatory response being elicited. The nuclear structure alteration in apoptotic cells is induced by endonuclease DNA cleavage that results in the generation of large 50–300 kb fragments. This produces the characteristic DNA "ladders" of apoptosis as viewed on agarose gel electrophoresis.

Reliable methods have been developed that enable the rapid assessment of apoptosis on sections prepared from paraffin-embedded material, e.g., the TUNEL method for TdT-mediated dUTP-biotin nick-end labeling. The APO-BRDU kit utilizes the same principle. The enzyme TdT is used to catalyze a template-independent addition of bromolated deoxyribonucleotide triphosphates (Br-dUTP) to the 3′-hydroxyl ends of the numerous fragments of double- and single-stranded DNA present in apoptotic cells. This allows the labeling of the very high concentrations of 3′-OH ends that are localized in apoptotic bodies. Br-dUTP is claimed to be more readily incorporated into the genome of apoptotic cells than are deoxyribonucleotide triphosphates complexed to larger ligands like fluorescein, biotin, or digoxigenin. Although rather specific for cells undergoing apoptosis, these techniques may also label cells undergoing necrosis. However, this is seldom a problem since the distinction between focal apoptotic events and necrosis is fairly clear. The histologic features of apoptosis include cell shrinkage and loss of junctional contact resulting in a "halo" around the cell. The nucleus shows condensation and margination of the chromatin. This is followed by the fragmentation or "pinching off" of pieces of nuclear material, which are surrounded by cytoplasm with intact cytoplasmic organelles as shown at ultrastructural level. These apoptotic fragments of pyknotic nuclear material and cytoplasm are phagocytosed by adjacent cells or macrophages. Apoptotic cells have been called by various names in different tissues, including "Councilman bodies," "Civatte bodies," "necrobiotic cells," and "nuclear dust."

The BM-1 antibody is directed to the Lewis^y antigen, which has been identified phenotypically as a marker of specific types of cells, and possibly specific stages of differentiation. Lewis^y is totally absent at the morula stage, but is highly expressed on the blastocyst surface and has been shown to play a role in the implantation process. Lewis^y has been identified as a characteristic of cells undergoing apoptosis. In Lewis^y-positive areas of tissue sections, typical apoptotic morphological changes and DNA fragmentation were frequently observed in certain loci, although not all Lewis^y-positive cells showed such signs of apoptosis. Although the BM-1 antibody against the Lewis^y antigen is reputed to detect apoptotic cells, further studies to test its efficacy, including a comparative analysis with the in-situ end labeling techniques, is awaited.

Another method of detection of apoptotic bodies is the use of annexin V, which is a 35–36 kDa Ca^{2+}-dependent phospholipid-binding protein that has a high affinity for the membrane phospholipid phosphatidylserine (PS). In apoptotic cells, PS is translocated from the inner to the outer leaflet of the plasma membrane, thereby exposing PS to the external cellular environment and allowing its binding to annexin V. Binding to a signal system such as fluorescein isothiocyanate allows the easy identification of apoptotic cells (in frozen sections and cell preparations). Annexin V is thought to identify cells at an earlier stage of apoptosis than assays based on DNA fragmentation because externalization of PS occurs earlier than the nuclear changes associated with apoptosis.

Applications

BM-1 antibody may be applied to neoplasms in general to assess the apoptotic index, e.g., endometrial adenocarcinoma. Recently, apoptosis has been considered to be a key event in oncogenesis, e.g., apoptosis has been reported to be promoted by the p53 tumor-suppressor gene and inhibited by oncogene *BCL2*. Although apparent cell loss by apoptosis occurs in carcinomatous tissue, the physiological significance is unclear. BM-1 positivity has been found to be as high as 25–35% in T cells of lymph nodes of patients with AIDS-related complex (ARC), in contrast to healthy controls, which were less than 5%.

Comments

Strong BM-1 immunoreactivity is observed in the apical surface of tubular urothelium, and in basal cells (glandular foveoli) of gastric and esophageal mucosa, and these tissues may be employed as controls.

The optimal method for the identification of apoptotic cells depends on the experimental system and the mode of induction of apoptosis. The degree of DNA degradation can vary according to the cell type, the nature of the inducing agent, and the stage of apoptosis.

Several other methods of assessing apoptosis in paraffin-embedded sections are available, and these include cyclin D1, Bcl-2, MDM-2, p53, Fas (CD95), c-kit (CD117), and CD40L, some of which are of relevance as prognostic markers. Antibodies to all of these proteins are separately discussed under their respective headings. In addition, antibodies to Bcl-x, Bax, and Bak can also be used to study apoptosis.

The Bcl-x protein belongs to the Bcl-2 oncoprotein family, members of which function as apoptosis-protective proteins and are overexpressed in 60% of carcinomas and 50% of adenomas compared to normal epithelial cells of adjacent mucosa. The polyclonal antibody to Bcl-x is available through Dako (A3535).

The Bax protein belongs to a family of proteins that share homology with Bcl-2 oncoprotein in several highly conserved regions. Overexpression of Bax functions to promote cell death through apoptosis. It has been suggested that the relative expression of the different Bcl-2 family proteins controls the sensitivity of cells to apoptotic stimuli. A polyclonal anti-Bax is available through Dako (A3533) and is immunoreactive in paraffin sections following HIER. The protein is located in the cytoplasm and stains a granular, punctate pattern. The Bak protein is another member of the Bcl-2 family that functions in the regulation of apoptosis. The Bak protein binds Bcl-x and Bcl-2 and is thought to induce apoptosis by counteracting the apoptotic-protective effects of Bcl-x and Bcl-2. Altered levels of Bak expression have been reported in *H. pylori*-infected tissues, and it may have a role in the development of gastric mucosa-associated lymphoid tissue (MALT) lymphoma through its interaction with *Helicobacter*-induced expression of Bcl-x. Anti-Bak is available through Dako (A3538). These Bcl-2 family proteins have been employed as prognostic markers in a variety of epithelial and soft tissue tumors, with varying degrees of success.

The application of multiple methods, each based on a different feature of the apoptotic process, may provide more information about the cell population than any one method would give alone.

Selected references

Arends MJ, Wyllie AH. Apoptosis: mechanism and roles in pathology. *International Reviews in Experimental Pathology* 1991; 32: 223–54.

Bukholm IR, Bukholm G, Nesland JM. Reduced expression of both Bax and Bcl-2 is independently associated with lymph node metastasis in human breast carcinomas. *APMIS* 2002; 110: 214–20.

Evans JD, Cornford PA, Dodson A, *et al*. Detailed tissue expression of bcl-2, bax, bak, and bcl-x in the normal human pancreas and in chronic pancreatitis, ampullary and pancreatic ductal adenocarcinomas. *Pancreatology* 2001; 1: 254–62.

Kerr JFR, Wyllie AH, Currie AR. Apoptosis: a basic biological phenomenon with wide-ranging implications in tissue kinetics. *British Journal of Cancer* 1972; 26: 239–57.

Krajewska M, Moss SF, Krajewski S, *et al.* Elevated expression of Bcl-x and reduced Bak in primary colorectal adenocarcinomas. *Cancer Research* 1996; 56: 2422–7.

Kuwashima Y, Uehara T, Kishi K, *et al.* Proliferative and apoptotic status in endometrial adenocarcinoma. *International Journal of Gynecological Pathology* 1995; 14: 45–9.

Morgner A, Sutton P, O'Rourke JL, *et al.* Helicobacter-induced expression of Bcl-X(L) in B lymphocytes in the mouse model: a possible step in the development of gastric mucosa-associated lymphoid tissue (MALT) lymphoma. *International Journal of Cancer* 2001; 92: 634–40.

Nagata S, Golstein P. The Fas death factor. *Science* 1995; 267: 1445–9.

Raynal P, Pollard HB. Annexins. The problem of assessing the biological role for a gene family of multifunctional calcium and phospholipid-binding proteins. *Journal of Biological Chemistry* 1994; 265: 4923–8.

Sarkiss M, Hsu B, El-Naggar AK, McDonnell TJ. The clinical relevance and assessment of apoptotic cell death. *Advances in Anatomic Pathology* 1996; 3: 205–11.

Schelwies K, Sturm I, Grabowski P, *et al.* Analysis of p53/BAX in primary colorectal carcinoma: low BAX protein expression is a negative prognostic factor in UICC stage III tumors. *International Journal of Cancer* 2002; 99: 589–96.

Sjostrom J, Blomqvist C, von Boguslawski K, *et al.* The predictive value of bcl-2, bax, bcl-xL, bag-1, fas, and fasL for chemotherapy response in advanced breast cancer. *Clinical Cancer Research* 2002; 8: 811–16.

Trask DK, Wolf GT, Bradford CR, *et al.* Expression of Bcl-2 family proteins in advanced laryngeal squamous cell carcinoma: correlation with response to chemotherapy and organ preservation. *Laryngoscope* 2002; 112: 638–44.

Wyllie AH, Kerr JFR, Currie AR. Cell death: the significance of apoptosis. *International Reviews in Cytology* 1980; 68: 251–306.

NOTES

Arginase-1

Sources/clones

Abcam (ab60176), Novus Biologicals (CL0186), Santa Cruz Biotech (H-52), Sigma-Aldrich (AB1), Thermo Scientific/ Pierce Antibody Products (PA5–22009), Ventana (SP156).

Fixation/preparation

The antibody can be used in formalin-fixed paraffin-embedded tissue. Pretreatment of deparaffinized tissue sections with heat-induced epitope retrieval (HIER) is required.

Background

Arginase-1 is a binuclear manganese metalloenzyme that catalyzes the hydrolysis of arginine to ornithine and urea. In rats, arginase-1 is expressed in the periportal hepatocytes. In addition, arginase-1 has been shown to be a sensitive and specific marker of benign and malignant hepatocytes in human formalin-fixed paraffin-embedded tissue.

Applications

Arginase-1 is a sensitive and specific marker of hepatocytes and demonstrates diffuse cytoplasmic expression in both normal liver samples and in hepatocellular neoplasms, with patchy nuclear reactivity. It can be used to distinguish hepatocellular carcinomas (HCCs) from metastatic tumors in the liver, and its sensitivity has been shown to be consistently superior to that of Hep Par 1 within each grade of HCC. Its expression is specific to HCC, with no expression of arginase-1 noted in tumors mimicking an HCC in the liver, such as renal cell carcinomas (RCCs), melanomas, neuroendocrine tumors, adrenocortical carcinomas, and gastric adenocarcinomas. However, expression of arginase-1 has rarely been noted in metastatic carcinomas and cholangiocarcinoma in the liver.

Arginase-1 has been shown to be highly specific compared to other hepatocellular markers such as Hep Par 1 and glypican-3 in cytology specimens, and it should be used as a part of a panel of these three markers for the diagnosis of HCC. Conflicting results have been noted for expression of arginase-1 in pancreatic ductal adenocarcinoma.

Comments

Selected references

Fatima N, Cohen C, Siddiqui MT. Arginase-1: a highly specific marker separating pancreatic adenocarcinoma from hepatocellular carcinoma. *Acta Cytologica* 2014; 58: 83–8.

Radwan NA, Ahmed NS. The diagnostic value of arginase-1 immunostaining in differentiating hepatocellular carcinoma from metastatic carcinoma and cholangiocarcinoma as compared to HepPar-1. *Diagnostic Pathology* 2012; 7: 149.

Yan BC, Gong C, Song J, *et al.* Arginase-1: a new immunohistochemical marker of hepatocytes and hepatocellular neoplasms. *American Journal of Surgical Pathology* 2010; 34: 1147–54.

NOTES

Bcl-2

Sources/clones

Dako (124), Immunotech (124), Zymed (BCL2–100).

Fixation/preparation

Antibodies to Bcl-2 are reasonably robust and work very well on paraffin-embedded tissue. Staining is not too dependent on fixation protocols, and good results may be obtained with formalin-fixed, B5-fixed, methacarn-fixed, and fresh frozen tissues. Staining is significantly enhanced by the use of antigen retrieval with either microwave or pressure-cooking pretreatment. The Bcl-2 antibody may be used for labeling acetone-fixed cryostat sections or fixed cell smears.

Background

The *BCL2* gene was identified more than a decade ago with the discovery and analysis of the t(14;18)(q32;q21) translocation. This translocation occurs in 70–80% of follicular lymphoma, comprising juxtaposition of the *BCL2* gene with the immunoglobulin heavy chain (IgH) gene on chromosome 14q32. This results in an overexpression of the translocated *BCL2* allele induced by enhancers in the IgH region, although the translocation is not a prerequisite for Bcl-2 protein expression, since this occurs in many cases without this rearrangement. The Bcl-2 polypeptide is a 26 kDa protein that is found on intracellular (mitochondrial and nuclear) membranes and in the cytosol (on the smooth endoplasmic reticulum), rather than on the cell surface. *BCL2* is not an oncogene and has no effect on cell replication; Bcl-2 protein does, however, prevent cells from undergoing apoptosis, conferring a survival advantage on cells harbouring the t(14;18) translocation. In normal lymphoid tissue, Bcl-2 antibody reacts with small B lymphocytes in the mantle zone and many cells within T cell areas. In the thymus many cells in the medulla are stained, with weak/negative reaction in the cortex.

Applications

The initial diagnostic application of Bcl-2 immunostaining was for the distinction of reactive follicular lymphoid hyperplasia from follicular lymphoma. Positive staining is cytoplasmic in location. Follicular lymphomas show striking Bcl-2 expression in neoplastic follicles, while only isolated individual cells within the reactive follicle centers are positive (mostly T cells). This difference in staining pattern is not due to downregulation or decreased Bcl-2 mRNA, but largely to a post-translational mechanism that results in decreased protein levels. Furthermore, Bcl-2 protein expression is demonstrated in all grades of follicle center cell lymphomas in both small and large cells. Strongly Bcl-2+ lymphoid aggregates in the bone marrow of patients previously diagnosed with nodal follicular lymphoma are indicative of lymphoma involvement. However, there is no practical value in applying the Bcl-2 antibody for classification of a malignant lymphoid infiltrate, since many different lymphoma types can be Bcl-2-positive. Nevertheless, it has been demonstrated that non-Hodgkin lymphoma with Bcl-2 expression has a significantly higher relapse rate and a lower cause-specific survival than in those without. Bcl-2 immunostaining together with CD10, CD5, CD20, and CD23 has been shown to be useful in identifying follicular lymphoma in bone marrow biopsies.

Expression of Bcl-2 has been studied in many epithelial neoplasms, and attempts have been made to correlate Bcl-2 expression with survival. In general, better prognoses accompany Bcl-2+ neoplasms than Bcl-2– ones, with some prostatic cancers being the exception to the rule. A reciprocal relationship has been demonstrated between Bcl-2 reactivity and p53 overexpression in 65% of colorectal neoplasia, with a Bcl-2+/p53– subgroup showing a strong correlation with negative lymph node status, implying a less aggressive pathway of neoplastic transformation. A similar reciprocal relationship was shown in acute leukemias, whereas a dissociated immunoexpression of Bcl-2 and Ki-67 was demonstrated in endometrial benign and malignant lesions. Bcl-2 protein was also detected in all grades of cervical intraepithelial neoplasia (CIN), with a striking increase in the number of positive cells with increasing severity of CIN, in combination with a mild increase in staining intensity.

Bcl-2 expression has been demonstrated in 80% of synovial sarcoma, but was negative in leiomyosarcomas, malignant peripheral nerve sheath tumors, and fibrosarcomas. However, another study showed Bcl-2 protein expression in rhabdomyosarcomas and leiomyosarcomas, epithelioid leiomyomas, and leiomyomas. Bcl-2 family proteins have been shown to modulate radiosensitivity in malignant glioma cells.

Selected references

Bakhshi A, Jensen JP, Goldman P, et al. Cloning the chromosomal breakpoint of t(14;18) human lymphomas: clustering around J_h on chromosome 14 near a transcriptional unit on 18. *Cell* 1985; 41: 899–906.

Chetty R, Dada MA, Gatter KC. Bcl-2: longevity personified. *Advances in Anatomic Pathology* 1997; 4: 134–8.

Bcl-6

Sources/clones

Dako (PG-B6p), Novocastra (P1F6), Santa Cruz (C-19, N-3).

Fixation/preparation

The antibodies are applicable to formalin-fixed paraffin-embedded or frozen tissues. Pretreatment with EDTA and heat-induced epitope retrieval (HIER) is recommended.

Background

The *BCL6* gene was identified from translocations involving the 3q27 locus in diffuse large-B-cell lymphomas. The *BCL6* gene product is a 92–98 kDa nuclear phosphoprotein that is highly expressed in germinal center B cells and their neoplastic counterparts. Hence, Bcl-6 protein is expressed exclusively by follicular center B cells in reactive lymphoid tissue and lymphomas which are thought to arise from follicular center cells, namely, follicular lymphoma, Burkitt lymphoma, some diffuse large-B-cell lymphomas, and nodular lymphocyte-predominant Hodgkin disease (NLPHD). While the Bcl-6 protein was expressed in the L&H cells of NLPHD in the majority of cases, half of the cases of classic Hodgkin disease were also immunopositive for Bcl-6. Cases of primary cutaneous follicular lymphoma have also been characterized by expression of Bcl-6. Marginal zone/MALT lymphomas and mantle cell lymphomas are negative. However, 50% of high-grade MALT lymphomas demonstrate Bcl-6 immunoreaction similar to systemic diffuse large-B-cell lymphoma.

All primary mediastinal large-B-cell lymphomas have been demonstrated to express Bcl-6 protein, supporting a germinal center derivation. However, only 40% of T-cell-rich B-cell lymphomas were immunoreactive with Bcl-6. The diffuse large-B-cell cutaneous lymphomas that are AIDS-related have also been shown to express Bcl-6 in 50% of cases.

Applications

Bcl-6 in conjunction with CDw75 and CD10 is a reliable marker of follicular center B-cell derivation with a sensitivity of 100%.

Immunoexpression of Bcl-6 may be a useful marker to distinguish follicular center cell lymphoma from other diffuse small lymphocytic lymphomas. In follicular lymphoma, Bcl-6 is expressed in both the follicular and interfollicular neoplastic B cells, while in reactive lymphoid hyperplasia Bcl-6 expression is confined exclusively to the germinal centers. The combination of Bcl-6 and Bcl-2 immunostaining can help in distinguishing neoplastic from reactive follicles, as they stain Bcl-6+/Bcl-2+ and Bcl-6+/Bcl-2–, respectively. Bcl-6 also provides distinction between pseudo-growth centers and entrapped germinal centers, which are Bcl-6– and Bcl-6+, respectively. Bcl-6 expression may also be helpful in identifying main subsets of diffuse large-B-cell lymphomas, those of follicular center cell origin showing Bcl-6 immunoexpression.

Selected references

Onizuka T, Moriyama M, Yamochi T, *et al*. BCL-6 gene product, a 92- to 98-kDa nuclear phosphoprotein, is highly expressed in germinal center B cells and their neoplastic counterparts. *Blood* 1995; 86: 28–37.

Ye BH, Rao PH, Chaganti RS, Dalla-Favera R. Cloning of BCL-6, the locus involved in chromosome translocations affecting band 3q27 in B-cell lymphoma. *Cancer Research* 1993; 53: 2732–5.

NOTES

Ber-EP4

Sources/clones

Axcel/Accurate, Dako, Diagnostic Bioscience.

Fixation/preparation

Ber-EP4 can be used on formalin-fixed paraffin-embedded tissue sections. Prolonged formalin fixation can be deleterious to immunoreactivity, which is enhanced by HIER or by enzymatic predigestion with proteolytic enzymes such as trypsin and pronase. Ber-EP4 may also be used to label acetone-fixed cryostat sections and fixed cell smears. A major advantage of this antibody is its high sensitivity, allowing use at high dilutions.

Background

Ber-EP4 was raised against MCF-7 cells and is directed against two glycoproteins of 34 and 49 kDa present on the surface and in the cytoplasm of all epithelial cells with the exception of the superficial layers of squamous epithelia, hepatocytes, and parietal cells. Although it is not yet clear what antigen is recognized by the antibody, an absence of reactivity to keratins has been found in immunoblotting experiments. A positive reaction is seen in epithelial cells known to contain large amounts of the Ber-EP4 antigen, e.g., epithelial cells in the bile ducts and ducts of the epididymis.

Applications

Ber-EP4 shows a broad pattern of reactivity with human epithelial tissues from simple epithelia to basal layers of stratified non-keratinized squamous epithelium and epidermis (Appendix 1.21). In addition, most cases of carcinoma demonstrate immunoreaction with this antibody. The only adenocarcinomas that failed to react were of breast origin and kidney. 90% of biphasic synovial sarcoma are positive for Ber-EP4.

Focal expression of Ber-EP4 in the mesothelium of the peritoneum and the ovarian surface epithelium adjacent to endometriotic lesions suggests that the mesothelium possibly acquires characteristics of epithelial nature, supporting a metaplastic process of the peritoneal mesothelium in the pathogenesis of endometriosis.

Comments

Any attempt to use Ber-EP4 to help distinguish epithelial mesothelioma from adenocarcinoma should be accompanied by a panel of antibodies (Appendix 1.17) including CEA, Leu-M1, B72.3 (all three antibodies in combination were reported to distinguish over 90% of pulmonary adenocarcinomas from pleural mesotheliomas), and more recent additions to the panel include calretinin, cadherin, WT1, and CK5/6. In addition, anti-EMA has been shown to produce a distinctive pattern of membrane staining corresponding to the circumferential long microvilli, which are pathognomonic of malignant mesothelial cells.

Selected reference

Latza U, Niedobitek G, Schwarting R, *et al.* Ber-EP4: New monoclonal antibody which distinguishes epithelia from mesothelia. *Journal of Clinical Pathology* 1990; 43: 213–19.

NOTES

β-hCG (human chorionic gonadotropin)

Sources/clones

Biodesign ([427,681], [812,813], [827,829,830], [827,31], 2B1–3, ME.1, ME.106, ME.108, polyclonal), Biogenesis (2F4/3, BIO-BCG-001, BIO-BCG-005, BHCG-010, polyclonal), Biogenex (D7), Caltag Laboratories (2092), Dako, Fitzgerald (M15292, M15294, M94138, M94139, M94140, M94141, polyclonal), Immunotech (2B1.3), Sanbio/Monosan (2092), Zymed (ZMCG13, ZSH17).

Fixation/preparation

These antibodies are applicable both to formalin-fixed paraffin-embedded sections and to frozen sections. Neither enzyme digestion nor HIER appears to enhance immunoreactivity.

Background

Human chorionic gonadotropin (hCG) is a glycoprotein (40 kDa) comprising a protein core and a carbohydrate side chain. The molecule is composed of two dissimilar subunits – α and β. The α-subunit is indistinguishable immunologically from the α-subunit of pituitary glycoprotein hormones: luteinizing hormone (LH), follicle stimulating hormone (FSH), and thyroid-stimulating hormone (TSH). The β-subunits are different from each other and confer specificity. hCG, secreted in large quantities by the placenta, normally circulates at readily detectable levels only during gestation.

The monoclonal antibody (IgG) to β-hCG was produced by immunization with pure chorionic gonadotropin β-subunit. β-hCG is demonstrable in syncytiotrophoblasts of normal human placenta.

Applications

hCG is the most important marker of gestational trophoblastic cells, being present in syncytiotrophoblastic cells and cells of the intermediate trophoblast but absent in cytotrophoblast (Appendix 1.33, 1.34). In syncytiotrophoblast cells, hCG is demonstrable from the 12th day of gestation, reaches a peak at six weeks, and decreases thereafter; at term hCG is present only focally in these cells. In choriocarcinoma strong diffuse immunostaining for hCG occurs in syncytiotrophoblastic cells (and focal immunostaining for human placental lactogen). In contrast, placental site trophoblastic tumor shows focal hCG immunopositivity (and diffuse human placental lactogen immunoreaction) (Appendix 1.34).

β-hCG expression in non-trophoblastic tumors may indicate aggressive behavior of the tumor. It is worth noting that hCG may be demonstrated in about 15% of patients with hepatocellular carcinoma. hCG may be demonstrated in the trophoblast-like cells which develop in undifferentiated carcinoma of the endometrium; however, the presence of recognizable glandular structures and the lack of the biphasic pattern of alternating rows of syncytial and cytotrophoblasts rule out the possibility of choriocarcinoma.

hCG has also been demonstrated in poorly differentiated areas with cells resembling syncytiotrophoblasts in three women with serous papillary or mucinous adenocarcinomas of the ovary. In dysgerminomas, there are individual or collections of syncytiotrophoblastic giant cells that contain/produce hCG.

Serum hCG is a promising tumor marker of gastrointestinal malignancies, and a monoclonal antibody applied to gastrointestinal malignancies showed staining in gastric carcinomas (60%), pancreatic carcinomas (55%), and extrahepatic cholangiocarcinomas (35%). By comparison, a polyclonal antibody showed a higher frequency of positivity but the staining was diffuse. Positive immunostaining for β-hCG with a monoclonal antibody has also been suggested to be of prognostic relevance in colorectal carcinoma, especially when employed in combination with serum levels of the hormone.

Selected reference

Bellisario R, Carlsen RB, Bahl OP. Human chorionic gonadotropin. Linear amino acid sequence of the α subunit. *Journal of Biological Chemistry* 1973; 248: 6796–809.

BOB-1

Sources/clones

Cell Marque (rabbit monoclonal antibody SP92).

Fixation/preparation

This antigen is preserved in formalin-fixed paraffin-embedded tissue.

Background

The B-cell-specific octamer-binding protein-1 (BOB-1), also known as OBF-1 or OCA-B, is a B-lymphocyte-specific transcriptional coactivator that interacts with the OCT1 and OCT2 transcription factors in B cells, to transactivate immunoglobulin genes. As a transcription factor, BOB-1 is predominantly expressed in the nucleus, although in strongly BOB-1-expressing cell populations, such as plasma cells, there is frequently detectable BOB-1 protein at low level in the cytoplasm. BOB-1 is expressed in a similar distribution as its partner gene *OCT2*, in all mature B-lymphoid cells from naïve B cells through plasma cells. While OCT2 appears to be lymphoid-specific, it is not B-cell-specific, and expression has been described in thymic T cells as well as cases of anaplastic large-cell lymphoma.

Applications

Unlike OCT2, which is normally expressed in neuronal tissue and some histiocytes, as well as aberrantly expressed in some large T-cell lymphomas, definitive BOB-1 expression in non-B-lineage tissues of either benign or neoplastic type has not been reported, although expression has been induced by various external means in several neoplastic cell lines.

Because of its relative B-cell specificity, BOB-1 can be a useful marker of B-lineage in poorly differentiated B-cell non-Hodgkin lymphomas (B-NHLs) such as plasmablastic lymphomas and primary effusion lymphomas (PELs). In such specimens, detection of convincing BOB-1 expression often will go along with PCR identification of a clonal immunoglobulin gene rearrangement, which may be sufficient to confirm B-lineage, although it should be noted that these transcriptional factors and clonal immunoglobulin gene rearrangements have also been reported in acute myeloid leukemias/myeloid sarcomas.

In addition to its application to confirm B-lineage in B-NHL and plasma cell neoplasms (PCNs), BOB-1 immunohistochemistry plays an important role in the diagnosis of Hodgkin lymphoma. Specifically, nearly all cases of classic Hodgkin lymphoma (CHL) express either no nuclear BOB-1 or extremely weak BOB-1, in contrast to all other B-lymphoid neoplasms, including B-NHL, PCN, and nodular lymphocyte-predominant Hodgkin lymphoma (NLPHL, the major morphologic differential with CHL). In those CHL cases in which nuclear BOB-1 is expressed, its coactivating factor OCT2 should be either negative or minimally expressed.

Selected references

Advani AS, Lim K, Gibson S, *et al.* OCT-2 expression and OCT-2/BOB.1 co-expression predict prognosis in patients with newly diagnosed acute myeloid leukemia. *Leukemia and Lymphoma* 2010; 51: 606–12.

Kim U, Qin XF, Gong S, *et al.* The B-cell-specific transcription coactivator OCA-B/OBF-1/Bob-1 is essential for normal production of immunoglobulin isotypes. *Nature* 1996; 383: 542–7.

NOTES

Brachyury

Sources/clones

Abcam: mouse monoclonal (1H9A2), rabbit polyclonal
Acris antibodies GmbH: rabbit polyclonal
Antibodies-online: goat polyclonal (AA 2–202)
Atlas Antibodies: rabbit polyclonal
Biorbyt: rabbit polyclonal
E-bioscience: mouse monoclonal (X1AO2)
Fitzgerald Industries International: rabbit polyclonal
GeneTex: mouse monoclonal (1H9A2)
LifeSpan BioSciences: mouse monoclonal (1H9A2), rabbit polyclonal
Novus Biologicals: rabbit polyclonal
R&D Systems: goat polyclonal
Santa Cruz Biotechnologies: goat polyclonal (N-19, C-19)
John's laboratory: mouse monoclonal
Thermo Scientific: mouse monoclonal (1H9A2), rabbit polyclonal

Fixation/preparation

Most of these antibodies are validated in formalin-fixed paraffin-embedded tissue. Please refer to vendor instructions for specific antigen retrieval requirements.

Background

Brachyury is a 47 kDa embryonic transcription factor encoded by the *T* gene. It binds to specific DNA regions near the palindromic sequence TCACACCT (T-site) through the T-box in its N-terminus. Brachyury functions during embryogenesis to regulate midline development by establishing the anterior–posterior axis through the regulation of genes involved in mesoderm formation and differentiation. It is expressed in notochord-derived cells. Variations in the *T* gene in humans are associated with neural tube defects and chordomas.

Chordomas are slow-growing malignant neoplasms with epithelioid and chondroid morphology that arise in the central axial skeleton, thought to derive from notochordal remnants. These tumors harbor a variety of chromosomal aberrations that result in gain of the T locus and overexpression of brachyury, which plays a major role in tumorigenesis and proliferation.

Expression of brachyury has also been identified in some epithelial tumors and in cancer-derived stem cells.

Applications

Brachyury is expressed in virtually all nuclei of chordomas and is extremely useful in the differential diagnosis between chordoma and other chondroid neoplasms, including low-grade chondrosarcoma of the skull base, chordoid meningiomas, myxoid chondrosarcoma, and others. Sensitivity and specificity are extremely high, and it is maintained after tissue decalcification. In addition, brachyury can contribute to the detection of extra-axial skeletal chordomas and the rare soft tissue chordomas.

Cytoplasmic staining of stromal cells has been reported in hemangioblastoma, a benign neoplasm of uncertain histological origin frequently seen in the central nervous system in patients with von Hippel–Lindau syndrome, and it may contribute to the differential diagnosis of this tumor as well.

Selected references

Barresi V, Vitarelli E, Branca, G, *et al*. Expression of brachyury in hemangioblastoma: potential use in differential diagnosis. *American Journal of Surgical Pathology* 2012; 36: 1052–57.

Lauer SR, Edgar MA, Gardner JM, Sebastian A, Weiss SW. Soft tissue chordomas: a clinicopathologic analysis of 11 cases. *American Journal of Surgical Pathology* 2013; 37: 719–26.

B Sangoi AR, Dulai MS, Beck AH, Brat DJ, Vogel H. Distinguishing chordoid meningiomas from their histologic mimics: an immunohistochemical evaluation. *American Journal of Surgical Pathology* 2009; 33: 669–81.

CA125

Sources/clones

Dako (OC125), Immunotech (Ov185).

Fixation/preparation

Monoclonal anti-CA125 (M11) can be used on formalin-fixed paraffin-embedded tissue sections. The deparaffinized tissue sections must be treated with heat (in citrate buffer or Dako Target Retrieval Solution) prior to the immunohistochemical staining procedure.

Background

CA125 was discovered with a monoclonal screen for tumor-specific antigens of hybridomas derived from mouse lymphocytes immunized to an ovarian cell culture line, OVCA433. The *MUC16* gene is a strong candidate for the CA125 antigen, and a partial cDNA was recently cloned. Transfection of this partial cDNA into two CA125-negative cell lines resulted in synthesis of CA125. The antigen is located on the surface of ovarian tumor cells with essentially no expression in normal adult ovarian tissue. Significantly, CA125 is also found in sera of patients with ovarian, pancreatic (about 50%), liver, colon, and other (22–32%) adenocarcinomas. Although CA125 is not specific for ovarian carcinoma, it nevertheless does correlate directly with disease status. Similar to other tumor markers, CA125 is also expressed normally in fetal development: the antigen has been localized to the amnion celomic epithelium and derivatives of Müllerian epithelium. In adult tissue, the monoclonal antibody OC125 reacted with the epithelium of the fallopian tube, endometrium, endocervix, apocrine sweat glands, and mammary glands.

Presently, little is known of the structure of this extracellular matrix molecule, nor is there any indication of its function. It appears to be part of a large-molecular-weight mucin-like glycoprotein complex that can be resolved to a 200–250 kDa species on gel electrophoresis. Although the antigen is thought to contain a carbohydrate component, the antigenic epitope recognized by OC125 is considered to be peptide in nature.

Applications

The most important property of CA125 is that it is regularly expressed on the tumor cell surface of serous cystadenocarcinoma of the ovary (>95%), while no expression is detected in mucinous cystadenocarcinomas. The following have also been found to stain positively with CA125: colonic adenocarcinoma, breast carcinoma, uterine papillary serous carcinoma, thyroid follicular adenoma, transitional cell carcinoma of the bladder, uterine adenomatoid tumor, lung bronchoalveolar carcinoma, endometrioid carcinoma of the ovary, and squamous cell carcinoma of the penis (Dako specifications). Employed in an appropriate panel, CA125 is useful for the separation of colonic carcinoma from ovarian endometrioid carcinoma in the pelvis (Appendix 1.14). Similarly, when used with other markers, it may be useful in distinguishing renal clear cell carcinoma from clear cell carcinomas of the ovary and other Müllerian tumors, the latter being CA125-positive.

A mesothelioma that demonstrated both serum and immunohistochemical positivity with CA125 has been reported. This indicates that CA125 cannot reliably distinguish between metastatic serous epithelial tumors of the peritoneum and mesothelioma. In occult nodal metastasis in endometrial carcinoma, CA125 was found on macrophages in the lymph nodes, raising doubts as to the specificity of some antibodies to CA125.

Comments

The major role of CA125 in immunohistology is in the identification of metastatic serous carcinoma of the ovary. Primary serous cystadenocarcinoma of the ovary is the recommended positive control tissue for optimization of CA125.

Selected references

Bast RC, Feeney M, Lazarus H, *et al*. Reactivity of a monoclonal antibody with human ovarian carcinoma. *Journal of Clinical Investigation* 1981; 68: 1331-7.

Davis AM, Zurawski VR, Bast RC, Klug TL. Characterization of the CA 125 antigen associated with human epithelial ovarian carcinomas. *Cancer Research* 1986; 46: 6143-8.

Kuzuya K, Nozaki M, Chihara T. Evaluation of CA 125 as a circulating tumor marker for ovarian cancer. *Acta Obstetric et Gynecologica Japan*. 1986; 38: 949-57.

O'Brien TJ, Raymond LM, Bannon GA, *et al*. New monoclonal antibodies identify the glycoprotein carrying the CA 125 epitope. *American Journal of Obstetrics and Gynecology* 1991; 165: 1857-64.

N/97-Cadherin/E-Cadherin

Sources/clones

Monoclonal antibody anti-N-cadherin (clone 13A9) and anti-E-cadherin (clone E9). Accurate (6F9), American Research Products (6F9), Calbiochem (HybEcad#l), Eurodiagnostica/Accurate (5H9), Immunotech (67A4), Sanbio/Monosan/Accurate (5H9), Urodiagnostica/Accurate (5H9), Zymed (HECD1, ECCD1, ECCD2, SHE78–7).

Fixation/preparation

Initially applied primarily to frozen sections, both antibodies are now applicable to formalin-fixed paraffin-embedded tissue with heat pretreatment in citrate buffer.

Background

It has long been recognized that cancer cells have differences in their adhesive properties when compared with non-transformed cells. There is evidence that among the different cell adhesion molecules, the cadherin family of calcium-dependent cell–cell adhesion molecules and their associated proteins are indeed tumor suppressors. The cadherin family includes several distinctive members, two of which are E (epithelial)-cadherin, a 120 kDa protein expressed in epithelial cells and concentrated in cell–cell adherens junctions, and N (nerve)-cadherin, a 135 kDa protein expressed in nerve cells, developing skeletal muscle, embryonic and mature cardiac muscle cells, and pleural mesothelial cells. The *E-cadherin* gene (*CDH1*) is located on chromosome 16q22.1, a region frequently affected with loss of heterozygosity in sporadic breast carcinoma. During embryonic development, expression of distinctive members of the cadherin family determines the aggregation of cells into specialized tissues as they interact with identical cadherins within the same tissue. Hence, the mesoderm-derived mesothelial cells that form the pleura express N-cadherin, while epithelial cells of the lung express E-cadherin. Therefore, the development of well-characterized monoclonal antibodies that recognize N-cadherin without cross-reactivity with E-cadherin provided an opportunity for its application to immunohistology.

Applications

A high level of expression of N-cadherin was found in all mesotheliomas, and E-cadherin in all pulmonary adenocarcinomas, on fresh frozen sections. The same group of investigators subsequently confirmed these findings using antibodies to N-cadherin and E-cadherin that reacted with fixation and paraffin-embedding resistant epitopes in a series of malignant mesotheliomas and adenocarcinomas. Although one case of mesothelioma was negative for N-cadherin and one adenocarcinoma was weakly positive for N-cadherin (but strongly positive for E-cadherin), these antibodies appeared to offer a sufficient degree of sensitivity and specificity for use in the differential diagnosis of mesothelioma and adenocarcinoma.

The application of antibodies to N- and E-cadherin to ovarian epithelial tumors has revealed interesting findings. Both E- and N-cadherins were expressed in serous and endometrioid tumors, while mucinous tumors strongly expressed E-cadherin only. The expression of N-cadherin in serous and endometrioid tumors traces their origin to the mesoderm-derived ovarian surface epithelium. Another study demonstrated both E- and N-cadherins in benign but not malignant ovarian tumors, while only N-cadherin was present in borderline tumors. Further, negative E-cadherin ovarian carcinomas presented a shorter survival. E- and N-cadherin differential expression may be involved in ovarian carcinogenesis, and may have diagnostic and prognostic value.

Reduction in E-cadherin expression has been associated with lack of cohesiveness, high malignant potential, and invasiveness in epithelial neoplasms of the colon, ovary, stomach, pancreas, lung, breast, and head/neck. In contrast, N-cadherin has also been demonstrated in astrocytomas/glioblastomas and rhabdomyosarcomas. We have shown that the loss of E-cadherin, demonstrated by immunostaining, is associated with a loss of staining for β-catenin in infiltrating ductal carcinoma of the breast, and in src cell lines heralds a change from epithelial shapes to spindle forms. Downregulation of E- and β-cadherin was suggested to be predictive of nodal metastasis in breast cancer, and loss of E-cadherin is considered to be a fundamental defect in diffuse-type gastric carcinoma and infiltrating lobular carcinoma of the breast. Invasive lobular breast carcinomas, which are typically completely E-cadherin-negative, often show inactivating mutations in combination with loss of heterozygosity of the wild-type *CDH1* allele. Mutations were found at early noninvasive stages, thus associating *E-cadherin* mutations with loss of cell growth control and defining *CDH1* as the tumor suppressor for the lobular breast carcinoma subtype. Ductal breast carcinomas in general show heterogeneous loss of E-cadherin expression, associated with epigenetic transcriptional downregulation.

Comments

Malignant mesothelioma and colonic adenocarcinoma tissue are recommended for use as positive controls for N- and E-cadherin respectively. We have found trypsin predigestion followed by HIER to produce the greatest immunoreactivity for these antigens, particularly E-cadherin.

Selected references

Hedrick L, Cho KR, Vogelstein B. Cell adhesion molecules as tumor suppressors. *Trends in Cell Biology* 1993; 3: 36–9.

Madhavan M, Srinivas P, Abraham E, *et al.* Cadherins as predictive markers of nodal metastasis in breast cancer. *Modern Pathology* 2001; 14: 423–7.

Matsuura K, Kawanishi J, Jujii S, *et al.* Altered expression of E-cadherin in gastric cancer tissues and carcinomatous fluid. *British Journal of Cancer* 1992; 66: 1122–30.

CAIX

Sources/clones

Clone Ab1508: Abcam, Cambridge, MA
Clone NB100–417: Rabbit Polyclonal, Novus Biological, Littleton, CO
Clone TH22: Leica, Buffalo Grove, IL

Fixation/preparation

Standardized for formalin-fixed paraffin-embedded tissue.

Background

Clear cell renal cell carcinoma (CCRCC) is the most common primary renal cancer of adults. It comprises approximately 75% of all primary renal cancers and accounts for the majority of metastases of renal origin.

Understanding of the molecular biology of CCRCC has identified molecular targets for therapy and aided in the development of useful immunohistochemical assays. A defective von Hippel–Lindau (VHL)-hypoxia inducible factor (HIF) pathway is believed to play a major role in the etiopathogenesis of sporadic as well as VHL-syndrome-associated CCRCC. HIFs are constantly produced and degraded by cells under normoxic conditions via ubiquitination. Under normoxic conditions, protein VHL (pVHL) functions as a recognition subunit in an E3 ubiquitin protein ligase complex, targeting hydroxylated HIF-α for ubiquitin-mediated degradation. Loss of pVHL, as a result of *VHL* gene inactivation, mimics hypoxic conditions by preventing the degradation of HIF. Accumulation of HIF leads to activation of numerous downstream transcription factors. Carbonic anhydrase IX (CAIX), one of the four transmembrane members of the carbonic anhydrase family, is one such important downstream target. It regulates the intracellular and extracellular pH by transmembrane transportation of CO_2. It is thought to play a major role in the survival of rapidly proliferating tumors by efficiently controlling the intracellular and extracellular pH in an attempt to adapt to progressively hypoxic conditions.

CAIX expression has been found in a variety of other tumors. In the gynecological tract it is expressed in carcinomas involving the ovary and the cervix. Gastrointestinal tract tumors such as those involving esophagus and colorectal region show an increased expression of CAIX. In the genitourinary system, renal cancers and urothelial carcinomas show an upregulation. Other sites include carcinomas of nasopharynx, breast, and lung, and some soft tissue sarcomas.

Because CAIX is constitutively activated in CCRCC it is uniformly expressed over the entire tumor. In other tumors the upregulation of CAIX is secondary to true tumor hypoxia, and hence its expression is primarily seen in the perinecrotic region. Increased expression of CAIX is associated with resistance to therapy and a poor outcome. Thus CAIX is not only an excellent diagnostic tool but also a promising biomarker for prediction of outcomes.

Applications

CAIX expression in primary renal cell carcinoma

Accurate subclassification of primary renal cell carcinoma is often challenging, as increasing numbers of genetic subtypes with histologically overlapping features are recognized. Each of these distinct entities has a distinct biologic behavior. Accurate classification not only provides important information regarding the patient's potential clinical course but may also guide therapy and provide avenues for future research. CAIX is one such biomarker that is highly expressed in CCRCC and used to guide patient treatment. A high CAIX expression has been found to be associated with a better prognosis for patients who present with metastatic disease. In stage- and grade-matched patients, those with lower CAIX expression did worse than those with high CAIX expression. The expression of CAIX in CCRCC is inversely related to the Fuhrman grade. The higher the Fuhrman grade, the lower the expression of CAIX.

CCRCC, papillary renal cell carcinoma (PRCC), clear cell papillary renal cell carcinoma (CCPRCC), unclassified RCC, and Xp11.2-translocation RCC all reveal some degree of CAIX expression. Among these, a consistently high expression is seen in CCRCC and CCPRCC. The expression of CAIX in PRCC and Xp11.2-translocation RCC is focal or patchy. Chromophobe RCC and oncocytomas are mostly negative. This pattern of staining can be utilized in conjunction with additional immunohistochemical markers to accurately subclassify difficult cases, or support the histologic impression.

A panel with CK7, CAIX, and racemase, with or without CD10 and RCC, can be used to distinguish CCRCC, PRCC, and CCPRCC.

- CCRCC is strongly diffusely positive for CAIX, negative for CK7 and racemase.
- PRCC may be focally positive for CAIX, but strongly diffusely positive for CK7 and racemase.
- CCPRCC is positive for CK7 and CAIX, but negative for racemase.

In a workup of renal pelvic tumors where the differential diagnosis includes poorly differentiated RCC and urothelial carcinoma it should be remembered that CAIX expression is high in both CCRCC and urothelial carcinoma, and therefore this marker should not be used in this context.

Workup of metastatic CCRCC

Diagnosis of metastatic CCRCC can occasionally be challenging. This may be due to CCRCC presenting for the first time as a metastasis in a patient with no known history of a renal mass or a metastasis discovered in a patient who had a remote history of renal cancer. CCRCC are notorious for metastasis to unusual sites such as skin, salivary glands, thyroid gland, and stomach. In patients who have a history of RCC, the metastatic CCRCC may histologically differ from the primary. All these factors may be further compounded by the limited sampling obtained by a needle core biopsy or fine needle aspiration. An accurate and concise immunohistochemical panel is therefore an invaluable tool to reach the diagnosis of metastatic CCRCC.

Many renal markers are available for the evaluation of CCRCCs. Renal cell carcinoma antigen is considered a specific marker for primary renal neoplasms, particularly CCRCC and PRCC. However, the sensitivity of RCCa has been low. CAIX is found to be more sensitive than RCCa. PAX-2 in metastatic CCRCC has shown moderate sensitivity (47–85%) and high overall specificity (90–97%). PAX-8 is expressed in 97% of CCRCC and in general shows higher expression in all other subtypes of RCC when compared to PAX-2. In the correct context, use of PAX-8 will specify renal origin and CAIX may further help in subclassification as CCRCC.

CCRCC is the most common type of RCC to metastasize to thyroid, accounting for approximately 33% of all metastases in clinical material. Metastatic CCRCC to thyroid could be misinterpreted as a clear cell change in adenomatoid nodules, follicular adenomas, or parathyroid glands. PAX-8 is expressed by both thyroid and renal lineage cells, and therefore cannot be used in the differential diagnosis of primary thyroid lesions and metastatic RCC. An immunohistochemical panel with a negative for TTF-1 and thyroglobulin and a positive CAIX has been found to be 100% sensitive and specific for metastatic CCRCC in thyroid.

CAIX has emerged as an important marker for CCRCC in the workup of metastases, and in differentiating RCC subtypes. Additionally, CAIX is also emerging as an important biomarker for calculating prognosis and guiding therapy.

Selected references

Al-Ahmadie HA, Alden D, Qin LX, *et al*. Carbonic anhydrase IX expression in clear cell renal cell carcinoma. An immunohistochemical study comparing 2 antibodies. *American Journal of Surgical Pathology* 2008; 32: 377–82.

Bing Z, Lal P, Lu S, *et al*. Role of carbonic anhydrase IX, α-methylacyl coenzyme a racemase, cytokeratin 7, and galectin-3 in the evaluation of renal neoplasms: a tissue microarray immunohistochemical study. *Annals of Diagnostic Pathology* 2013; 17: 58–62.

Bui MH, Visapaa H, Seligson D, *et al*. Prognostic value of carbonic anhydrase IX and KI67 as predictors of survival for renal clear cell carcinoma. *Journal of Urology* 2004; 171: 2461–6.

Genega E, Ghebremichael M, Najarian R, *et al*. Carbonic anhydrase IX in renal neoplasms. Correlation with tumor type and grade. *American Journal of Clinical Pathology* 2010; 134: 873–9.

Stillebroer AB, Mulders PFA, Boerman OC, *et al*. Carbonic anhydrase IX in renal cell carcinoma: implications for prognosis, diagnosis and therapy. *European Urology* 2010; 58: 75–83.

Calcitonin

Sources/clones

Axcel/Accurate (polyclonal), Biodesign (polyclonal), Biogenesis (polyclonal, 115), Biogenex (polyclonal), Chemicon (polyclonal), Dako (polyclonal, CAL-3-F5), Fitzgerald (polyclonal), Immunotech (polyclonal), Sanbio/Monosan (polyclonal), Sera Lab (polyclonal), Zymed (polyclonal).

Fixation/preparation

These antibodies are applicable to formalin-fixed paraffin-embedded sections. HIER does not appear to enhance immunoreactivity but is not deleterious.

Background

CAL-3-F5 was raised against the synthetic peptide corresponding to the C-terminal portion of human calcitonin (aa 24–32). The polyclonal antibodies were raised in rabbits using synthetic human calcitonin (35 kDa). Molecular biology studies have shown that most regulatory peptides are cleavage products of larger precursor molecules. The structure of the calcitonin precursor was predicted from the nucleotide sequence of cloned cDNA prepared from the mRNA obtained from medullary thyroid carcinoma. In the human calcitonin precursor, calcitonin is flanked by two molecules: PDN (peptide-aspartic acid-asparagine), a 21-amino acid C-terminal flanking peptide, and a larger N-terminal peptide. Calcitonin gene-related peptide (CGRP)-α is also encoded by the calcitonin gene and is produced as a result of differential RNA processing. The differential production of CGRP and calcitonin from the calcitonin gene is regulated in a tissue-specific manner, with CGRP being produced in nervous tissue and calcitonin in thyroid C cells. However, both CGRP and calcitonin are found in normal, hyperplastic, and neoplastic C cells in humans, although the immunohistochemical pattern of localization is different for individual antigens.

Applications

Antibodies to calcitonin are useful to identify normal, hyperplastic, and neoplastic C cells. Medullary thyroid carcinoma (MTC) occurs both in a sporadic and inherited form, with a biological behavior between that of anaplastic and differentiated thyroid carcinomas. Given the morphologic heterogeneity of MTC, both in histological structure (solid, trabecular, or insular) and in cellular patterns (spindle, polyhedral, angular, or round), as well as the description of papillary, follicular, clear cell, and anaplastic variants, the role of antibodies to calcitonin becomes crucial in making the correct diagnosis. In series of 60 and 25 cases, all MTC demonstrated immunoreaction with antibodies to calcitonin. It has also been suggested that calcitonin-rich tumors appeared to have a better prognosis than calcitonin-poor neoplasms. However, subsequent studies were at a variance with these observations. Studies have also shown sporadic MTC to be a more life-threatening neoplasm than MTC occurring in the setting of MEN IIa syndrome, while those in MEN IIb syndrome were most aggressive.

Antibodies to calcitonin are also useful to identify the concept of C-cell hyperplasia in benign and malignant thyroid glands. A novel application of immunostaining in forensic science has also been proposed: immunoreactivity for calcitonin in thyroid C cells was consistently lost 13 days following death, providing a means of delimiting the time of death.

Comments

Antibody to calcitonin is a compulsory addition to any immunohistochemical histopathology laboratory for the diagnosis of MTC. Normal parafollicular C cells are suitable as positive control tissue.

Selected references

Allison J, Hall L, MacIntyre I, Craig RK. The construction and partial characterisation of plasmids containing complementary DNA sequences to human calcitonin precursor polyprotein. *Biochemistry Journal* 1981; 199: 725–31.

Saad MF, Ordonez NG, Guido JJ, Samaan NA. The prognostic value of calcitonin immunostaining in medullary carcinoma of the thyroid. *Journal of Clinical Endocrinology and Metabolism* 1984; 59: 850–6.

h-Caldesmon

Sources/clones

Dako (h-CD).

Fixation/preparation

h-CD requires microwave HIER in citrate buffer. Some workers have combined this with pepsin pretreatment.

Background

Caldesmon is a protein that binds to calmodulin, tropomyosin, and actin and is thought to play an important role in the regulation of smooth muscle contraction. It exists in two isoforms: 1-CD (70–80 kDa) and high-molecular-weight caldesmon (h-CD: 120–150 kDa). Although 1-CD is present in many cells, h-CD is exclusively expressed in vascular and visceral smooth muscle cells and in myoepithelial cells.

h-CD is expressed intensely and extensively in tumors with smooth muscle differentiation – leiomyomas, leiomyosarcomas, angiomyomas, and glomus tumors – whereas rhabdomyosarcomas, malignant fibrous histiocytomas, desmoids, and inflammatory myofibroblastic tumors are negative for h-CD. In addition, h-CD has not been found in vascular pericytes and myofibroblasts (around ulcers and granulomas). Although non-neoplastic myoepithelial cells are immunopositive for h-CD, tumors with a myoepithelial cell participation (pleomorphic adenomas, chondroid syringoma, myoepithelioma, and epimyoepithelial carcinoma) are negative for h-CD.

Endometrial stromal sarcomas are negative with h-CD, while uterine cellular leiomyomas showed a heterogeneous but intense pattern of immunoreactivity with h-CD. As the converse is generally true for CD10, the combined use of these two markers may serve to distinguish leiomyosarcoma from endometrial stromal neoplasms. This specificity of h-CD for smooth muscle tumors has also been demonstrated in soft tissue tumors; however, it should be noted that this marker has shown significant variability in expression. Leiomyosarcomas confined to peripheral soft tissue were all negative for h-CD.

Applications

h-CD appears to be useful in distinguishing smooth muscle tumors (h-CD+) from tumors with myofibroblastic and myoepithelial differentiation (h-CD–). However, its expression is not consistent, and peripheral soft tissue leiomyosarcomas appear to show low immunoexpression. The other major application pertains to the differential diagnosis between cellular leiomyoma (h-CD+) and endometrial stromal tumors, although the latter may show focal muscle differentiation.

Selected reference

Hisaoka M, Wei-Qi S, Jian W, et al. Specific but variable expression of h-caldesmon in leiomyosarcomas. An immunohistochemical reassessment of a novel myogenic marker. *Applied Immunohistochemistry and Molecular Morphology* 2001; 9: 302–8.

NOTES

Calponin

Sources/clones

Accurate (CP-93), Dako (Calponin, N3), Novocastra (CALP), Sigma (CP-93).

Fixation/preparation

These antibodies are applicable to formalin-fixed paraffin-embedded tissue sections. A heat-induced epitope retrieval (HIER) system with additional enzyme digestion is required.

Background

Calponin is a 34 kDa smooth muscle-specific protein implicated in the regulation of smooth contraction as a result of its ability to inhibit actin-activated MgATPase of smooth muscle myosin. Calponin is a calmodulin-negative, F-actin-negative and tropomyosin-negative binding protein.

Calponin has been demonstrated in all periacinar and periductal myoepithelial cells of normal salivary glands, being negative in acinar/ductal epithelial cells. There is calponin immunoexpression in 98% of pleomorphic adenomas, reacting to almost all myoepithelial cells, including 60% of modified and 30% of transformed myoepithelial cells. Calponin was the most sensitive marker of neoplastic myoepithelium. This sensitivity has also been demonstrated in myoepithelial carcinomas, which show up to 75% calponin immunopositivity.

In mesenchymal tumors, calponin immunoexpression has been demonstrated in benign smooth muscle tumors from various locations, and in retroperitoneal and uterine leiomyosarcomas. However, caution is advised as calponin also reacted with myofibroblasts, both reactive and in myofibroblastic lesions.

Myofibrosarcomas may also be highlighted with calponin. The demonstration of calponin in 85% of angiomatoid fibrous histiocytomas is further confirmation of the myoid phenotype of these tumors. About 80% of neurothekeomas, including cellular and mixed variants, have been shown to express calponin.

Applications

Within the established panel of muscle markers, including S100 protein, calponin is probably the most sensitive marker for myoepithelial cells. However, caution is advised, as myofibroblasts may also be immunopositive.

Selected references

Miettinen MM, Sarloma-Rikala M, Kovatich AJ, Lasota J. Calponin and h-caldesmon in soft tissue tumors: consistent h-caldesmon immunoreactivity in gastrointestinal stromal tumors indicates traits of smooth muscle differentiation. *Modern Pathology* 1999; 12: 756–62.

Savera AT, Gown AM, Zarbo RJ. Immunolocalization of three novel smooth muscle-specific proteins in salivary gland pleomorphic adenoma: assessment of the morphogenetic role of myoepithelium. *Modern Pathology* 1997; 10: 1093–100

NOTES

Calreticulin

Sources/clones

Abcam (ab2907, ab22683), Bio-Rad (1G11-1A9), EMD Millipore (06-661), Enzo Life Sciences (FMC75), GeneTex (GTX20004, GTX42683), LSBio (LS-C41535), Novus Biological (NBP2-33524), SIGMA (C4606), StressMarq (SPC122A), Proteintech (10292-1-AP), ThermoFisher (Pa3-900, PA1-902A).

Fixation/preparation

Fresh frozen tissue and cytologic preparations, and formalin-fixed paraffin-embedded tissue.

Background

Calreticulin (CALR) is a multifunctional protein of 417 amino acids (molecular weight 48 kDa), and consists of three domains: a 180 aa N-terminal globular region, a 111 aa P- or proline-rich domain, and a 109 aa C-terminus. It acts as a major $Ca2+$-binding (storage) protein in the lumen of the endoplasmic reticulum and sarcoplasmic reticulum. It is also a molecular chaperone and is involved in protein folding events. It is also found in the nucleus, suggesting that it may have a role in transcription regulation. CALR can play a role as modulator of the regulation of gene transcription by nuclear hormone receptors. It interacts with the DNA-binding domain of NR3C1 and mediates its nuclear export. The amino terminus of CALR interacts with the DNA-binding domain of the glucocorticoid receptor and prevents the receptor from binding to its specific glucocorticoid response element.

Applications

CALR mutations are associated with primary myelofibrosis and essential thrombocythemia. All *CALR* mutations lead to a frameshift generating a new 36 amino-acid C-terminus, which can be identified by immunohistochemistry using a monoclonal antibody (CAL2). Therefore, the lack of *CALR* mutation demonstrates negative staining. Specificity is 100%, sensitivity 82–91%, positive predictive value 100%, and negative predictive value 90–95%. *CALR* may be useful together with other markers in the diagnosis of upper urothelial carcinomas. It is also overexpressed in adrenocortical carcinomas, ductal breast carcinomas, and lung cancer cells.

Comments

CALR is expressed in the endoplasmic reticulum lumen: cytoplasm and cytosol and cell surface. It may be secreted into the extracellular space and extracellular matrix. It is also present in the cell surface (T cells) and associated with the lytic granules in cytolytic T lymphocytes.

Selected references

Andrici J, Farzin M, Clarkson A, *et al*. Mutation specific immunohistochemistry is highly specific for the presence of calreticulin mutations in myeloproliferative neoplasms. *Pathology* 2016; 48: 319–24.

Kabbage M, Trimeche M, Bergaoui S, *et al*. Calreticulin expression in infiltrating ductal breast carcinomas: relationships with disease progression and humoral immune responses. *Tumour Biology* 2013; 34: 1177–88.

NOTES

Calretinin

Sources/clones

Biogenesis (polyclonal), Chemicon (polyclonal AB149), Novocastra (mouse anti-human 1568), Swart (Ab7696 raised against human recombinant calretinin), Zymed (prediluted polyclonal).

Fixation/preparation

These antibodies are applicable to formalin-fixed paraffin-embedded sections. Pretreatment of tissue sections with citrate buffer in a microwave oven or with 0.01% pronase in phosphate-buffered saline at room temperature increases calretinin immunoreactivity.

Background

Calretinin is a calcium-binding protein of 29 kDa. It is a member of the large family of EF-hand proteins, to which the S100 protein also belongs. EF-hand proteins are characterized by a peculiar amino acid sequence that folds up into a helix-loop-helix that acts as a calcium-binding site. Calretinin contains six such EF-hand stretches. The calretinin gene was initially isolated from a cDNA clone from the chick retina, and it is abundantly expressed in central and peripheral neural tissues, particularly in the retina and in neurons of the sensory pathways. Although the function of calretinin is unknown, a possible role as a calcium buffer has been postulated. Consistent calretinin immunoreactivity has been found in a variety of normal tissues including mesothelial cell lining of all serosal membranes, eccrine glands of skin, convoluted tubules of kidney, Leydig and Sertoli cells of the testis, epithelium of rete testis, endometrium and ovarian stromal cells, and adrenal cortical cells.

The consistent calretinin immunoreactivity (using Ab7696) in normal and hyperplastic mesothelial cells led to its establishment as a reliable positive marker for mesothelial differentiation. Exhibiting a sensitivity close to 100%, immunoreactivity was observed in the majority of tumor cells in epithelioid, biphasic, and sarcomatoid mesotheliomas, with focal positivity in about 10% of adenocarcinomas metastatic to serous membranes. An alternative antibody to calretinin (AB149) demonstrated calretinin immunopositivity in both mesotheliomas and adenocarcinomas following a heat-induced antigen retrieval system. Using the same antibody to calretinin, another group demonstrated immunopositivity in about 42% of mesotheliomas with a diffuse distribution in the majority of cases but only approximately 6% of adenocarcinomas with a weak or moderate staining pattern. Hence, while specificity with the calretinin antibody AB149 was high, sensitivity was low; in contrast, the anti-calretinin antibody 7696 demonstrated both high specificity and sensitivity. Similar findings have also been demonstrated with the anti-calretinin polyclonal antibody from Zymed.

Immunocytochemical analysis of cytologic specimens from serous effusions has been shown to demonstrate positive immunoreaction in all cases of mesothelioma.

As calretinin is expressed abundantly in neurons of the central and peripheral nervous system, neoplasms exhibiting neuronal differentiation also demonstrate immunoreactivity with calretinin.

Applications

Calretinin represents one of the more sensitive and specific markers for mesothelial differentiation available to date. Applicable to both histologic and cytologic material, it is recommended for inclusion in a panel of antibodies when investigating the differential diagnosis between epithelioid mesothelioma and adenocarcinoma. The E-cadherin/calretinin combination has been shown to demonstrate both high specificity and high sensitivity in distinguishing between mesothelioma and metastatic adenocarcinoma, with E-cadherin highlighting the latter. A note of caution is that calretinin decorates both normal/hyperplastic and neoplastic mesothelial cells and therefore does not distinguish between reactive and neoplastic mesothelial cells.

Calretinin is particularly useful for distinguishing central neurocytoma from oligodendroglioma, being negative in the latter. It has a wider potential application in distinguishing between brain tumors with glial and neuronal differentiation.

Calretinin is a sensitive marker of ovarian sex cord–stromal tumors and may be of value in this diagnostic setting as part of a larger panel. In ovarian sex cord–stromal tumors, strong calretinin immunostaining is seen in all hilus cell tumors and in the Leydig cell component of Sertoli–Leydig cell tumors; and staining is absent in fibrothecomas and granulosa cell tumors.

Calretinin has been shown to be an important diagnostic marker for both solid and cystic ameloblastomas, and helpful in the differential diagnosis of unicystic ameloblastomas. Although immunopositivity has been demonstrated in mast cell lesions of the skin, the cost-effectiveness has been questioned, in view of the availability of less expensive special stains. Demonstration of calretinin-positive cells in biphasic synovial sarcomas has been largely confirmed to the spindle cells with a focal distribution, raising a cautionary note in the differential diagnosis of pleural-based malignancies and underscoring the role of an antibody panel in such investigations. Positive expression of calretinin in neoplastic cells of cardiac myxoma supports the concept that myxoma cells may originate from endocardial sensory nerve tissue.

Comments

Calretinin immunoexpression involves both the nucleus and cytoplasm. An often useful "built-in" positive control in test sections is adipocytes. Purkinje cells of mature cerebellum may be used as controls. Biogenesis polyclonal antiserum (1741-1007) cross-reacts with rat, monkey, guinea pig, cow, mouse, and chick calretinin.

Selected references

Barberis MCP, Faleri M, Veronese S, *et al.* Calretinin: a selective marker of normal and neoplastic mesothelial cells in serous effusions. *Acta Cytologica* 1997; 41: 1757–61.

Cao QJ, Jones JG, Li M. Expression of calretinin in human ovary, testis, and ovarian sex cord–stromal tumors. *International Journal of Gynecologic Pathology* 2001; 20: 346–52.

Dei Tos AP, Doglioni C. Calretinin: a novel tool for diagnostic immunohistochemistry. *Advances in Anatomic Pathology* 1998; 5: 61–6

Candida albicans

Sources/clones

Biogenex (monoclonal antibody 1B12).

Fixation/preparation

Antigen retrieval involving microwave treatment of specimens in citrate buffer is required for formalin-fixed paraffin-embedded (FFPE) tissue sections.

Background

The diagnosis of oral candidiasis requires the sampling of the mucosal surface for the culture and identification of *Candida* species. In chronic hyperplastic candidiasis, the fungal hyphae of *Candida* species invade the superficial layers of the epithelium, making diagnosis difficult on candidal culture alone. Hence, biopsy of such lesions for microscopic examination is essential for diagnosis. Staining with periodic acid-Schiff (PAS) or methenamine-silver stains detects hyphal structures consistent with *Candida* species in formalin-fixed tissue sections. However, these stains do not permit identification of individual *Candida* species. Further, the variable sensitivity of *Candida* to antifungal agents makes identification of the infecting species important.

The mouse monoclonal antibody (1B12) was raised against the high-molecular-weight mannoproteins of *Candida albicans* (Biogenex). This antibody is species-specific.

Identification of the infecting species is not only important for therapeutic purposes, but may help clarify the association of chronic hyperplastic candidiasis with the development of squamous cell carcinoma.

Applications

The ability of monoclonal antibody 1B12 to identify *Candida* hyphae penetrating lesional tissue in chronic candidiasis provides an opportunity to enhance our understanding of the role of *Candida* species in this form of oral candidiasis.

Selected references

Monteagudo C, Marcilla A, Mormeneo S, Llombart-Bosch A, Sentandreu R. Specific immunohistochemical identification of *Candida albicans* in paraffin-embedded tissue with a new monoclonal antibody (1B12). *American Journal of Clinical Pathology* 1995; 103: 130–5.

Williams DW, Jones HS, Allison RT, Potts AJ, Lewis MA. Immunocytochemical detection of *Candida albicans* in formalin fixed, paraffin embedded material. *Journal of Clinical Pathology* 1998; 51: 857–9.

NOTES

Carcinoembryonic antigen (CEA)

Sources/clones

Accurate (C234, 12–140–10, MIC0101), Axcel/Accurate (A5B7, polyclonal), Biodesign (ME.104, CEJ 065, MAM6, 9207, 9201, 9203, polyclonal), Biogenesis (6.2, 1G9/9,10, MAC601, polyclonal), Biogenex (SP-651, TF3H8–1), Biosource, Calbiochem, Caltag Laboratories (CEA6.2), Cymbus Bioscience (85A12), Dako (11–7, polyclonal), EY Labs, Fitzgerald (M94129, M94130, M94131, M94132, M 2103124, M2103125, polyclonal), Immunotech (FJ95, CEJ 065), Immunotech SA (F023C5), Novocastra (85A12, 12–140–10), Oncogene (TF3H8), Shandon Lipshaw (CEJ065), Sigma Chemical (C6G9), Zymed (ZCEA1, COL-l).

Fixation/preparation

This antibody can be used on formalin-fixed paraffin-embedded tissue sections. Prolonged fixation in buffered formalin may destroy the epitope. Antibody to CEA may also be used for frozen sections. Trypsinization is essential for antigen unmasking. HIER does not appear to enhance staining.

Background

CEA consists of a heterogeneous family of related oncofetal glycoproteins (approximately 200 kDa molecular weight) which is secreted into the glycocalyx surface of gastrointestinal cells. CEA was first described in 1965 as a specific antigen for adenocarcinoma of the colon and the digestive tract of a 2–6-month-old fetus. The monoclonal antibody to CEA was raised using tumor cells derived from a hepatic metastasis of colonic carcinoma. CEA is a complex glycoprotein; hence, even after purification some degree of molecular heterogeneity exists. Therefore antibodies to CEA, particularly polyclonal, commonly react against a nonspecific cross-reactive antigen (NCA) located in normal colon and granulocytes. Because of the cross-reactivity of most heterologous anti-CEA antisera with NCA, the results obtained when polyclonal anti-CEA antibody was used have been questioned. The anti-NCA reactivity of anti-CEA antibody is demonstrated with positive immunoreaction in polymorphonuclear leukocytes and macrophages, since the cells lack CEA antigen but contain NCA. Therefore it is recommended that positive results obtained with a polyclonal anti-CEA antibody, without preabsorption with NCA, be interpreted as being nonspecific. Even monoclonal antibodies to CEA may cross-react with other molecules of the CEA family, including NCA. Therefore, each antibody needs to be evaluated to avoid nonspecific results.

Applications

CEA is found in several adenocarcinomas, such as colon, lung, breast, stomach, and pancreas. Over 70% of adenocarcinomas from a variety of organs are CEA-positive, with no evidence of expression of CEA by neoplastic cells in malignant mesothelioma. Hence, expression of CEA by adenocarcinomas and their absence in mesothelioma represents a valuable marker in the discrimination of mesotheliomas from morphologically similar adenocarcinomas involving any organ. However, it should be stressed that such results are dependent on individual antibody evaluation. Occasional hyaluronate-rich epithelial mesotheliomas may produce false positivity with CEA, although this staining can be abolished by hyaluronidase digestion prior to immunoprocessing. CEA is the best single marker in separating adenocarcinoma from mesothelioma: positive with 97% specificity and sensitivity for adenocarcinoma; negative with 97% specificity and sensitivity for mesothelioma (Appendix 1.17). Polyclonal CEA is also useful for the demonstration of bile canaliculi in hepatocytes and the cells of hepatocellular carcinoma, both in cytologic preparations and in tissue sections (Appendix 1.8). Although the presence of bile canaliculi is specific for hepatocytes, its sensitivity is low.

Comments

The fact that no single antibody is sufficiently specific and sensitive for the distinction of mesothelioma from adenocarcinoma necessitates the use of a panel of antibodies comprising a broad-spectrum cytokeratin, monoclonal CEA, Leu-M1, and BER-EP4, which allows for confident differentiation of these tumors in approximately 90% of cases. The addition of calretinin, CK5/6, D2-40, and WT1 to the panel increases the diagnostic accuracy. Colonic carcinoma is the favored positive control tissue for antibodies against CEA.

Selected reference

Robb JA. Mesothelioma versus adenocarcinoma: false-positive CEA and Leu-M1 staining due to hyaluronic acid. *Human Pathology* 1989; 20: 400.

Catenins α, β, γ

Sources/clones

α-Catenin: Becton Dickinson (1G5), Transduction Laboratories

β-Catenin: Transduction Laboratories, Zymed (5H10)

γ-Catenin: Becton Dickinson (10C4), Transduction Laboratories

Fixation/preparation

HIER is necessary for the immunoreactivity of these antibodies in fixed paraffin-embedded sections. Immunoreactivity is preserved in frozen sections and cell preparations.

Background

There is currently a great deal of interest in the adhesion molecules and their expression and localization. Cell-to-cell adhesion plays a major role not only in embryogenesis but also in the intercellular adhesion of cancer cells and hence their motility and metastasis. The transmembrane molecule E-cadherin is considered to be one of the key molecules in the formation of the intercellular junctional complex and establishment of polarity in epithelial cells. The cytoplasmic domain of E-cadherin in adherens junctions interacts via intracellular catenins with the actin-based cytoskeleton and includes fodrin, whereas the extracellular domain is involved in homotypic cell-to-cell adhesion through the formation of a molecular zipper complex. The integrity of the E-cadherin adhesion system has been shown to be disturbed or disrupted in experimental and human carcinomas, and reduced expression of E-cadherin induces dedifferentiation and invasiveness in tumor cells.

Catenins, the α-subunit (102 kDa), β-subunit (88 kDa), and γ-subunit (82 kDa), are a group of proteins that interact with the intercellular domain of E-cadherin, resulting in complexes of E-cadherin/β-catenin/α-catenin or E-cadherin/γ-catenin/α-catenin. α-Catenin shows sequence homology to vinculin and interacts with the actin cytoskeleton, either directly or indirectly via α-actinin; β-catenin is the vertebrate homolog of the *Drosophila* segment polarity gene *armadillo*; and γ-catenin is identical to plakoglobin and is also found in desmosomes. The regions of both α- and β-*catenin*, located on 5q21–22 and 3p21, have been shown to be involved in the development of certain tumors, and reduced expressions of both α- and β-catenin have been described in various tumors including breast carcinoma. Besides adhesion functions, β-catenin binds to adenomatous polyposis coli (APC) protein, a putative tumor suppressor. *APC* mutation disturbs the equilibrium and levels of free β-catenin in the cell, and may have a role in tumorigenesis. β-catenin has recently been shown to have a function in signal transduction when bound with members of the Tcf-LEF family of DNA-binding proteins. In src cell lines, the loss of E-cadherin is associated with loss of immunostaining for β-catenin and heralds a change in morphology from epithelial to spindled shapes. Somatic mutations of the β-catenin and APC genes are associated with nuclear translocation of β-catenin in both sporadic and familial adenomatous polyposis (FAP)-associated breast fibromatosis. The nuclear accumulation of β-catenin has also been shown in sporadic basal cell carcinoma, desmoid-type fibromatosis, and pancreatic solid-pseudopapillary neoplasms.

Applications

Although currently not of diagnostic importance, the expression of the catenin proteins and their localization are potentially important markers to predict motility and invasiveness of epithelial neoplasms. Our studies suggest that the detachment of β-catenin from the cell membrane heralds the breakdown of the cadherin–catenin–fodrin–cytoskeletal complex both in vitro and in vivo. The loss of cell-to-cell adhesion is concomitant with a change in cell shape, from epithelioid to fibroblastoid.

Comments

The monoclonal antibodies from Transduction Laboratories are immunoreactive in routinely fixed paraffin-embedded tissue section, but only following HIER in citrate buffer.

Selected references

Birchmeier W, Behrens J. Cadherin expression in carcinomas: role in the formation of cell junctions and the prevention of invasiveness. *Biochemia Biophysiology Acta* 1994; 1198: 11–26.

Hinck L, Nathke IS, Papkoff J, Nelson WJ. Dynamics of cadherin/catenin complex formation: novel protein interactions and pathways of complex assembly. *Journal of Cell Biology* 1994; 125: 1327–40.

CD1

Sources/clones

Accurate (WM35-la), Becton Dickinson (Leu-5), Biogenesis (DMC1), Biogenex (T6-la), Bioprobe, Biosource (BB5), Boehringer Mannheim (YIT6), Coulter (T6), Cymbus Bioscience (CBNT6-la), Dako (NA1/34), Immunotech (010, CD1a), Oncogene, Sanbio (66–11-C7), Sera Lab (CD1), Serotec (4A76, NAI-34-la).

Fixation/preparation

Fresh frozen tissues. CD1a (clone 010) is effective in paraffin-embedded tissues, immunoreactivity enhanced by HIER.

Background

Human CD1 genes are a family of five non-polymorphic genes that, although homologous to both class I and II major histocompatibility complex genes, map to chromosome 1. Four isoforms of the CD1 proteins have been clustered, namely CD1a, -b, -c, and -d. They are expressed on the surface of cells in association with β2-microglobulin and may function as nonclassical antigen-presenting molecules. While CD1 genes have been found in a wide variety of vertebrates, they have shown differences in size and complexity in different mammals. Most CD1 molecules can be separated into two groups based mainly on homology of nucleotide and amino acid sequences. Group 1 includes the human CD1a, -b, and -c proteins, which are the classic CD1 antigens first identified on human thymocytes and now recognized on a variety of specialized antigen-presenting cells, including dendritic cells in lymphoid and non-lymphoid tissues. These proteins can also be induced in vitro on virtually all circulating human monocytes by exposure to granulocyte-macrophage-CSF, suggesting that they might be upregulated on tissue macrophages in many inflammatory lesions. The group 2 CD1 proteins include the human CD1d and mouse CD1, which so far have been found to be most prominently expressed by gastrointestinal epithelia and B lymphocytes.

CD1a, -b, and -c are expressed in about 70% of all thymocytes, predominantly the cortical thymocytes. CD1 is not expressed in early thymocytes or by mature resting or activated T lymphocytes. This distribution is reflected by neoplastic populations of T cells in that precursor T-ALL/LBLs expressing cortical or immature phenotypes are CD1-positive, in contrast to those with prothymocyte or medullary thymocyte phenotypes. All post-thymic or Tdt-negative T-cell neoplasms such as T-CLL, T-PLL, Tγ-lymphoproliferative disorder, Sézary syndrome, cutaneous T-cell lymphoma, and node-based T-cell lymphoma are consistently negative for CD1.

Applications

CD1a, CD1b, and CD1c antigens are membrane glycoproteins with molecular weights of 49 kDa, 45 kDa, and 43 kDa, respectively. Their expression on thymocytes and also on a variety of antigen-presenting cells including Langerhans cells and interdigitating dendritic cells makes detection, particularly of CD1a, useful in the diagnosis of Langerhans cell histiocytosis, and in the classification of thymomas and malignancies of T-cell precursors.

CD1a is a specific marker for Langerhans cells. Thymic lymphocytes that are CD1-positive represent cortical thymocytes. Myeloid leukemias, some B-cell malignancies, and dendritic cells in most peripheral cutaneous T-cell lymphomas are also positive.

Comments

Antibodies to CD1a are useful in diagnosis of Langerhans cell histiocytosis and in the classification of thymomas, especially when used in combination with the PE-35 antibody that reacts with a variety of epithelia including the medullary epithelium of the thymus and malignancies of T-cell precursors. While most of the antibodies available are only reactive in fresh frozen tissues, clone 010 is reactive in paraffin sections following heat-induced epitope retrieval (HIER) and is available through Immunotech. S100 positivity has been employed as the conventional marker to distinguish between Langerhans histiocytosis and non-Langerhans histiocytosis, but it is now clearly recognized that abnormal histiocytes may stain for this marker, so CD1a staining becomes an important diagnostic discriminator.

Selected references

Boumsell L. Cluster report: CD1. In Knapp W, Dorken B, Gilks W, *et al.*, eds. *Leucocyte Typing IV: White Cell Differentiation Antigens*. Oxford: Oxford University Press, 1989, pp. 251–4.

Krenacs L, Tiszalvicz LT, Krenacs T, Boumsell L. Immunohistochemical detection of CD1A antigen in formalin-fixed and paraffin-embedded tissue sections with monoclonal antibody 010. *Journal of Pathology* 1993; 171: 99–104.

Porcelli SA, Modlin RL. CD1 and the expanding universe of T cell antigens. *Journal of Immunology* 1995; 55: 3709–10.

CD2

Sources/clones

Becton Dickinson (Leu-5, S5.2), Biodesign (BH1), Boehringer Mannheim (MT26), Caltag Labs (Gil), Coulter (6F10.3, T11, 39C15), Cymbus Bioscience (GJ12), Dako (MT910), Immunotech (39C1.5), Novocastra (X1X8), Ortho (OKT2), Pharmingen (RPA2.10), Sanbio (MEM65), Serotec (MCA651), Zymed (RPA2.10).

Fixation/preparation

Fresh frozen tissue, fresh air-dried cell preparations.

Background

Human T lymphocytes were initially distinguished from B lymphocytes by their ability to produce spontaneous rosettes with sheep red blood cells, a phenomenon mediated by the CD2 molecule, a glycosylated transmembrane receptor molecule also referred to as Ti1 antigen or leukocyte function-associated antigen 3 (LFA-3). Three functionally important epitope groups have been defined on the human CD2 molecule, designated $T11_1$, $T11_2$, and $T11_3$ (CD2R). $T11_1$ is the epitope responsible for E-rosetting, and T-cell stimulation through this epitope is mediated by an IL-2-dependent pathway. Stimulation of the $T11_2$ and $T11_3$ epitopes occurs via an alternative pathway.

CD2 is one of the earliest T-cell lineage-restricted antigens to appear during T-cell differentiation, and only rare CD2+ cells can be found in the bone marrow. It is found in all T lymphocytes and natural killer cells but not in B cells or any other cell population. CD2 binds to its counter-receptor CD58 (LFA-3), a member of the Ig gene superfamily, which locates on the surface of target cells. CD2 binding to LFA-3 activates T cells and may also have a role in prothymocyte homing, as it is known to mediate thymocyte–thymic epithelium adhesion. Although it is known that CD2 appears after CD7 but before CD1, its temporal relationship with CD3 is less definite, with some recent evidence suggesting that CD3 appears in the cytoplasm before CD2.

Applications

CD2 can be considered a pan-T-cell antigen and is therefore useful for the identification of virtually all normal T lymphocytes. It is also very useful in the assessment of lymphoid malignancies as it is expressed in the majority of precursor and post-thymic lymphomas and leukemias and is not expressed by B neoplasms. As with other pan-T-cell antigens, CD2 may be aberrantly deleted in some neoplastic T-cell populations, especially peripheral T-cell lymphomas. Rarely, sIg+ B-cell neoplasms have been described to form spontaneous E-rosettes, but these reactions are not mediated via the CD2 receptor.

Comments

CD2 antibodies can be used for identification of lymphomas and leukemias of T-cell origin. Positive-staining cells include thymocytes (95%), mature peripheral T cells (almost all), NK cells (80–90%), and thymic B cells (50%). Currently, the majority of monoclonal antibodies available are reactive only in fresh frozen tissue. Clones MCA651 (Serotec) and 6F10.3 (Beckman/Coulter) are claimed to be immunoreactive in fixed sections, and it has been shown that some of the other antibody clones may be reactive in tissues fixed with special fixatives such as non-aldehyde fixatives containing zinc salts or formal dichromate, and with an appropriate antigen retrieval and signal amplification system.

Selected references

Gonzalez L, Anderson I, Deane D, et al. Detection of immune system cells in paraffin wax-embedded ovine tissues. *Journal of Comparative Pathology* 2001; 125: 41–7.

Knowles DM. Lymphoid cell markers: their distribution and usefulness in the immunophenotypic analyses of lymphoid neoplasms. *American Journal of Surgical Pathology* 1985; 9 (Suppl.) 85–108.

CD3

Sources/clones

Accurate (CLBT3, T3, UCHT1), Becton Dickinson (Leu-4), Biodesign, Biogenex (CD3, 12F6), Bioprobe, Boehringer Mannheim (4B5), Coulter (T3, CD3), Dako (T3-4B5, UCHT1), Novocastra (UCHT1), Ortho (OKT3), Pharmingen (HIT3A), Sanbio (MEM57), Serotec, Zymed (SPV-T36). Polyclonal CD3 antisera from Dako, Serotec, Bioprobe/Tha.

Fixation/preparation

The monoclonal antibodies are immunoreactive only in fresh frozen section and cell preparations, whereas polyclonal antisera will react in fixed paraffin-embedded tissue, but only following HIER or prolonged enzyme digestion.

Background

The CD3 antigen consists of five structurally distinct membrane glycoproteins of molecular weight 20–28 kDa assembled as a complex comprising extracellular, transmembrane, and intracellular domains. It is non-covalently associated with the polymorphic T-cell receptor (TCR)-α/β or, alternatively, the TCR-γ/δ heterodimer. Stimulation of the CD3 complex results in T-cell proliferation, release of cytokines, and display of nonspecific cytotoxicity, properties requiring the participation of accessory cells. It is believed that the CD3 complex is responsible for mediating signal transduction to the internal environment upon antigenic recognition by the TCR, although the actual mechanisms of T-cell activation following antigen binding to the TCR are not known.

CD3 is present in the cytoplasm prior to its detection on the cell surface of thymocytes, and more than 95% of thymocytes bear surface and/or cytoplasmic CD3. The antigen is one of the earliest to be expressed in T-cell differentiation and begins during the prothymocyte stage prior to entrance into the thymus. It is a T-cell-specific surface marker normally present in resting and activated T lymphocytes. Cytoplasmic CD3 expression is lost as common thymocytes differentiate into medullary thymocytes, and the antigen is found only on the cell surface in postcortical T cells but not in B cells, monocytes/macrophages, myeloid cells, or any other cell type except for weak expression in Purkinje cells of the cerebellum. CD3δ and CD3ε proteins are detectable in the cytoplasm of virtually all surface CD3-negative acute lymphoblastic leukemias (ALLs), including those that have not yet rearranged their TCR-β genes, supporting the contention that CD3 gene transcription is one of the earliest events to occur in T-cell ontogeny, beginning prior to its entrance into the thymus. The polyclonal anti-CD3 may produce weak staining of squamous epithelium and Hassal's corpuscles in the thymus, but this lacks the distinct membrane ring-like pattern seen in T cells and may represent weak cross-reactivity.

Applications

CD3 is the most specific T-cell antibody. It is therefore a useful marker to distinguish precursor T-cell acute lymphoblastic leukemia/lymphoblastic lymphoma from their B-cell counterparts and acute myeloid leukemia. CD3 is a pan-T-cell lineage-restricted antigen that is useful for labeling both neoplastic and non-neoplastic T cells, and surface CD3 is expressed by all categories of post-thymic T-cell lymphomas as well as lymphoblastic lymphoma but not lymphomas of B-cell lineage. CD3 may be aberrantly deleted in some peripheral T-cell lymphomas. The majority of anti-CD3 monoclonal antibodies including Leu-4 and UCHT1 recognize epitopes mapping to the CD3ε subunit. Positive-staining cells are thymocytes, peripheral T cells, NK cells, and also Purkinje cells of the cerebellum.

Comments

The appropriate antibody should be used for cytocentrifuge preparations, as monoclonal antibody OKT3 detects surface CD3 but not the cytoplasmic antigen in cytocentrifuge preparations. Monoclonal antibodies Leu-4 and UCHT1 detect cytoplasmic CD3 in cytocentrifuge preparations, and many other antibodies are not reactive at all in such preparations. The polyclonal CD3 antibody is a useful reagent for paraffin-embedded sections as well as cytocentrifuge smear especially following heat-induced epitope retrieval (HIER). It is reactive against both normal and neoplastic T cells. CD3 is absent in a subpopulation of T-cell neoplasms including cases of mycosis fungoides, pleomorphic small-cell lymphoma, pleomorphic medium- and large-cell lymphoma, and anaplastic large-cell lymphoma. This may reflect aberrant gene expression by the malignant T cells with loss of the antigen at the outset; alternatively, deletion may occur during the process of large-cell transformation as seen in anaplastic large-cell lymphoma.

Selected references

Cabecadas JM, Isaacson PG. Phenotyping of T cell lymphomas in paraffin sections – which antibodies? *Histopathology* 1991; 19: 419–24.

Campana D, Thompson JS, Amlot P, *et al*. The cytoplasmic expression of CD3 antigen in normal and malignant cells of the T lymphoid lineage. *Journal of Immunology* 1987; 138: 648–55.

Chetty R, Gatter K. CD3 structure, function, and role of immunostaining in clinical practice. *Journal of Pathology* 1994: 173; 303–7.

CD4

Sources/clones

Becton Dickinson (Leu-3), Biotest (T4, TT1), Dako (MT310), Immunotech (BL4, 13B8.2), Novocastra (IF6), Sanbio (BL-TH4, MEM115), Sera Lab, Serotec (B-A1, B-F5, B-B14, 13B8.2), Pharmingen (RM-4-4, RM-4-5), Zymed (IF6).

Fixation/preparation

Paraffin-embedded sections, fresh frozen tissue, and cell preparations.

Background

After the discovery that lymphocytes could be divided into B cells and T cells, discrete subsets of T cells functioning as helper, suppressor, and cytotoxic cells were recognized. The CD4 molecule is a non-polymorphic glycoprotein belonging to the Ig gene superfamily that is expressed on the surface membrane of a functionally distinct subpopulation of T cells, mutually exclusive of the CD8 molecule. The CD4 molecule is a 55 kDa glycoprotein with five external domains, each homologous to an Ig light chain variable region, a transmembrane domain, and a highly conserved intracellular domain. The CD4 gene has been mapped to the short arm of chromosome 12.

The CD4 molecule acts as a co-receptor with the TCR complex and appears to bind to the non-polymorphic region of the MHC class II molecule and may serve to increase the avidity of cell-to-cell interactions. The CD4 molecule also serves as a receptor for the human immunodeficiency virus on T cells, monocytes/macrophages, and some neural cells.

The CD4 antigen, like CD8, appears at the common thymocyte stage of T-cell differentiation and is expressed in about 80–90% of normal thymocytes. CD4 thus marks helper/inducer T cells and is expressed in 55–65% of mature peripheral T cells. It should be noted that the phenotypic–functional association of CD4 to helper and CD8 to suppressor/cytotoxic function is not universal. Subpopulations of suppressor or cytotoxic T cells can be identified among CD4+ T cells. Although it is also expressed on monocytes/macrophages, Langerhans cells and other dendritic cells, B cells do not express CD4.

Applications

The CD4 antibody is useful for the identification of T helper/inducer cells and plays an important role in the immunophenotyping of reactive lymphocytes and in lymphoproliferative disorders. The majority of peripheral T-cell lymphomas are derived from the helper T-cell subset, so most post-thymic T-cell neoplasms are CD4+CD8−. Tγ lymphoproliferative disease is an exception where the proliferative cells are CD4−CD8+. As with other T-cell antigens, CD4 may be aberrantly deleted in neoplastic T cells, and the evaluation of such tumors therefore requires the application of a panel of markers in order to identify tumors with such anomalous antigenic expression. CD4 immunostaining is seen in thymocytes (80–90%), mature T cells (65%, T helper and CD4/CD8 thymocytes), macrophages, Langerhans cells, dendritic cells, granulocytes, and acute myeloid leukemia cells.

Comments

Anti-CD4 antibodies are mostly immunoreactive only in fresh frozen tissue sections and fresh cytologic preparations. In the latter preparations, fixation in 10% buffered formalin or in 0.1% formal saline produces consistent immunostaining, especially if heat-induced epitope retrieval (HIER) is employed. As many phagocytic histiocytes and dendritic cells are also CD4-positive, interpretation of frozen section staining is difficult.

Clone IF6 is immunoreactive in fixed paraffin-embedded sections but the use of 1% or greater of hydrogen peroxide to block endogenous peroxidase is detrimental to staining with this antibody, and if blocking is necessary it should be done before unmasking with 0.5% H_2O_2/methanol for 10 minutes. Fixation in formal dichromate was claimed to improve immunoreactivity in paraffin sections of bovine tissue.

OPD4 (CD45RA) was initially claimed to be specific for CD4+ T cells, but this has not been proven to be so, and OPD4 labels both CD4– and CD8+ cells.

Selected reference

Brady RL, Barclay AN. The structure of CD4. *Current Topics in Microbiology and Immunology* 1996; 205: 1–18.

CD5

Sources/clones

Ancell (UCHT2), Becton Dickinson (Leu-1), Biodesign (BL1a, UCHT2), Biogenex (T1), Bioprobe (T1), Coulter (T1), Cymbus Bioscience (UCHT2), Dako (DK23), Novocastra (NCL-CD5, NCL-CD5-4C7), Oncogene (UCHT2), Sanbio (BL-TP), Sera Lab (UCHT2), Serotec, Sigma, and Pharmingen (UCHT2).

Fixation/preparation

Fresh or frozen tissue for most antibodies. Clone NCL-CD5-4C7 is immunoreactive in fixed paraffin-embedded sections following antigen retrieval at 98 °C.

Background

The CD5 molecule is a transmembrane glycoprotein of 67 kDa, with the typical tripartite structure of a signal peptide. The human CD5 has a sequence similar to that of the Ly-1 antigen in mouse, and both are distantly related members of the immunoglobulin superfamily of genes. CD5 is expressed on both T and some B lymphocytes. It is weakly positive in the most immature T-cell precursors which are CD34-positive, with the intensity of expression increasing with maturation. CD5 expression is first seen in intrathymic T-cell progenitors (CD5+/CD34+) which differentiate into CD3+/CD4+/CD8+ T cells. This antigen is expressed in the majority of T cells with only as many as 11% of CD4+ lymphocytes being CD5-negative. Two-thirds of these CD5− cells are αβ T-cell receptor-positive cells and one-third are γδ T-cells. Anti-CD5 antibodies have been shown to prolong the proliferative response of anti-CD3 activated T lymphocytes by enhancing signal transduction by the T-cell receptor antigen, a process associated with increased IL-2 production and increased IL-2 receptor expression by the T cells. The CD5 antigen may also act as a signal transducing molecule in a manner independent of CD3. It has also been suggested that the B-cell surface protein CD72 (Lyb-2) is the ligand or counterstructure for CD5, and that occupancy of CD72 by anti-CD72 antibodies, and possibly CD5-positive T cells, enhances IL-4-dependent CD23 expression on resting B lymphocytes.

When CD5 is expressed on B lymphocytes, it is usually weakly staining compared to the strong expression of mature T lymphocytes. This weak expression makes precise identification of the CD5+ and CD5− B-cell populations difficult. CD5+ B-cells (B-l cells) are first seen in the peritoneal and pleural cavities of the fetus at gestation week 15. The cells become prominent in the fetal spleen with 60% or more of splenic B cells expressing the antigen. At birth, about 68% of cord blood B cells and approximately half of the peripheral blood B lymphocytes are CD5-positive, and this level drops dramatically in the peripheral blood, to near adult levels, within the first year of life. Between 15% and 25% of peripheral blood B lymphocytes in adults are positive for CD5.

There is some suggestion that CD5+ B-lineage represents a distinct subpopulation. Although both CD5+ and CD5− B cells produce immunoglobulin, upon activation CD5+ cells selectively produce primarily IgM antibodies, while CD5− B cells make primarily IgG antibodies, an observation made in cord blood. CD5+ B cells have also been reported to be associated with usually low-affinity, polyreactive antibody production, often called auto-antibodies. About 50% of auto-antibody-associated cross-reactive idiotype-bearing B lymphocytes are CD5-positive. It is possible that some of these differences may be due to lineage differences or simply secondary to some type of B-cell activation, and this requires further investigation.

Applications

CD5 is a fairly specific and sensitive marker of T-cell lineage. Almost 85% of T-cell acute lymphoblastic leukemias

(T-ALL) are CD5-positive, and lack of CD5 expression in T-ALL in patients with a white cell count of less than 50,000/ml is reported to be associated with a worse prognosis than corresponding patients with CD5+ T cells. CD5 expression has been reported in 3–10% of cases of acute myeloid leukemia. As CD5 is a pan-T-cell marker, it is not surprising that the majority of T-cell malignancies (76%) are CD5-positive. In peripheral T-cell lymphomas, including cutaneous T-cell lymphomas, the loss of CD5 expression can be employed to support a diagnosis of malignancy. In cutaneous T-cell lymphoma, CD5 is not as frequently lost when compared to loss of CD7.

With B-cell neoplasms, CD5 expression has been considered an almost defining characteristic of many entities. Chronic lymphocytic leukemia (CLL) is the most common CD5+ B-cell malignancy. It is assumed that the small population of CD5+ B cells found in normal healthy adults, and prominent in cord blood, is the non-neoplastic counterpart of this type of CLL. B-cell CLL is also associated with poly-specific antibodies or auto-antibodies, and frequently expresses cross-reactive idiotypes. Over 90% of cases of typical CLL are CD5-positive. CD5 expression may be lost when the large-cell lymphoma of Richter's syndrome supervenes in CD5+ CLL.

Unlike small lymphocytic lymphoma (SLL) and mantle cell lymphoma, with rare exceptions, monocytoid B-cell lymphoma and low-grade B-cell lymphoma of mucosa-associated lymphoid tissue are usually CD5-negative, a feature which can be employed to distinguish the small B-cell lymphoid neoplasms (Appendix 2.8). CD5+ B cells have been reported to be increased in some patients with monoclonal gammopathy of undetermined significance and in cases of multiple myeloma.

De novo expression of CD5 in diffuse large B-cell lymphoma has been shown to be an indicator of poor prognosis associated with a centroblastic phenotype, interfollicular growth pattern, and intravascular or sinusoidal infiltration.

CD5+ neoplastic cells have been found in cases of thymic carcinomas and some cases of atypical thymomas but not in typical thymomas. Carcinomas of the lung, breast, esophagus, stomach, colon, and uterine cervix have been reported to be all CD5-negative.

Positive staining for CD5 is seen in almost all T cells and most T-cell malignancies, B cells of the mantle zone of the spleen and lymph node and the corresponding mantle cell lymphomas, B cells in peritoneal and pleural cavities, B-cell small-cell lymphomas, and hairy cell leukemia.

Comments

Most publications indicate that the CD5 antigen is only demonstrable in fresh and frozen tissues, but we have successfully demonstrated CD5 using Leu-1 antibody following microwave epitope retrieval with TUR. One antibody to CD5 (clone NCL-CD5) was claimed to be immunoreactive in paraffin-embedded tissues following steam-heat-induced antigen retrieval, but in a study of 12 CD5+ malignancies, only one, a small-cell lymphoma, was positive in fixed tissues. Clone NCL-CD5–4C7 shows good immunoreactivity in fixed paraffin-embedded sections following antigen retrieval at 98 °C.

Selected reference

Arber DA, Weiss LM. CD5: a review. *Applied Immunohistochemistry* 1995; 3: 1–22.

CD7

Sources/clones

Becton Dickinson (Leu-9), Biodesign (WT1, WM31, 8H8.1), Biogenesis (WM31), Coulter (3A1), Cymbus Bioscience (WM31), Dako (DK24), GenTrak, Immunotech, Oncogene U3A1E), Sanbio (WT1), Sera Lab and Serotec (B-F12, B-5, HNE51).

Fixation/preparation

Fresh frozen tissue and fresh cytologic preparations.

Background

CD7 antigen is a cell surface glycoprotein of 40 kDa expressed on the surface of immature and mature T cells, and natural killer cells. It is a member of the immunoglobulin gene superfamily and is the first T-cell lineage-associated antigen to appear in T-cell ontogeny, being expressed in prethymic T-cell precursors (preceding CD2 expression) and myeloid precursors in fetal liver and bone marrow, and persisting in circulating T cells. While its precise function is not known, there is a suggestion that the molecule functions as an Fc receptor for IgM.

Applications

CD7 is the most consistently expressed T-cell antigen in lymphoblastic lymphomas and leukemias. It is specific for T-cell lineage and is therefore a useful marker in the identification of such neoplastic proliferations. In mature post-thymic T-cell neoplasms, it is the most common pan-T antigen to be aberrantly absent, and its absence in a T-cell population is a useful pointer to a neoplastic conversion.

CD7 is immunoexpressed on 85% of mature peripheral T cells, the majority of post-thymic T cells, NK cells, some myeloid cells, T-cell acute lymphoblastic leukemia/lymphoma, acute myeloid leukemia (especially M4/5), and chronic myeloid leukemia. Interestingly, CD7 is conspicuously absent in adult T-cell leukemia/lymphoma and is not expressed in Sézary cells.

Comments

Current antibodies are not immunoreactive in fixed tissues. One antibody to CD7 (clone CBC.37) was reported to be immunoreactive in fixed paraffin-embedded sections.

Selected references

Lazarovits AI, Osman N, Le Feuvre CE, et al. CD7 is associated with CD3 and CD45 in human T cells. *Journal of Immunology* 1994: 153; 3956–66.

Saati TA, Alibaud L, Lamant L, et al. A new monoclonal anti-CD7 antibody reactive in paraffin sections. *Applied Immunohistochemistry and Molecular Morphology* 2001; 9: 289–96.

NOTES

CD8

Sources/clones

Becton Dickinson (Leu-2), Biodesign (UCHT4, CD8.C12, B9.11, B9.2), Biogenesis (T80C), Biogenex (T8), Biotest (Tu 102), Dako (DK25, C8/144B), Novocastra (1A5, 4B11), Pharmingen (RPA-Y8), Research Diagnostics (CLB-T8/4, UCHT4), Sanbio (MEM31, BL-T58/2), Sera Lab (UCHT4), Serotec (BHT, MF8).

Fixation/preparation

Fresh frozen section and fresh cytological preparations. Clones C8/144B and 1A5 are immunoreactive in fixed paraffin-embedded tissue sections following HIER.

Background

Like CD4, the CD8 molecule is composed of non-polymorphic glycoproteins, belonging to the Ig superfamily, that are expressed on the surface membrane of mutually exclusive, functionally distinct T-cell populations. The CD8 molecule is a 34 kDa glycoprotein that forms disulfide-linked homodimers and homomultimers on the cell surface of peripheral T cells, the CD8 gene being linked to the κ locus on chromosome 2. The CD8 molecule comprises an external domain and highly conserved transmembrane and intracellular domains; the external domain shows striking homology with other members of the Ig gene superfamily. The CD8 molecule functions as a TCR co-receptor on suppressor/cytotoxic T cells and recognizes foreign antigens as peptides presented by MHC class I molecules. In the thymus, the CD8 molecule forms complexes with the CD1 glycoprotein, an MHC class I-like molecule. CD8 appears to bind to the non-polymorphic regions of MHC class I molecules and may thus serve to enhance the avidity of cell-to-cell interactions. Both CD4 and CD8 antigens appear during the common thymocyte stage of T-cell differentiation, and CD8 is expressed by about 80% of normal thymocytes. Thereafter, CD4 and CD8 are retained by those maturing thymocytes destined to become helper/inducer and suppressor/cytotoxic T cells respectively, CD8 being expressed by about 25–35% of peripheral T cells, specifically of the suppressor/cytotoxic subset. In addition, about 30% of NK cells express low levels of CD8. This phenotypic–functional association is not universal, and subpopulations of suppressor/cytotoxic T cells can be identified among CD4-positive cells.

Applications

As with the CD4 marker, CD8 has an important role in the immunophenotypic analysis of reactive and neoplastic populations of T cells, being used to identify a mature T-cell subset with suppressor/cytotoxic function. Like the CD4 marker, CD8 may also be aberrantly deleted from neoplastic T cells. The CD8 antigen is expressed on T-cell lymphoblastic lymphomas.

A hypopigmented form of mycosis fungoides has been shown to frequently express a CD8+ phenotype.

Between 25% and 35% of mature peripheral T cells stain for CD8, these mostly being cytotoxic T cells. CD8 positivity is also seen in NK cells, including 30% that are CD3-negative, and 70–80% of cortical thymocytes.

Comments

The development of clones C8/144B and 1A5, which are immunoreactive in fixed paraffin-embedded sections, has allowed the study of CD8+ T cells in a variety of diseases including the inflammatory dermatoses, cutaneous T-cell lymphomas, gastrointestinal diseases and colorectal carcinoma, and neuronal destruction.

Selected references

Eichmann K, Boyce NW, Schmidt UR, Jonsson JI. Distinct functions of CD8 (CD4) are utilised at different stages of T lymphocyte differentiation. *Immunological Reviews* 1989; 109: 39–75.

Martz E, Davignon D, Kurzinger K, Springer TA. The molecular basis for cytotoxic T lymphocyte function: analysis with blocking monoclonal antibodies. *Advances in Experimental Medicine and Biology* 1982; 146: 447–465.

Parnes JR. Molecular biology and function of CD4 and CD8. *Advances in Immunology* 1989; 44: 265–311.

CD9

Sources/clones

Biodesign (ALB6, MM2/57), Cymbus Bioscience (MM2/57), GenTrak, Immunotech (ALB6), Novocastra (72F6), Research Diagnostics (MM2/57), Sanbio (CLB/CD9), Sera Lab (FMC56, FMC8), Serotec (MM 2/57).

Fixation/preparation

Fresh frozen tissue and cytologic preparations, and formalin-fixed paraffin-embedded tissue.

Background

The CD9 antigen is a cell surface glycoprotein (p24) of 24 kDa belonging to the tetra-membrane-spanning protein family (tetraspanins), coded by chromosome 12. The antigen is present on pre-B cells, monocytes, and platelets and has protein kinase activity. The majority of mature peripheral blood or lymphoid tissue B cells or other normal circulating hematopoietic cells other than platelets do not express it. It is present on activated T cells, mast cells, and some dendritic reticulum cells. CD9 also regulates motility in a variety of cell lines and appears to be an important regulator of Schwann cell behavior in the peripheral nervous system.

Applications

The expression of CD9 in malignant cells is complex and not strictly lineage-, activation-, or differentiation-associated. It is found in more than 75% of precursor B-cell ALL/LBL, about 50% of B-cell CLL, and some better-differentiated B-cell neoplasms such as prolymphocytic leukemia and multiple myeloma as well as some T-cell lymphomas and acute myeloid leukemias. Other B-cell lymphomas, including centrocytic lymphoma, follicle center cell lymphoma, and Burkitt lymphoma, may also express this antigen, and there is also variable expression on neuroblastomas and some epithelial tumors. CD9 immunoexpression has been claimed to indicate a favorable prognosis in breast carcinoma, although at least one study has shown no benefit. Anti-CD9 antibodies were found to specifically inhibit the transendothelial migration of melanoma cells, and the protein immunostaining was suggested to be useful in the differential diagnosis of papillary renal cell carcinoma and collecting duct carcinomas, and also in distinguishing between chromophobe and conventional renal cell carcinomas, CD9 being consistently positive in papillary and chromophobe carcinomas.

Comments

Expressed on pre-B cells, B-cell subset, T cells, macrophages, platelets, eosinophils, basophils, megakaryocytes, endothelial cells, brains, peripheral nerves, vascular smooth muscle, cardiac muscle, and epithelial cells. Because of its expression by a wide spectrum of B- and T-cell neoplasms, this marker has limited application in the phenotypic analysis of hematopoietic neoplasms. It may have other diagnostic applications in non-hematopoietic tumors discussed above. The Novocastra 72F6 clone is employed in paraffin-embedded sections with retrieval in EDTA at pH 8.0.

Selected references

Carbone A, Poletti A, Manconi R, et al. Heterogenous in situ immunotyping of follicular dendritic reticulum cells in malignant lymphomas of B cell origin. Cancer 1987; 60: 2919–26.

Lardelli P, Bookman MA, Sundeen J, et al. Lymphocytic lymphoma of intermediate differentiation: Morphologic and immunophenotypic spectrum and clinical correlations. American Journal of Surgical Pathology 1990; 14: 752–63.

San Miguel JF, Caballero MD, Gonzalez M, et al. Immunological phenotype of neoplasms involving the B cell in the last step of differentiation. British Journal of Haematology 1986; 62: 75–83.

NOTES

CD10 (CALLA)

Sources/clones

Accurate, Biodesign (ALBl, ALB2), Coulter (J5), Cymbus Bioscience (Mem 78), Dako (SS2/36), GenTrak, Immunotech (ALB1, ALB2), Novocastra (56C6), Research Diagnostics (MEM 78, J-149), Sanbio (MEM 78, BFA.11), Sera Lab (B-E3) and Serotec.

Fixation/preparation

With the exception of clone 56C6, current antibodies are mostly immunoreactive only in fresh frozen tissue.

Background

The common acute lymphoblastic leukemia antigen (CALLA) is a 100 kDa single chain glycoprotein whose sequence is virtually identical to that of neutral endopeptidase (NEP-24.11 enkephalinase). It is a metalloenzyme that requires zinc as a cofactor and is thought to inactivate regulatory peptides favoring cell differentiation. It was originally defined by hetero-antiserum raised in rabbits by immunization with cells of a "non-B, non-T"-cell acute lymphoblastic leukemia (ALL). CD10 is present on the cell surface of stem cells in the bone marrow and fetal liver that are also TdT- and HLA-DR antigen-positive.

Applications

CD10 was originally used as a specific marker for non-B-, non-T-cell ALL. It is expressed in approximately 75% of precursor B-cell ALL and more than 90% of cases of myelogenous leukemia in lymphoid blast crisis, but CD10 is not a leukemia-specific antigen, nor is it B- or T-cell lineage-restricted. The antigen is found on variable proportions of cells making up T-cell ALL/LBL, Burkitt lymphoma, follicular lymphoma, and multiple myeloma. In addition, CD10 is expressed on the renal glomerular and tubular cells, fibroblasts, bile canaliculi, melanoma cell lines, and various other epithelial cells. More recent applications of CD10 include the staining of endometrial stroma, including endometrial stromal nodules and endometrial stromal sarcoma, so that it can be used as a discriminator from histologic mimics such as uterine cellular leiomyoma and leiomyosarcoma, adult granulosa cell tumor, and undifferentiated endometrial carcinoma, the latter staining diffusely for α-smooth muscle actin (α-SMA), and desmin, α-inhibin, and cytokeratins respectively.

There is suggestion that CD10 immunostaining in large B-cell lymphoma correlates with prognosis. CD10 immunoreactivity is significantly stronger in follicular lymphoma compared to hyperplastic follicles, so this antigen has been used to distinguish the two forms of lymphoid nodules. Interestingly, CD10 positivity has been demonstrated in the neoplastic T cells of 90% of cases of angioimmunoblastic lymphoma but not in other peripheral T-cell lymphomas. The antigen has also been shown in melanoma cells, renal cell carcinoma, and mesenchymal cells of the skin including tumors such as dermatofibroma, dermatofibrosarcoma protuberans, neurofibromas, and as many as 47% of malignant melanoma cases. The demonstration of CD10 immunoexpression in myoepithelial cells of the breast suggested that it might be an alternative to smooth muscle actin as a marker of such cells, particularly as the latter stains normal vessels and spindled stromal cells. CD10 immunoexpression has also been employed to stain the canaliculi in 60% of hepatocellular carcinomas studied, but no staining was seen in cholangiocarcinomas or metastatic carcinoma.

Comments

Clone 56C6 is the most immunoreactive antibody for paraffin sections and requires HIER for enhancement. Paraffin section immunostaining correlates well with flow cytometric analysis, and decalcification does not appear to affect immunoreactivity. Retrieval at 120 °C produces the best results. While CD10 is neither lineage-specific nor tumor-restricted, it remains a useful marker, especially in the analysis of childhood ALL/LBL and follicular lymphomas.

CD10 is localized to cell membranes and cytoplasm of hematolymphoid cells, and rarely Golgi staining is seen.

Selected references

Anderson KC, Bates MP, Slaughtenhoupt BL, *et al.* Expression of human B cell associated antigens on leukemias and lymphomas: a model of B cell differentiation. *Blood* 1984; 63: 1424–33.

Chu P, Arber D. Paraffin section detection of CD10 in 505 non-hematopoietic neoplasms: frequent expression in renal cell carcinoma and endometrial stromal sarcoma. *American Journal of Clinical Pathology* 2000; 113: 374–82.

Chu P, Chang KL, Weiss LM, Arber DA. Immunohistochemical detection of CD10 in paraffin sections of hematopoietic neoplasms. A comparison with flow cytometry detection in 56 cases. *Applied Immunohistochemistry and Molecular Morphology* 2000; 8: 257–62.

McCluggage WG, Sumathi VP, Maxwell P. CD10 is a sensitive and diagnostically useful immunohistochemical marker of normal endometrial stroma and of endometrial stromal neoplasms. *Histopathology* 2001; 39: 273–8.

CD11

Sources/clones

CD11a

Ancell (38), Biodesign (MEM 25, SPV-L7), Cymbus Bioscience (38), Dako (MHM24), GenTrak, Immunotech (25.3), Pharmingen (2D7), Sanbio (MEM 25), Serotec (B-B15).

CD11b

Ancell (44), Biodesign (44, Bear-1), Biogenex, Boehringer Mannheim, Cymbus Bioscience, Dako (2LPM19c), GenTrak, Immunotech (Bear-1), JapanTanner, Pharmingen (Ml/70), Research Diagnostics (CD44), Sanbio (Bear-1), Sera Lab (44), Serotec (ED7).

CD11c

Ancell (3.9), Becton Dickinson (Leu-M5), Biodesign (FK24, BU15), Cymbus Bioscience, Dako (KB90), GenTrak, Immunotech (BU15), Oncogene (3.9), Research Diagnostics (CD39), Sanbio (FK24), Sera Lab (FK24), Serotec (3.9).

Fixation/preparation

Current antibodies are only immunoreactive in fresh frozen tissue.

Background

Each of the CD11 subtypes represents a different α-chain which forms one of the β2 family of integrin adhesion receptors when linked non-covalently to β2 (CD18) to form a heterodimer. CD11a, leukocyte function-associated antigen (LFA-1), with a molecular weight of 180 kDa, is present on B cells, T cells, NK cells, monocytes, granulocytes, megakaryocytes, and activated platelets. CD11b (Mac-1), the C3bi receptor, has a molecular weight of 165 kDa and it is present on granulocytes, monocytes and some histiocytes. CD11c, which has a molecular weight of 150 kDa, is present on monocytes, tissue macrophages, granulocytes, some suppressor/cytotoxic T cells, and a subset of B cells. It is usually positive on true histiocytic malignancies and some B-cell lymphomas including hairy cell leukemia and monocytoid B-cell lymphoma.

CD11/CD18 integrins have a function in intercellular communication between lymphocytes and between lymphocytes and endothelial cells. The interaction between leukocytes and endothelial cells involves CD11/CD18 integrins which bind to intercellular adhesion molecules ICAM-1 (CD45) and ICAM-2.

Applications

Currently, the diagnostic applications for this marker are very limited, and available antibodies are reactive only in frozen sections. Differential expression of CD11a (LFA-1) has been described in small-cell lymphocytic lymphoma and CLL and has been used to account for the difference in peripheral blood involvement in these entities, but the findings require confirmation. In the immunophenotypic separation of monocytoid B-cell lymphoma from other small-cell lymphomas such as plasmacytoid small-cell lymphoma, CLL, and mantle cell lymphoma, CD11c has been suggested to be a useful discriminant, being more frequently expressed in monocytoid lymphoma.

CD11a is found on all leukocytes. CD11b is found on granulocytes, macrophages, NK cells, follicular dendritic cells, myeloid cells, and some B and T lymphocytes. Hairy cell leukemia expresses this antigen. CD11c stains 50% of activated CD4+/CD8+ T cells, granulocytes, lymphocytes, macrophages, and NK cells. In B-CLL expression is associated with good prognosis, and it is expressed in virtually all cases of hairy cell leukemia.

Selected reference

Chadburn A, Inghirami G, Knowles DM. Hairy cell leukemia-associated antigen LeuM5 (CD11c) is preferentially expressed by benign activated and neoplastic CD8 cells. *American Journal of Pathology* 1990; 136: 29–37.

CD15

Sources/clones

Accurate (C3D-1), Becton Dickinson (Leu-M1), Biodesign (B428, 80H5, G15), Biogenex (Tu9), Cymbus Bioscience (28), Dako (C3D-1), Immunotech (80H5), Novocastra, Research Diagnostics (28), Sanbio (BL-G15), Sera Lab (MC-1), Serotec (NH6, B-H8).

Fixation/preparation

Fresh frozen tissue and formalin-fixed paraffin-embedded tissue. Muramidase pretreatment increases reactivity, particularly in acute myeloid leukemia.

Background

A variety of antibodies to CD15 have been generated in different ways, but they appear to have similar immunoreactivity patterns. Some antibodies were developed by immunization and screening against human hematopoietic cell lines and were originally felt to be specific for myeloid leukemias, while others were developed from specific human and mouse carcinoma cell lines and were later found to react with granulocytes and a variety of human carcinomas. The antibodies are mostly of IgM isotype and have the common property of being able to recognize a specific sugar sequence that occurs in the glycolipid lacto-N-fucopentaose III ceramide and is also found in several glycolipids such as glycoproteins. The sugar sequence is referred to as X hapten or Le^x, and its highly immunogenic nature in mice has led to the production of several IgM monoclonal antibodies to the CD15 cluster. The lacto-N-fucopentaose III has been identified in human milk and is virtually absent in benign human epithelium. A related substance, lacto-N-fucopentaose II, is present in many benign human epithelial cells. The glycolipid lacto-N-fucopentaose III has a structure similar to the Lewis blood group antigens. The CD15 antigen exists in a sialylated or unsialylated form, the former requiring prior digestion with muramidase to enable detection. Mature granulocytes and monocytes express the unsialylated molecule.

Applications

CD15 antibodies react with mature neutrophils, and generally the reactivity is less with the less mature forms of the granulocyte series. Normal bone marrow myeloblasts are negative, and some promyelocytes may not stain. Paraffin-embedded cells show both membrane and cytoplasmic staining. Normal platelets, red blood cells, and B lymphocytes are routinely negative, as are the vast majority of T lymphocytes. Mitogen-activated lymphocytes show positivity with the Leu-M1 antibody, and these are mostly T lymphocytes of the T4 subset. While some T8+ cells also express the antigen, a longer period of stimulation was needed to induce this finding.

In leukemia, CD15 antibodies react with all neoplastic myeloid and monocytic proliferations, although there is a variable pattern with different antibodies (Appendix 2.5). CD15 positivity is reported to be lost in cases of relapsed acute myeloid leukemia (AML), correlating with a poorer survival. Almost all cases of chronic myeloid leukemia (CML) have demonstrated the presence of CD15 while in chronic phase. Approximately 16% of cases of acute lymphoblastic leukemia (ALL) demonstrate the co-expression of at least one myeloid antigen, and up to 50% of such cases are reportedly CD15-positive, although the range of positivity is between 2% and 6%. CD15 expression is highest in common acute lymphoblastic leukemia antigen (CALLA)-negative cases, which generally have a worse prognosis than cases of CALLA-positive ALL.

CD15 expression is very helpful in the diagnosis of Hodgkin disease, as almost all the CD15 antibodies available react with Reed–Sternberg cells and the mononuclear variants (Appendix 2.3). Characteristically, the staining is membranous with globular, juxtanuclear staining of the

Golgi complex. The cytoplasmic membrane staining has been confirmed by ultrastructural studies, and lysosomal granules contiguous with perinuclear vesicles representing the Golgi apparatus are also stained. Reed–Sternberg cells and atypical mononuclear variants in Hodgkin disease of mixed-cellularity, nodular sclerosing, and lymphocyte-depleted type show staining with CD15 antibodies. However, lymphocyte-predominant Hodgkin disease is CD15-negative, particularly in the nodular and in some cases of the diffuse subtype. Digestion with neuraminidase has been reported to result in staining of the L&H cells in lymphocyte-predominant Hodgkin disease, although the staining has been described to be less intense and predominantly cytoplasmic in distribution. Similarly, enzyme pretreatment has been reported to produce positivity in T-cell lymphomas mostly of the mature phenotype, particularly in advanced-stage mycosis fungoides. A smaller percentage of low-grade B-cell lymphomas have also been reported to be CD15-positive. CD15 is a useful marker for granulocytic sarcoma, staining the majority of cases.

While CD15 expression has been widely employed for the confirmation of the diagnosis of Hodgkin disease, little is known of the role of the CD15 antigen in the pathobiology of the disease and its prognostic relevance, if any. It has been shown that CD15 expressed in its non-sialylated form (clones Leu-M1 and 80H5) and the absence of sialylated CD15 (FH6 and CSLEX1) expression on Reed–Sternberg cells correlated with favorable outcome. There was also preferential expression of sialyl-CD15, notably in bone marrow metastases, so it was suggested that in the progression of Hodgkin disease towards a widely disseminated form the Lewis^x moiety of the antigen acquires sialyl-group, conferring on the tumor cells the capacity to metastasize.

Strong CD15 positivity has been found in carcinomas from a wide variety of sites. It is employed in a panel for the discrimination of adenocarcinoma from malignant mesothelioma, the latter being generally CD15-negative. However, it should be noted that this is not an absolute discriminator, as CD15 may be immunoexpressed in as many as 6% of mesotheliomas. Cytomegalovirus-infected cells have also been found to react with CD15 antibodies, predominantly with cytoplasmic staining. The combination of immunostaining with cytokeratin, HBME, CD57, or CD15 is said to be a sensitive and specific test for papillary thyroid carcinoma, allowing separation from reactive thyroid nodules.

Comments

CD15 antibodies are particularly useful for the identification of Reed–Sternberg cells, especially when they are employed in a panel that includes CD45 (LCA), Reed–Sternberg cells showing the characteristic membranous and Golgi staining for CD15 and negative staining for CD45 (Appendix 2.3). It is also a useful discriminant when used in an appropriate panel for the separation of adenocarcinoma from malignant mesothelioma, since adenocarcinomas and the antibodies label the myeloid cells of granulocytic sarcoma whereas CD15 is mostly negative in mesothelioma. Staining is enhanced with microwave epitope retrieval using a citrate buffer, and enzyme digestion should not be performed when CD15 antibodies are employed for the identification of Reed–Sternberg cells and adenocarcinomas.

Positive staining is seen in myeloid cells (90%), activated B and T cells (including infectious mononucleosis), Reed–Sternberg cells, 20% of T-cell lymphomas, 5% of B-cell lymphomas, and 50% of carcinomas. No staining is seen in erythroid cells, platelets, or ALL.

Selected reference

Aber DA, Weiss LM. CD15: a review. *Applied Immunohistochemistry* 1993; 1: 17–30.

CD19

Sources/clones

Accurate (B19, CLB/B4/1, FMC63, polyclonal), Becton Dickinson (SJ25C1), Biodesign (BC3), Biogenex (B4), Biosource (BC3, SJ25C1), Caltag Laboratories (SJ25C1), Coulter (B4), Cymbus Bioscience (RFB9, SJ25-C1), Dako (HD37), Immunotech (386.12, J4.119), Novocastra (4G7/2E, FMC63), Pharmingen (B43, HIB19), Sanbio/Monosan (SJ25C1), Sera Lab, Sigma Chemical (SJ25C1), Zymed (SJ25-C1).

Fixation/preparation

The majority of these antibodies are only applicable to cryostat sections, although they may be used in acetone-fixed cryostat sections and smears. They are not suitable for formalin-fixed paraffin-embedded sections.

Background

The CD19 gene (along with CD20 and CD22) encodes transmembrane proteins with at least two extracellular immunoglobulin-like domains that are of vital importance to B-cell function. Similar to the immunoglobulin genes, they are expressed in a lineage-specific and developmentally regulated manner. In normal cells, CD19 antigen (90 kDa polypeptide) ($\beta 2$ integrin) is the most ubiquitously expressed protein in the B-lymphocyte lineage. CD19 expression is induced at the point of B-lineage commitment during the differentiation of the hematopoietic stem cell. Its expression continues through pre-B-cell and mature B-cell differentiation, being downregulated during terminal differentiation into plasma cells. Furthermore, CD19 expression is maintained in neoplastic B cells, enhancing its diagnostic usefulness. Since CD19 is not expressed in pluripotent stem cells, it has become the target for a variety of immunotherapeutic agents.

Applications

B43 monoclonal antibody recognizes the same surface epitope as several other anti-CD19 monoclonal antibodies. Using clone B43 to test for CD19 expression on 340 leukemias and 151 malignant lymphomas, CD19 was shown to be the most reliable B-lineage surface marker. The advantage of immunodetection of CD19 expression is that B-lineage leukemias and lymphomas rarely lose the epitope. Furthermore, CD19 is not expressed on myeloid, erythroid, megakaryocytic, or multilineage bone marrow progenitor cells.

Comments

Although most B cells carry the CD19 antigen, the use of anti-CD19 is restricted to cryostat sections and therefore not useful in routine diagnostic histopathology practice.

CD19 is the first antigen to be expressed on B cells after HLA-DR. Positive staining is seen in pre-B cells, B cells, and follicular dendritic cells. Plasma cells are negative.

Selected references

Kehrl JH, Riva A, Wilson GL, Thevenin C. Molecular mechanisms regulating CD19, CD29 and CD22 gene expression. *Immunology Today* 1994; 15: 432–6.

Scheuermann RH, Racila E. CD19 antigen in leukemia and lymphoma diagnosis and immunotherapy. *Leukemia and Lymphoma* 1995; 18: 385–97.

NOTES

CD20

Sources/clones

Becton Dickinson (Leu-16), Biodesign (BB6), Biogenesis (MEM97), Biogenex (L260), Coulter (B1), Cymbus Bioscience (MEM97, BC1), Dako (L26), Immunotech (L26, HRC20-B9E9), Monosan (MEM-97), Sanbio (MEM97), Sera Lab (BC1), Serotec (B>B6, BC1), Signet, Novocastra, Pharmingen (2H7), Zymed (L26).

Fixation/preparation

All the available antibodies to CD20 react in paraffin and frozen sections and can be used to label cells in suspension. Immunoreactivity is enhanced by heat-induced antigen retrieval but not proteolytic digestion.

Background

The CD20 molecule is one of the best markers of B-cell lineage. It is a membrane-embedded, nonglycosylated phosphoprotein which appears in early pre-B cells and throughout their maturation into late pre-B cells. It is expressed on the surface of all mature B lymphocytes but not in secreting plasma cells. The CD20 gene is a single copy gene located on chromosome 11q12–q13, near the site of the t(11;14)(q13;q32) translocation which is commonly noted in mantle zone lymphoma. The complete gene is 16 kbp long and comprises eight exons, with six exons encoding the protein.

The exact function of the CD20 molecule is unknown, but it is involved in the regulation of B-cell activation, proliferation, and differentiation. Certain anti-CD20 antibodies trigger resting B cells to enter the cell cycle and induce IgM production, while other antibodies to CD20 can inhibit B-cell activation.

The CD20 antigen appears on the cell surface after light chain gene rearrangement and before the expression of intact surface Ig, remaining throughout the course of B-cell development, and it is lost only prior to plasma cell differentiation. While it is expressed on both resting and activated B cells, its expression is about fourfold greater in the latter.

Virtually all lymphoid cells in the germinal center express CD20, besides CD19, CD22, and other pan-B-cell antigens, and CD20 and CD19 are also expressed by cells of the mantle zone, but at a lesser intensity. In the thymus, CD20 stains medullary B cells and cells within the epithelial meshwork of the thymic parenchyma. Cortical cells are negative for this antigen.

Weak expression of CD20 may be seen in a subpopulation of T cells but the antigen is not expressed in normal myeloid, erythroid, monocytic, or mesenchymal cells. Antigen-presenting dendritic cells in the blood do not stain for CD20, and the antigen is not expressed in cells of the normal skin or adnexal structures.

Applications

CD20 is the most useful marker for neoplasms of B-cell derivation and is almost always expressed in B-cell lymphomas of small-cell type, prolymphocytic leukemia, follicular center cell lymphomas, large- or small-cell types of both diffuse and follicular patterns, monocytoid lymphomas, mantle cell lymphomas, hairy cell leukemias/lymphomas, and immunoblastic lymphomas. Originally, it was thought that neoplastic plasma cells mirrored the lack of expression in benign plasma cells, but it has been shown that up to 20% of cases of myeloma may immunoexpress CD20. The staining of CD20 in chronic lymphocytic leukemia/small-cell lymphoma may be weak and often not in all cells. It has not been shown to stain the neoplastic cells in T lymphomas. While CD20 has great diagnostic utility, it is of no prognostic relevance. Homogeneous staining for CD20 in bone marrow lymphoid aggregates is more common in neoplastic aggregates than in benign ones and may be a useful discriminator in such settings.

About 10–20% of lymphoblastic lymphomas are non-T-cell lineage and express B-cell antigens, about half the latter group expressing CD20.

In Hodgkin disease, 60–100% of cases of the nodular lymphocyte-predominant subtype show CD20 staining of the L&H malignant cells. Up to 20% of Reed–Sternberg cells of classic Hodgkin disease may stain for CD20, but this finding is not associated with different clinical outcomes after treatment with equivalent regimens.

Occasional cases of acute myeloid leukemia and extramedullary myeloid tumors may show aberrant expression of CD20, but this is estimated to involve only 3% of cases, with no correlation between any lymphoid antigen expression and morphology. In the case of chronic myeloid leukemia, about 25–30% of the cases that show blastic transformation display lymphoid differentiation by morphology, cytochemistry, and immunophenotyping. The lymphoid cells usually display the immunophenotype of precursor B cells, including the expression of CD20 as well as other B-cell antigens such as CD10, CD19, increased TdT, and rearranged immunoglobulin genes. Follicular dendritic cells, 40% of pure B ALL/LBL, and 80% of lymphocyte-predominant Hodgkin disease may show reactivity for CD20, which may also be weakly expressed in benign and neoplastic T cells in immunofluorescence labeling. As 90% of B cell lymphomas express CD20 in vivo, ablation of malignant B cells may be achieved using antibodies directed to the CD20 antigen. Immunoreactivity for CD20 has been observed in the epithelial cells of a subset of thymomas and seems to correlate with spindling of the neoplastic cells.

Comments

Antibodies to CD20 are mostly reactive in formalin-fixed paraffin-embedded tissues, and this is by far the best marker for B lymphocytes (Appendix 2.1), with a sensitivity of 95% and specificity of 100%. The pattern of staining is membranous and continuous. It may be accompanied by nuclear, paranuclear, and diffuse cytoplasmic staining but this should be generally weak. Heat-induced epitope retrieval (HIER) has been reported to produce nucleolar staining. Very rare cases of low-grade B-cell lymphomas may not stain for CD20 and may express CD43 in paraffin sections, suggesting an erroneous interpretation of T-cell lineage. However, an awareness of this and the proper use of antibody panels will avoid such pitfalls. Clone L26 is the most commonly used of the CD20 antibodies.

CD20 is immunoexpressed on most B cells (after CD19 and CD10 expression and before CD21/22 and surface immunoglobulin expression), retained on mature B cells until plasma cell development; also follicular dendritic cells, 90% of B-cell lymphomas, 40% of pre-B ALL/LBL; 80% of lymphocyte-predominant Hodgkin disease; and weakly expressed on benign and neoplastic T cells. As many as 20% of cases of myeloma may express CD20. CD20 is generally not expressed on non-hematopoietic cells, most T cells, and non-neoplastic plasma cells. Aberrant focal expression of CD20 on thymoma cells has been described. The staining is membranous and dendritic in outline, and together with the presence of lymphoid cells with immature phenotype CD1a+, CD2+, CD99+, and TdT+ has been employed for the identification of thymoma.

Immunoexpression may be reduced in tissues fixed in Zenker's solution and following decalcification. Trypsinization may similarly reduce immunoreactivity, but heat-induced antigen retrieval is useful.

Selected reference

Chang KL, Arber DA, Weiss LM. CD20: a review. *Applied Immunohistochemistry* 1996; 4: 1–15.

CD21

Sources/clones

Coulter (B2), Dako (1F8), Immunotech (BL13).

Fixation/preparation

CD21 is applicable to formalin-fixed paraffin-embedded tissue sections. Enzymatic digestion with proteolytic enzyme trypsin is essential for positive immunoreaction, but HIER produces significant enhancement of immunoreactivity. CD21 may also be used for labeling acetone-fixed cryostat sections or fixed cell smears.

Background

CD21 antigen (CR2) (isotype: IgG1κ) represents the purified receptor of the C3d fragment of the third complement component from human tonsils. This membrane molecule is a glycoprotein of molecular weight 145 kDa and is involved in the transmission of growth-promoting signals to the interior of the B cell. CD21 also functions as a receptor for Epstein–Barr virus. 1F8 reacts with an epitope localized on trypsin fragments of CR2 of molecular weights 95, 72, 50, 32, and 28 kDa. The 28 kDa and 72 kDa fragments of CR2 contain the binding site for the C3d receptor.

The CD21 antigen is a restricted B-cell antigen expressed on mature B cells. The antigen is also present on follicular dendritic cells (FDCs), the accessory cells of the B zones (Appendix 2.7). 1F8 labels B cells moderately and demonstrates FDCs strongly on cryostat sections. However, on paraffin sections, B-cell immunoreaction is abolished while the FDCs remain highlighted, similar to the cryostat sections. Hence, in normal and reactive lymph nodes, tonsils, and extranodal lymphoid tissue, the antibody demonstrates the FDC meshwork remarkably clearly defined in the germinal centers.

Applications

On paraffin sections, antibodies to the CD21 antigen are useful to demonstrate FDC meshwork in lymphoid proliferations where the germinal centers may be ill-defined and difficult to delineate morphologically, e.g. HIV lymphadenopathy. In the early stages of progressive generalized lymphadenopathy (PGL, stage I), the large geographic reactive germinal centers may occupy large areas of the lymph node, giving an appearance of effacement of the architecture. Similarly, in the late stage of PGL (stage III), the atrophic germinal centers are not easily definable.

The demonstration of the nodular dense FDC meshwork of follicular lymphomas is also a potential application of the CD21 antibody. Similarly, the follicular/nodular architecture of nodular lymphocyte-predominant Hodgkin disease may be highlighted. Residual germinal centers that have been colonized in low-grade B-cell MALT lymphomas may also be demonstrated with antibody to CD21, which reveals an expanded and dense FDC meshwork. Nodal mantle cell lymphoma and multiple lymphomatous polyposis are characterized by the presence of a monotonous small lymphoid B-cell population, and interspersed cells with "naked" nuclei (FDCs), which is helpful in distinguishing this lymphoma from other low-grade B-cell lymphomas.

The demonstration of an FDC meshwork is also characteristic of peripheral T-cell lymphomas of angioimmunoblastic lymphadenopathy (AILD) type. The FDC meshwork in AILD is typically around hyperplastic venules.

The diagnosis of angiofollicular lymph node hyperplasia or Castleman's disease (hyaline vascular type) may also benefit from highlighting the follicles with anti-CD21. Dysplastic FDCs have been demonstrated in association with Castleman's disease of the hyaline vascular type, and these are thought to be the precursor to FDC tumors. Again the characteristic dendritic processes in FDC tumors are well demonstrated with CD21 antibodies. Recent findings of chromosomal aberrations involving 12q13–15 targeting the gene *HMGIC*, a member of the high mobility group (HMG) protein family, suggests that FDC proliferation in the hyaline vascular type of Castleman's disease is clonal.

Comments

Although sometimes patchy and focal, positivity with the paraffin section-reactive CD21 is essential for the diagnosis of FDC tumors, which are probably underdiagnosed through under-recognition. CD35 generally produces stronger staining of FDC sarcomas compared to antibodies to CD21. Both antibodies benefit from heat-induced antigen retrieval.

Selected reference

Bagdi E, Krenacs L, Krenacs T, *et al*. Follicular dendritic cells in reactive and neoplastic lymphoid tissues: a reevaluation of staining patterns of CD21, CD23, and CD35 antibodies in paraffin sections after wet heat-induced epitope retrieval. *Applied Immunohistochemistry and Molecular Morphology* 2001; 9: 117–24.

CD23

Sources/clones

Accurate, Biodesign (BB-10, 9P.25), Biotest (TU1), Cymbus Bioscience, Dako (MHM6), GenTrak, Immunotech (9P25), Novocastra (1B12, Tul), Pharmingen (B3B4), RDI (TU1), Sanbio (BL-C/B8), Serotec (B-G6, BSL-23), www.bindingsite.co.uk (BU38).

Fixation/preparation

With exception of clones MHM6, Tul, and 1B12, other available antibodies are immunoreactive only in fresh frozen sections and fresh cytologic preparations. Immunoreactivity in fixed paraffin-embedded sections follows heat-induced antigen retrieval.

Background

The antigen is an integral membrane glycoprotein of molecular weight 45–60 kDa. The CD23 antigen has been identified as a low-affinity receptor for IgE, and it may be involved in the regulation of IgE production as well as being a receptor for lymphocyte growth factor. Following cross-linkage of antigen and Ig, CD23 becomes expressed and serves as an autocrine stimulus driving B-cell proliferation. CD23 appears on B cells within 24 hours following a variety of stimuli. Surface CD23 has a half-life of only 1–2 hours and is shed in the form of soluble fragments of varying molecular weight that display the autocrine promoting activity. Two species of CD23 have been described, FcεRIIa and FcεRIIb, differing in the N-terminal cytoplasmic region and sharing the same C-terminal extracellular region. FcεRIIa is strongly expressed on IL-4-activated B cells and weakly on mature B cells; it also stains some dendritic reticulum cells, which probably acquire the antigen from neighboring B cells. FcεRIIa is not found on circulating B cells, and its expression can only be induced on surface IgMD-positive cells and not on those B cells that have lost IgD, undergone isotype switch, and express IgG, IgA, or IgE. FcεRIIb is expressed weakly on a range of cell types including monocytes, eosinophils, platelets, some T cells, and NK cells. IL-4-treated monocytes show stronger staining. CD23 is strongly expressed on EBV-transformed lymphoblastoid B-cell lines. The aberrant expression of CD23 in B CLL appears to be the result of deregulation of Notch2 signaling; members of the Notch family encode transmembrane receptors that modulate differentiation, proliferation, and apoptotic programs of many precursor cells including hematopoietic progenitors.

Applications

CD23 is found in most low-grade B-cell lymphomas and in Reed–Sternberg cells in Hodgkin disease. Activated B cells within germinal centers express CD23 in high density, but mantle zone (resting) B cells are negative or only stain weakly. The majority of B-cell CLLs and a variable proportion of B-cell non-Hodgkin lymphomas are CD23-positive, whereas mantle cell lymphomas are generally negative, so that this marker is useful when applied with other markers to separate the small-cell lymphomas (Appendix 2.8). Precursor B-cell and T-cell ALL/LBL, acute myeloid leukemia, chronic myeloid leukemia, and post-thymic T-cell neoplasms are CD23-negative. The marker is upregulated by EBV infection.

Comments

CD23 negativity is rare in typical B-cell CLL/SLL, so it is an important marker for the distinction of small-cell lymphomas (Appendix 2.8). CD23 is positive on activated mature B cells expressing IgM or IgD, monocytes/macrophages, T-cell subsets, eosinophils, Langerhans cells, follicular dendritic cells, and B-cell CLL/SLL. Mantle cells do not stain for CD23.

Selected references

Armitage RJ, Goff LK. Functional interaction between B cell subpopulation defined by CD23 expression. *European Journal of Immunology* 1988; 18: 1753–60.

DiRaimondo F, Albitar M, Huh Y, *et al.* The clinical and diagnostic relevance of CD23 expression in the chronic lymphoproliferative disease. *Cancer* 2002; 94: 1721–30.

CD24

Sources/clones

Biodesign (ALB9), Cymbus Bioscience (ALB9), Dako (SN389), Immunotech (ALB9), RDI (ALB9), Serotec (ALB9).

Fixation/preparation

Current antibodies are reactive in fresh frozen sections and cell preparations only.

Background

Antibodies to CD24 react with a 42 kDa single chain cell surface sialoglycoprotein which is expressed throughout B-cell differentiation but, like other pan-B-cell antigens, is lost following activation and before the secretory (plasma cell) stage. CD24 is not entirely restricted to B cells and is expressed on granulocytes, interdigitating cells, renal epithelial cells, as well as some benign and malignant epithelial tumors. CD24 can function as a ligand for β-selectin and may have a role in the lung colonization of human tumors, and through glycolipid-enriched membrane fractions it may mediate intracellular signaling and apoptosis in human B lymphocytes. CD24 has adhesion molecule functions and promotes invasion of glioma cells in vivo. In breast carcinoma, the binding of tumor cells to platelets and the rolling of these cells on endothelial β-selectin facilitates metastasis.

Applications

CD24 is expressed on the majority of precursor B-cell ALL/LBLs and by virtually all mature, TdT-negative, surface membrane immunoglobulin (SIg)-positive and SIg-negative B-cell non-Hodgkin lymphoma. It is not found in multiple myeloma or on benign and neoplastic T cells. Anti-CD24 has been used for purging bone marrow of B-ALL cells in autologous bone marrow transplantation.

CD24 is abundantly expressed on breast cancer cell lines and tumor tissues and has been suggested as a possible marker for breast carcinoma, with cytoplasmic expression in carcinoma cells compared to apical expression in benign cells.

CD24 is positive on all B cells, granulocytes, kidney cells, epithelial cells, both benign and malignant, most pre-B ALL/LBL and virtually all B-cell lymphomas. It is not expressed on plasma cells, myeloma, T cells, monocytes, red blood cells, and platelets.

Selected reference

Abramson CS, Kersey JH, LeBien TW. A monoclonal antibody (BA-1) reactive with cells of human B lymphocyte lineage. *Journal of Immunology* 1981; 126: 83–8.

NOTES

CD25

Sources/clones

Abcam (rabbit monoclonal), GenWay Biotech (mouse monoclonal), LifeSpan BioSciences (mouse monoclonal), Novus Biological (mouse monoclonal), Thermo Scientific (mouse monoclonal), Vector Laboratories (4C9, mouse monoclonal).

Fixation/preparation

The antigen is preserved in formalin-fixed paraffin-embedded tissue.

Background

The CD25 antigen is the α-chain of the interleukin-2 receptor (IL2R-α). It is a transmembrane protein that forms a complex with the β- (CD122) and γ-subunits to form a high-affinity receptor for IL-2. CD25 is expressed on a variety of normal hematopoietic cell types, including activated lymphocytes, monocytes, and a subset of myeloid precursors. The neoplastic cells in certain hematopoietic neoplasms also characteristically express CD25. In addition, abnormalities of IL2R-α expression have been demonstrated in patients with autoimmune diseases such as rheumatoid arthritis, systemic lupus erythematosus, diabetes mellitus, scleroderma, and Crohn's disease as well as other conditions like sarcoidosis, chronic allograft rejection, and graft-versus-host disease. Consequently, anti-CD25 antibodies have been used to treat an array of clinical conditions, including CD25-expressing lymphomas and leukemias, autoimmune diseases, and allograft rejection.

Applications

In non-neoplastic lymph nodes, CD25 will highlight scattered, activated lymphocytes and macrophages within the interfollicular areas, comprising less than 1% of overall lymphocytes. The number of CD25+ cells is reportedly increased in cases of progressively transformed germinal centers and dermatopathic lymphadenitis. The proportion of CD25+ lymphocytes in reactive inflammatory infiltrates in the skin is variable, with percentages ranging from 5% to 50% reported in the medical literature.

While CD25 is expressed in lymphocytes and macrophages in reactive and inflammatory conditions, there are certain T-cell malignancies that characteristically express CD25, including adult T-cell leukemia/lymphoma (ATLL) and anaplastic large-cell lymphomas. Adult T-cell leukemia/lymphoma is a subtype of mature T-cell lymphoma whose pathogenesis is etiologically linked to the human T-cell lymphotropic virus (HTLV-1). The neoplastic cells in ATLL express CD2 and CD5, often downregulate surface expression of CD3 and T-cell receptor-β, and frequently show aberrant loss of CD7. The most characteristic immunophenotypic feature of the neoplastic cells is strong expression of CD25. CD25 expression is distinctive but not unique to ATLL. CD25 can be expressed in other T-cell neoplasms, although often at a lower level than what is characteristically seen in ATLL. Anaplastic large-cell lymphoma, including both ALK-positive and ALK-negative subtypes, also frequently express strong CD25 (~60–70%).

CD25 is also essential in the diagnostic workup of certain B-cell neoplasms. Hairy cell leukemia (HCL) is an indolent mature B-cell neoplasm that primarily involves the bone marrow and spleen. While the cytomorphology of the neoplastic cells and the patterns of tissue involvement are useful, the diagnosis requires immunophenotypic studies to identify the classic hairy cell leukemia profile: expression of CD25, CD103, and CD123 with strong co-expression of CD19, CD20, CD22, and CD11c. Flow cytometry's ability to assess the intensity of antigen expression is very useful in making the diagnosis of HCL; however, when fresh tissue is not available, immunohistochemical evaluation of CD25, in conjunction with a panel of other immunohistochemical stains such as CD103, CD123, annexin A1, etc., can be diagnostic. Evaluation of CD25 expression is particularly important to exclude a diagnosis of hairy cell leukemia-variant (HCL-v), a provisional diagnostic entity in the 2008 WHO classification. HCL-v morphologically resembles hairy cell leukemia, but expresses a variant immunophenotype, with absence of CD25. This distinction is important, as cases of HCL-v are resistant to conventional hairy cell leukemia therapies.

CD25 is also expressed in other B-cell neoplasms, including lymphoplasmacytic lymphomas, follicular lymphoma, chronic lymphocytic leukemia/small lymphocytic lymphoma, and diffuse large B-cell lymphomas. While expression of CD25 in these entities is not diagnostic, the demonstration of CD25 positivity may have prognostic and therapeutic implications in some B-cell neoplasms.

The neoplastic Reed–Sternberg cells in classic Hodgkin lymphoma also often express CD25. Interestingly, Epstein–Barr virus (EBV) enhances CD25 expression on infected cells (including Reed–Sternberg cells in a subset of classic Hodgkin lymphoma) through the NFκB pathway in EBV-related lymphomas. While demonstration of CD25 positivity is seldom evaluated in the diagnostic workup of Hodgkin lymphoma, it may represent a potential therapeutic target.

CD25 expression has diagnostic and prognostic implications in myeloid neoplasms. Systemic mastocytosis is a clonal mast cell neoplasm characterized by abnormal mast cell accumulations in extracutaneous organs. Specific criteria for the diagnosis of systemic mastocytosis have been described by the WHO, including one major criterion (multifocal, dense infiltrates of ≥15 mast cells in the bone marrow or other extracutaneous organs) and four minor criteria (>25% of mast cells within the bone marrow exhibiting atypical morphology, detection of an activating point mutation at codon 816 of KIT, aberrant expression of CD2 and/or CD25 by the atypical mast cells, and total serum tryptase ≥20 ng/mL). The diagnosis of a systemic mastocytosis can be made when the major criterion and one minor criterion or at least three minor criteria are present. Immunohistochemical staining with CD25 can therefore be very useful in the diagnostic workup of suspected mastocytosis patients, particularly when specimens are not obtained for flow cytometry.

CD25 expression has been demonstrated by flow cytometry in both acute myeloid leukemias and acute lymphoblastic leukemias, is often associated with a poor outcome, and is associated with the presence of the t(9;22) in B-cell acute lymphoblastic leukemia. However, CD25 immunohistochemistry currently has a limited, if any, role in acute leukemia prognostication.

Regulatory T cells (Tregs) are a subset of T cells that play a pivotal role in the maintenance of immunological self-tolerance and immune homeostasis. Tregs are involved in both normal and pathologic suppression of immune reactivity with important implications for the development of autoimmune diseases and anti-tumor immunity. There are several subpopulations of Tregs, although many studies focus on the Treg subset defined by expression of CD4, FoxP3, and CD25. The clinical significance of regulatory T cells has been investigated in hematologic neoplasms, solid tumors, and many inflammatory/autoimmune conditions; however, the implications of increased Tregs are beyond the scope of this chapter.

In terms of non-hematopoietic applications, CD25 is reportedly a marker of bile canaliculus, with similar levels of expression noted in normal and diseased liver tissues; however, CD25 immunohistochemistry is not widely used in the workup of non-hematopoietic neoplasms.

Selected references

Baumgartner C, Sonneck K, Krauth MT, *et al*. Immunohistochemical assessment of CD25 is equally sensitive and diagnostic in mastocytosis compared to flow cytometry. *European Journal of Clinical Investigation* 2008; 38: 326–35.

Cerny J, Yu H, Ramanathan M, *et al*. Expression of CD25 independently predicts early treatment failure of acute myeloid leukemia (AML). *British Journal of Haematology* 2013; 160: 262–6.

Fujiwara S, Muroi K, Hirata Y, *et al*. Clinical features of de novo CD25+ diffuse large B cell lymphoma. *Hematology* 2013; 18: 14–19.

Fujiwara S, Muroi K, Tatara R, *et al*. Clinical features of de novo CD25-positive follicular lymphoma. *Leukemia and Lymphoma* 2014; 55: 307–13.

Konoplev S, Medeiros LJ, Bueso-Ramos CE, Jorgensen JL. Immunophenotypic profile of lymphoplasmacytic lymphoma/Waldenström macroglobulinemia. *Hematopathology* 2005; 124: 414–20.

Lu ZH, Chen W, Ju CX, *et al*. CD25 is a novel marker of hepatic bile canaliculus. *International Journal of Surgical Pathology* 2012; 20: 455–61.

O'Malley DP, Chizhevsky V, Grimm KE, Hii A, Weiss LM. Utility of BCL2, PD1, and CD25 immunohistochemical expression in the diagnosis of T cell lymphomas. *Applied Immunohistochemistry and Molecular Morphology* 2014; 22: 99–104.

Swerdlow SH, Campo E, Harris NL, *et al*. *WHO Classification of Tumours of Haematopoietic and Lymphoid Tissues*. Lyon: IARC Press, 2008.

CD30 (Ki-1)

Sources/clones

Accurate (Ki-1, Ber-H2), Biodesign (HRS4), Bioprobe (IC-88), Cymbus Bioscience (Ki-1), Dako (Ber-H2, Ki-l), Diagnostic Biosystems (Ki-1, Ber-H2), Immunotech (HRS4, Ki-1), Serotec.

Fixation/preparation

The Ki-1 antibody produces membrane staining only in frozen sections and does not stain paraffin-embedded tissues. Ber-H2 labels an epitope that survives routine fixation and processing.

Background

The first CD30 antibody generated was called Ki-1 and was thought to be specific for Reed–Sternberg cells. The Ki-1 antibody recognizes an intracellular protein and a membrane-bound glycoprotein that are apparently not related. The membrane-bound glycoprotein is often referred to as the true CD30 antigen. It has a molecular weight of 105–120 kDa and is phosphorylated at serine residues and contains an N- and O-glycosidyl bound carbohydrate portion. The extracellular domain of CD30 shows significant homology with members of the tumor necrosis factor/nerve growth factor receptor superfamily. The human CD30 gene has been localized to the short arm of chromosome 1 at 1p36, a band frequently involved in neoplastic disorders. Deletions, duplications, translocations, and inversions of this band have been observed in non-Hodgkin lymphomas, and abnormalities of the short arm of chromosome 1 have been described in Hodgkin disease. 1p36 is also the location for the TNF receptor-2 gene and appears to be a preferential site for integration of viruses such as the Epstein–Barr virus.

CD30 appears to be a lymphoid activation antigen, and its expression can be induced on B and T lymphocytes in vitro by a number of stimuli, which include viruses and lectins.

CD30 may act as a receptor whose ligand is a cytokine. Recombinant CD30L exhibits pleiotropic cytokine activities, with CD30L inducing proliferation of activated T cells in the presence of an anti-CD3 co-stimulus and enhancing the proliferation of a Hodgkin cell line, HDLM2. CD30L mRNA expression can be induced on T cells and macrophages, suggesting that a variety of autocrine and paracrine mechanisms may be operative. Immunoelectron microscopic studies have localized the antigen in the cytoplasm and in association with the nuclear envelope, chromatin structures, and nucleoli.

Applications

CD30 antibodies do not react against any resting peripheral blood cells. *Staphylococcus*-stimulated B lymphocytes and phytohemagglutinin-stimulated T lymphocytes become CD30-positive, and expression of the antigen can be induced by activating T-helper lymphocytes with autologous and allogeneic stimulator cells. The antigen is also expressed in Epstein–Barr virus-transformed B cells and human T-lymphotrophic virus-transfected T-cell lines. Activated T cells express CD38, CD71, CD25, epithelial membrane antigen, HLA-DR, and CD15 together with α-1-antitrypsin and CD11C prior to the expression of CD30. Scattered large B and T cells localized around lymphoid follicles and at the margin of germinal centers show CD30 positivity in normal and reactive lymph nodes. These cells may also co-express Ki-67 nuclear antigen, indicating their proliferating state. Similarly, macrophages which are generally negative for CD30 may become CD30-positive in conditions such as miliary tuberculosis, sarcoidosis, and other granulomatous reactions such as cat scratch disease and toxoplasmosis. Ber-H2 may also label a subpopulation of plasma cells. Among non-hematopoietic tissues, exocrine pancreatic cells, some cerebral cortical neurons, and Purkinje cells may be positive for CD30.

Initially, Hodgkin disease was the only neoplasm that was CD30-positive. About 90% of non-lymphocyte-predominant Hodgkin disease are positive for CD30, and the staining pattern is membranous, often with a strong paranuclear globule in the region of the Golgi body and weaker cytoplasmic staining (Appendix 2.3). In frozen sections, Ber-H2 produces stronger staining than Ki-1, and staining is also stronger in frozen sections than in paraffin sections. A variable degree of positivity was reported in the L&H cells of lymphocyte-predominant Hodgkin disease (LPHD). About 25% of cases were said to show positivity in paraffin sections, the staining being generally weaker and limited usually to the cell membrane. A study of 16 cases of nodular LPHD showed that CD30 remains negative in L&H cells even after enhanced antigen retrieval methods and advocates the use of the marker to distinguish nodular LPHD from classic Hodgkin disease.

CD30 expression is a characteristic of anaplastic large-cell lymphoma (ALCL), which is defined in part by its nearly constant CD30 positivity. The pattern of staining is similar to that seen in Reed–Sternberg cells and may be expressed by ALCLs of both T- and B-cell lineage as well as "null" cell types. The small-cell variant of ALCL is prone to leukemic presentation, and a discordant expression of CD30 and ALK protein has been found in such cases. Peripheral blood cells were negative for CD30 and ALK protein which were expressed on bone marrow tumor cells. CD30 expression, however, is not limited to ALCL and may be found in other types of non-Hodgkin lymphoma. In one study of about 500 cases of non-Hodgkin lymphomas, 36 cases of lymphomas other than ALCL were CD30-positive. The expression of CD30 is highest in immunoblastic lymphomas, and among the T-cell lymphomas both mycosis fungoides and other types of peripheral T-cell lymphomas (including AILD-like T-cell lymphoma, so-called Lennert's lymphoma, and HTLV-I-positive T-cell leukemia/lymphoma) may show a relatively high incidence of CD30 positivity. It has been suggested that primary CD30+ lymphomas, particularly primary cutaneous lymphomas, have a better prognosis than their CD30– counterparts. However, the expression of CD30 in cutaneous lymphomas which arise in patients with a preceding history of another lymphoma may have a particularly poor prognosis. The expression of CD30 in lymphomatoid papulosis and regressing atypical histiocytosis has suggested a close relationship between these disorders and cutaneous CD30+ ALCL. These three lesions may represent a spectrum, with their histologic and clinical characteristics determined by the degree of biological aggressiveness of the neoplasm and the host immune defenses. Prognosis in primary cutaneous T-cell lymphomas is determined by the expression of CD30, those expressing the antigen having excellent prognosis with five-year survival of 96% compared to 15–21% in CD30– cases.

Occasional cases of plasmacytomas and myelomas may show CD30 positivity. Hairy cell leukemia is consistently negative for CD30, and Langerhans cell histiocytosis is also CD30-negative. Staining has also been reported to be negative in three cases of dendritic reticulum cell sarcoma, and the expression in true histiocytic tumors is not known. CD30 positivity has not been reported in cases of leukemia.

CD30 positivity has been reported in embryonal carcinomas and in the embryonal elements of mixed germ cell tumors, and, less commonly, has been observed in pancreatic and salivary gland carcinomas. CD30 expression in metastatic deposits of embryonal carcinoma may be lost following chemotherapy. The combination of CD30 and CD117 (c-kit) staining has been advocated for the distinction of embryonal carcinoma from seminoma, these tumors staining CD30+/CD117– and CD30–/CD117+ respectively. Occasionally, other paraffin-embedded carcinomas and malignant lymphomas may show weak, diffuse cytoplasmic staining, and CD30 positivity has more uncommonly been observed in mesenchymal tumors including leiomyoma, leiomyosarcoma, rhabdomyosarcoma, synovial sarcoma, giant cell tumor of tendon sheath, malignant fibrous histiocytoma, osteogenic sarcoma, Ewing's sarcoma, malignant schwannoma, ganglioneuromas, and aggressive fibromatosis. Occasional lipoblasts in liposarcoma may show positivity.

Comments

Ber-H2 staining is enhanced by microwave epitope retrieval in citrate buffer with or without enzyme pretreatment. Because it is expressed in stimulated B- and T-lymphoid cells, Ber-H2 should not be employed as a primary marker of Reed–Sternberg cells. However, it should be used in a panel for the identification of ALCL, bearing in mind that such tumors may be CD45-negative and EMA-positive, an immunophenotype that may be mistaken for carcinoma. From a practical standpoint, ALCLs do not express cytokeratin.

Staining is membranous, frequently accompanied by staining of the Golgi. Cytoplasmic staining per se should not be considered as positive. CD30 expression is seen in granulocytes, plasma cells, activated B, T, and NK cells, lymphocytes infected with HIV, HTLV-1, EBV, HHV-8, and hepatitis B, Reed–Sternberg cells, 90% of anaplastic large-cell lymphomas, lymphomatoid papulosis, peripheral T-cell lymphomas, and embryonal carcinoma. The available antibodies may not be immunoreactive in B5 fixed tissue.

Selected references

Awaya N, Mori S, Takeuchi H, *et al.* CD30 and the NPM-ALK fusion protein (p80) are differentially expressed between peripheral blood and bone marrow in primary small cell variant of anaplastic large cell lymphoma. *American Journal of Hematology* 2002; 69: 200–4.

Berney DM, Shamash J, Pieroni K, Oliver RT. Loss of CD30 expression in metastatic embryonal carcinoma: the effect of therapy? *Histopathology* 2001; 39: 382–5.

Chang KL, Arber DA, Weiss LM. CD30: a review. *Applied Immunohistochemistry* 1993; 1: 244–55.

NOTES

CD31

Sources/clones

Accurate (JC70A, CLB-HEC75), Becton Dickinson (L133.1), Biogenex (9G11), Coulter (56E), Dako (JC/70A), Monosan (CLB-58, VM64), Novocastra (HC1.6), Pharmingen (2ET, M290, WM59), Research Diagnostics, Sanbio (VM64).

Fixation/preparation

Antibodies to CD31 are generally immunoreactive in fixed paraffin-embedded tissue sections as well as fresh cell preparations and cryostat sections. HIER enhances immunoreactivity, and if this is employed, enzyme predigestion is not necessary.

Background

CD31 is a 130 kDa glycoprotein, also designated platelet endothelial cell adhesion molecule 1 (PECAM-1), that is normally expressed on endothelial cells and circulating and tissue-phase hematopoietic cells, including platelets, monocytes/macrophages, granulocytes and B cells. This antigen is also expressed in sinusoidal endothelial cells in the liver, lymph node, and spleen. The same endothelial cells display variable staining with *Ulex europaeus* agglutinin 1 (UEA-1) and for von Willebrand factor (factor VIII-related protein), indicating that the sinusoidal endothelium differs from other vascular endothelium. CD31 does not label connective tissue, basement membrane, squamous epithelium, or adnexal structures of the skin. The exact function of CD31 has not been fully elucidated, but it appears to mediate platelet adhesion to endothelial cells and may promote vascular adhesion of leukocytes.

Applications

The main application of CD31 is as a marker of both benign and malignant endothelial cells. CD31 is an apparently more sensitive marker than CD34, von Willebrand factor, or UEA-1 as a marker of malignant vascular endothelium. Despite the earlier suggestion that CD31 is specific for vascular endothelium, with no expression by lymphangiomas, we clearly showed that there was distinct staining for CD31 in all 19 cases of lymphangioma studied, albeit of lesser intensity than that observed in vascular endothelium. Indeed, the endothelial cells of blood and lymphatic vessels share many common antigens such as CD34, von Willebrand factor, and UEA-1 and none provides absolute distinction between the two types of vessels. In the light of these findings, claims that Kaposi's sarcoma shows vascular endothelial differentiation or derivation will need to be reassessed. CD31 is thus employed as a marker of endothelial cells in the evaluation of tumor angiogenesis.

While CD31 is only occasionally found in Ewing's sarcoma/peripheral neuroendocrine tumors, it has been consistently found in small lymphocytic lymphoma and lymphoblastic lymphoma and less often in mantle cell and follicular center cell lymphomas. Rhabdomyosarcomas and desmoplastic small round cell tumors do not express the antigen.

Comments

Some form of HIER should be used with anti-CD31 to produce optimal immunoreactivity in fixed tissue sections (we employ microwave-stimulated HIER in citrate buffer). CD31 is useful as part of the panel for the identification of epithelioid and spindled tumors in the skin and soft tissue (Appendix 1.23, 1.24). The antigen is localized to the cell membrane, with some weaker staining of the cytoplasm. CD31 is expressed on macrophages, granulocytes, T/NK cells, endothelium, and in epithelioid hemangioendothelioma. CD31 is also expressed on megakaryocytes.

Selected references

Albelda SM, Muller WA, Buck CA, Newman PJ. Molecular and cellular properties of PECAM-1 (endoCAM/CD31): a novel vascular cell–cell adhesion molecule. *Journal of Cell Biology* 1991; 114: 1059–61.

DeYoung BR, Wick MR, Fitzgibbon JF, *et al.* CD31: an immunospecific marker for endothelial differentiation in human neoplasms. *Applied Immunohistochemistry* 1993; 1: 97–100.

Stokinger H, Gadd SJ, Eher R, *et al.* Molecular characterization and functional analysis of the leukocyte surface protein CD31. *Journal of Immunology* 1990; 145: 3889–97.

Suthipintawong C, Leong AS-Y, Vinyuvat S. A comparative study of immunomarkers for lymphangiomas and hemangiomas. *Applied Immunohistochemistry* 1995; 3: 239–44.

Teo NB, Shoker BS, Jarvis C, *et al.* Vascular density and phenotype around ductal carcinoma in situ (DCIS) of the breast. *British Journal of Cancer* 2002; 86: 905–11.

CD33

Sources/clones

Leica (Novacastra) (PWS44, mouse monoclonal IgG2b).

Background

CD33 is a sialoadhesin that belongs to the immunoglobulin supergene family. It includes extracellular, transmembrane, and intracellular domains, and is involved in binding of carbohydrates and other lectins. CD33 is post-translationally modified by N-linked glycosolation. It is a pan-myeloid antigen, universally expressed on myeloid progenitors, monocytes/macrophages, and both mature and immature granulocytes. CD33 is not thought to be expressed in non-hematopoietic cells.

Applications

In any normal tissue that contains a monocyte/macrophage cell population, CD33 immunohistochemistry should identify these cells. For example, the sinusoidal histiocytes of both liver and spleen would be expected to be uniformly positive with this antibody. Similarly, CD33 should be uniformly expressed by normal mature and immature myeloid cells in the bone marrow, and in any other tissues with significant infiltration by such cells, including granulocytes. In our experience, the highest levels of CD33 expression on normal myeloid cell populations are seen on monocytes/macrophages and mast cells. Normal granulocytes characteristically have lower-level CD33 expression than other myeloid cells. Presumably due to polymorphisms in the CD33 gene, a small number of patients show significantly lower CD33 expression than the majority.

CD33 is expressed to varying extents on all myeloid neoplasms, with the following themes: (1) CD33 expression tends to be particularly high in neoplastic monocyte populations, including chronic myelomonocytic leukemia (CMML) and acute myeloid leukemia (AML) with monocytic differentiation; (2) CD33 is highly expressed in mast cell neoplasms; (3) CD33 expression is much more variable in other myeloproliferative neoplasms, myelodysplastic syndromes, and the myelodysplastic/myelproliferative overlap syndrome known as atypical chronic myeloid leukemia; (4) CD33 is highly expressed in acute promyelocytic leukemia; (5) CD33 is low to very low in AML bearing the t(8;21); (6) CD33 is frequently aberrantly co-expressed in B-lymphoblastic leukemia/lymphoma (B-LBL), particularly B-LBL bearing the t(9;22); (7) CD33 is often expressed at very low level in normal plasma cells, and at an increased level in plasma cell neoplasms.

CD33 assessment is not only important for assigning lineage to cells of interest, but also represents a potential therapeutic target. The initial anti-CD33 antibody–drug conjugate, in which the conjugate was a toxin known as caleachiamycin, has been withdrawn from the market in the US, although it continues to be used in Europe. Note that new anti-CD33 therapies are being developed and tested to succeed the initial anti-CD33 therapy.

Selected references

Bovio I, Allan RW. The expression of myeloid antigens CD13 and/or CD33 is a marker of ALK+ anaplastic large cell lymphomas. *American Journal of Clinical Pathology* 2008; 130: 628–34.

Golay J, Di Gaetano N, Amico D, *et al.* Gemtuzumab ozogamicin (Mylotarg) has therapeutic activity against CD33 acute lymphoblastic leukaemias in vitro and in vivo. *British Journal of Haematology* 2005; 128: 310–17.

Hoyer JD, Grogg KL, Hanson CA, Gamez JD, Dogan A. CD33 detection by immunohistochemistry in paraffin-embedded tissues: a new antibody shows excellent specificity and sensitivity for cells of myelomonocytic lineage. *American Journal of Clinical Pathology* 2008; 129: 316–23.

Jilani I, Estey E, Huh Y, *et al.* Differences in CD33 intensity between various myeloid neoplasms. *American Journal of Clinical Pathology* 2002; 118: 560–6.

Kaleem Z, White G. Diagnostic criteria for minimally differentiated acute myeloid leukemia (AML-M0). Evaluation and a proposal. *American Journal of Clinical Pathology* 2001; 115: 876–84.

Larson RA, Sievers EL, Stadtmauer EA, *et al.* Final report of the efficacy and safety of gemtuzumab ozogamicin (Mylotarg) in patients with CD33-positive acute myeloid leukemia in first recurrence. *Cancer* 2005; 104: 1442–52.

Robillard N, Wuillème S, Lodé L, *et al.* CD33 is expressed on plasma cells of a significant number of myeloma patients, and may represent a therapeutic target. *Leukemia* 2005; 19: 2021–2.

Shin YK Choi EY, Kim SH, *et al.* Expression of leukemia-associated antigen, JL1, in bone marrow and thymus. *American Journal of Pathology* 2001; 158: 1473–80.

CD34

Sources/clones

Becton Dickinson (MY 10), Biodesign (QBEND/10), Biogenex (QBEND/10), Cymbus Bioscience, Dako (BIRMA-K3), GenTrak, Immunotech (QBEND/10, IMMU133.3), Oncogene, PerSeptive, RDI (9BI-3c5, ICH3), Selinus (BI-3C5), Sera Lab (BI-3C5), Serotec (QBEND/10).

Fixation/preparation

Antibodies are immunoreactive in fixed tissue, and staining is significantly enhanced by HIER.

Background

The CD34 antigen is a 110 kDa heavily glycosylated transmembrane protein of generally unknown function. Some evidence suggests that CD34 might play a role in cell adhesion, with the highly glycosylated molecule allowing it to act as a ligand for lectins. In this way, CD34+ hematopoietic precursors might bind to lectin-expressing cells of the bone marrow stroma. The CD34 antigen was originally defined by monoclonal antibody MY10 raised against the human myeloid leukemia cell line KG1a. The gene for CD34 has been localized to chromosome 1 in the region of 1q32, and the DNA sequence demonstrates no homology with any previously known human genes.

The CD34 antigen is present on ~1% of normal bone marrow mononuclear cells including hematopoietic precursors/stem cells. Thus, antibodies to CD34 can be used to purify the CD34+ stem cell population from CD34- malignant cells. The CD34+ bone marrow population contains not only hematopoietic stem cells but also more mature lineage-committed precursor cells for the erythroid, myeloid, and lymphoid lineages. Included among these CD34+ cells are stromal cells necessary for the appropriate bone marrow environment for hematopoiesis.

The demonstration of CD34 on immature leukemias and vascular neoplasms has been the main contribution to its diagnostic utility. Besides bone marrow stem cells and normal endothelial cells, the antigen is found on cells in the splenic marginal zone, and in dendritic interstitial cells around vessels, nerves, hair follicles, muscle bundles, and sweat glands in a variety of tissues and organs. CD34+ cells appear in the peripheral blood after treatment with chemotherapy or cytokines. In blood vessel endothelium the antigen may be absent from large veins and arteries and from sinuses in the placenta and spleen. It is expressed on the luminal surface and membrane processes that interdigitate between endothelial cells. In new vessels such as in tumors, the location of the antigen is altered, and it is found on the abluminal microprocesses of such vessels.

Among the hematopoietic neoplasms, CD34 is seen in the immature leukemias such as acute lymphoblastic leukemia (ALL) of both T-cell and B-cell lineage, and acute myeloblastic leukemia. In myelodysplastic syndromes the expression of CD34 has been shown to be predictive of transformation and poor survival outcome. There is some confusion over the value of CD34 as a prognostic parameter in the leukemias. Some studies have suggested that its expression is a poor prognosticator in AML, whereas it is a marker of good prognosis in childhood ALL, probably those restricted to B-cell lineage – all these studies being performed with flow cytometry analysis.

Applications

The expression of CD34 is retained in malignant endothelial cells, so it is a good marker for vascular tumors (Appendix 1.16, 1.23, 1.24, 1.26). The endothelial cells of both vascular and lymphatic vessels express the antigen. There is variable staining for CD34 in smooth muscle cells and their tumors. Antibodies to CD34 label gastrointestinal stromal tumors (GIST) very strongly (Appendix 1.29). Epithelioid smooth muscle tumors stain less frequently, but the marker may serve as a useful discriminator from epithelial tumors, which are generally negative for CD34. The antigen is displayed by nerve sheath tumors, although in some series both neurofibromas and schwannomas failed to stain. In the latter, staining may be mainly in the Antoni B areas. While the staining in malignant nerve sheath tumors is largely negative, some series report a high frequency of reactivity, suggesting that CD34 may be a useful inclusion in the diagnostic panel for such tumors, as S100 and CD57 are negative in such tumors. Epithelioid sarcoma shows staining for CD34, and the marker is invariably found in solitary fibrous tumors and dermatofibrosarcoma protuberans, two tumors which are generally distinguished from their histologic mimics by the absence of specific markers. Recently, CD34 was also demonstrated in 4 of 12 cases of angiomyofibroblastomas. Interestingly, reactivity for CD34 was found in giant cell fibroblastomas and one Bednar tumor, supporting the relationship of both tumors to dermatofibrosarcoma protuberans.

CD34 stains a stromal fibrocyte which functions as a matrix-producing cell and possibly as an antigen-presenting cell capable of priming naïve T cells in situ, and which may have an important role in host response to tissue damage. Loss of this stromal CD34+ fibrocyte has been observed in invasive breast cancer and in ductal carcinoma in situ with the appearance of smooth muscle actin-positive myofibroblasts, whereas benign lesions of the breast and normal breast stroma contain CD34+ fibrocytes but no smooth muscle positive myofibroblasts. The expression of a common vimentin+/CD34+/Bcl-2+/CD99+ phenotype in spindle cell lipoma-like tumor, solitary fibrous tumor, and myofibroblastoma of the breast suggests a common histogenesis.

CD34 is also a useful marker for early myeloid cells and hence stains granulocytic sarcoma.

Comments

Much of the earlier controversy concerning the staining of CD34 in spindle cell tumors was due to the sensitivity of the staining technique. CD34 staining is greatly enhanced by HIER, especially microwave-induced techniques. Although CD34 is widely employed for labeling vascular endothelial cells for the enumeration of vessels in neoplasms, the staining of stromal fibrocytes makes the use of other endothelial markers such as CD31 preferable. Nonetheless, CD34 can be employed as a useful substitute for CD31 in antibody panels for the identification of epithelioid and spindled tumors in the skin and soft tissue (Appendix 1.23, 1.24).

CD34 is expressed on hematopoietic progenitor cells, leukemic blasts, vascular and lymphatic endothelial cells, 40% of acute myeloid leukemias, and 75% of pre-B acute lymphoblastic leukemia.

Selected references

Greaves MF, Brown J, Molgaard HV, et al. Molecular features of CD34: a hematopoietic progenitor cell-associated molecule. *Leukemia* 1992; 1: 31–6.

Ramani P, Bradley NJ, Fletcher CMD. QBEND/10, a new monoclonal antibody to endothelium: assessment of its diagnostic utility in paraffin sections. *Histopathology* 1990; 17: 237–42.

CD35

Sources/clones

Dako (Ber-MAC-DRC, To5), Immunotech (J3D3).

Fixation/preparation

This antibody can be used on formalin-fixed paraffin-embedded tissue section. Enzymatic digestion with proteolytic enzymes (e.g., pronase) for antigen retrieval must be performed for optimum immunoreaction. HIER enhances immunoreactivity, especially when Target Retrieval Solution is employed. The CD35 antibody may also be applied to acetone-fixed cryostat sections or fixed cell smears.

Background

Dako-CD35 (isotype: IgG1κ) reacts with a formalin-resistant epitope of the receptor for the C3b fragment of the third component of human complement. This receptor, which is often referred to as CR1, consists of a single glycoprotein chain with a molecular weight of approximately 220 kDa. The antigen has been designated CD35 in the system for classifying human leukocyte antigens and is therefore equivalent to To5.

In frozen sections of normal tissues, Dako-CD35 shows immunostaining of B-cell follicles of lymphoid tissue. The most strongly labeled cells within B-cell follicles are follicular dendritic cells (FDCs), but mantle zone lymphoid cells also immunoreact to a lesser degree. The C3b receptor on epithelial cells of renal glomeruli may also be clearly demonstrated with this antibody. Further, enzyme-treated, routinely processed paraffin sections show strong immunoreaction of FDCs in lymphoid tissue (both nodal and extranodal). The well-defined dense meshworks of FDCs in germinal centers are well demonstrated with this antibody.

Applications

Immunohistological analyses of FDCs in paraffin sections are confined to the demonstration of FDC meshworks in reactive and neoplastic lymphoid tissue. In this regard identical immunoreaction of the dendritic cell processes of FDC are demonstrated with antibodies to both CD21 and CD35. Hence, the application of antibody to CD35 in surgical pathology (being similar to CD21) remains largely for the demonstration of FDC meshworks in follicles of HIV lymphadenopathy, Castleman's disease, follicular lymphoma, follicular colonization by low-grade B-cell MALT lymphoma, and nodular lymphocyte-predominant Hodgkin disease. Demonstration of FDCs with CD35 antibody is also useful in mantle cell lymphoma and peripheral T-cell lymphoma AILD type. In contrast to follicular lymphomas, in which the lymphoma cells are encased within a network of proliferating FDCs, the network of FDCs in mantle cell lymphoma is loosely arranged. In angioimmunoblastic T-cell lymphoma, there is a pronounced proliferation of FDCs around postcapillary venules. CD35 has its greatest utility in the diagnosis of follicular dendritic cell tumors (see section on CD21) (Appendix 2.7).

The CNA.42 antibody is reactive in fixed paraffin-embedded sections and stains FDCs, but apparently identifying an antigen different from other known anti-FDC antibodies. The antibody also labels some T-cell lymphomas as well as a variety of soft tissue tumors and a proportion of carcinomas of the gastrointestinal tract and lung. Aberrant expression of CD35 is seen on mast cells in mastocytosis. The antigen is conserved in a wide spectrum of animal tissues other than humans.

Comments

In post-chemotherapy excision specimens, immunostaining with a CD21/CD35 antibody cocktail is useful to highlight dispersed small islands of residual tumor among the negative foamy histiocytes. Reactive germinal centers highlighted by antibodies to FDCs are ideal for use as positive control tissue.

CD35 is expressed on granulocytes, macrophages, B cells, T cells (10%), NK cells, follicular dendritic cells, glomerular podocytes, and some astrocytes.

Selected references

Badgi E, Krenacs L, Krenacs T, *et al.* Follicular dendritic cells in reactive and neoplastic lymphoid tissues: a reevaluation of staining patterns of CD21, CD23, and CD35 antibodies in paraffin sections after wet heat-induced epitope retrieval. *Applied Immunohistochemistry and Molecular Morphology* 2001; 9: 117–24.

Bettelheim P. M8, cluster report: CD35. In Knapp W, Dorken B, Gilks W, *et al.*, eds. *Leucocyte Typing IV. White Cell Differentiation Antigens*. Oxford: Oxford University Press, 1989, pp. 829–30.

CD38

Sources/clones

Accurate (BCAP38), Advanced Immunochemical (24G3), Biodesign (MIG-P12, T16), Biosource (BA6), Caltag Laboratories (BL-AC38, HIT2), Coulter (CD38, T16), Cymbus Bioscience (BA6), Dako (AT13/5), Immunotech (T16), Pharmingen (HIT2), Sanbio/Monosan (BL-D2, MIG-P12), Sanbio/Monosan/Accurate (BLD2), Sera Lab, Serotec (BA6, AT13/5, T16).

Fixation/preparation

Most antibodies are reactive in fixed paraffin-embedded sections, and HIER in Target Retrieval Solution enhances immunoreactivity.

Background

The CD38 molecule, initially described as T10, consists of a single chain of 46 kDa, spanning the membrane with its carboxyl terminus located in the extracellular compartment. CD38 has been one of the most elusive molecules within the family of leukocyte multilineage markers. It is expressed on different precursor cells, monocytes, activated T cells, and terminally differentiated B cells, including plasma cells. This transmembrane glycoprotein appears to mediate several diverse functions such as signal transduction, cell adhesion (including binding to endothelium), with an important role in lymphocyte homing, and cyclic adenosine diphosphate–ribose synthesis, but its activities remain elusive. Immunoreactivity for CD38 has also been described in a subset of pyramidal neurons and astrocytes, predominantly distributed in the perikarya and dendrites in association with rough endoplasmic reticulum, ribosomes, small vesicles, mitochondria, and cell membranes. CD38 has also been demonstrated in normal prostate epithelium within both basal and secretory epithelial cells, and appeared to be lost in some cases of prostatic carcinoma and hyperplasia, and in nonmalignant glands surrounding tumor. It was speculated that the role of CD38 in intracellular calcium mobilization may contribute to smooth muscle contraction and/or sperm motility. The ligand to CD38 is the adhesion molecule CD31.

Insulin secretion is one of the functions mediated by CD38. The molecule is the target of an autoimmune response, and serum auto-antibodies to CD38 have been detected in diabetic patients. Anti-CD38 auto-antibodies have been suggested to be a new diagnostic marker of β-cell autoimmunity in diabetes.

The source of the antigen for raising anti-CD38 specific monoclonal antibody was mainly preparations obtained from MLC cells, normal thymocytes, and the plasmacytoma cell line LP-1. This was used in the context of endometrial biopsy specimens to allow the definitive diagnosis of chronic endometritis to be made.

Applications

The expression of CD38 is not restricted to a specific lineage, nor to a discrete activation step. It is found on precursor cells in the bone marrow, activated cells (T and B blasts), terminally differentiated cells (such as plasma cells), monocytes, and most peripheral blood NK cells. CD4+/CD45RA+ cells also preferentially express CD38, but the antigen is not expressed by CD4+/CD45RO+ cells. From a practical standpoint, CD38 has been useful in the immunophenotyping of acute leukemias and in research into the role of activated T cells in immunodeficiency diseases and autoimmune diseases. It is a useful marker for plasma cells, as poorly differentiated plasma cells may mimic other blastic lymphoid cells and suboptimal cytomorphologic preservation may impede the accurate recognition of plasma cells. It has been employed to identify plasma cells in synovial biopsies, aiding in the differential diagnosis of early arthritis. CD38 is a better antibody than VS.38 when employed to identify plasma cells such as in the diagnosis of chronic endometritis, as the latter also stains stromal and endometrial cells, reducing its usefulness in this setting. CD38 shows strong labeling of plasma cells, enhancing their distinctive cytologic characteristics.

Selected references

Alessio M, Roggero S, Funaro A, *et al.* CD38 molecule: structural and biochemical analysis on human T lymphocytes, thymocytes, and plasma cells. *Journal of Immunology* 1990; 145: 878–84.

Dianzani U, Funaro A, DiFranco D, *et al.* Interaction between endothelium and CD4+CD45RA+ lymphocytes: role of the human CD38 molecule. *Journal of Immunology* 1994; 153: 952–9.

CD40

Sources/clones

Ancell (BEI), Biodesign (BL-C4), Caltag Laboratories (BLB40), Coulter/Immunotech (MAB89), Cymbus Bioscience (B-B20), Immunotec (MAB89), Pharmingen (5C3), Sanbio/Monosan (BL-C4), Sanbio/Monosan/Accurate (BLC4), Serotec (B-B20).

Fixation/preparation

The antigen is resistant to formalin fixation, with enhanced staining following heat-induced antigen retrieval at pH 8.0.

Background

CD40 is a 48 kDa integral membrane protein expressed by B lymphocytes, follicular dendritic cells, interdigitating reticulum cells, monocytes, epithelial cells, endothelial cells, and tumor cells including carcinomas, B-cell lymphomas/leukemia and Reed–Sternberg cells of Hodgkin disease. CD40 has been clustered as a member of the nerve growth factor (NGF)/tumor necrosis factor (TNF) receptor superfamily. Its corresponding counterstructure, the CD40 ligand (CD40L), is mainly expressed by activated CD4+ T cells and also some activated CD8+ T cells, basophils, eosinophils, mast cells, and stromal cells. CD40L shares significant amino acid homology with TNF, particularly in its extracellular domain, and is therefore viewed as a member of the TNF ligand superfamily.

The flurry of publications relating to CD40 suggests that this receptor may have a pivotal role in the function of B lymphocytes and their survival. Binding of CD40L+ T cells to CD40+ B cells is thought to play a major role in the T-cell-dependent B-cell activation, B-cell proliferation, Ig isotype switching, memory B-cell formation, and rescue of B cells from apoptotic death in germinal centers. Mutations of the CD40L gene have been associated with the X-linked hyper-IgM immunodeficiency syndrome, indicating the critical role of the CD40/CD40L interaction in the T-cell–B-cell interplay. Accordingly, expression of CD40 has been found in most of the B-cell neoplasms, Reed–Sternberg cells of Hodgkin disease, and some carcinomas. In contrast, functional CD40/CD40L interactions appear to be critical for cellular activation signals during immune responses and neoplastic tumor cell growth. Lack of this important interaction results in greatly reduced activation of CD4+ T cells, while successful interaction of these molecules results in full activation of T-cell effector functions such as help for B-cell differentiation and class switch, activation of monocytes and macrophages to produce lymphokines and to kill intracellular pathogens, and activation of autoreactive T cells to mount an autoimmune response. CD40 may also play a similar role in the transduction of regulatory signals for cell functions such as proliferation and differentiation in non-lymphoid cells, and it has a role in the binding of tumor cells to endothelium, cell migration, and enhancement of cell motility, so that it is of interest in tumor metastasis and prognostication.

Applications

The intense research interest in CD40 and its ligand has yet to be translated into diagnostic applications. Current uses of CD40 have mostly been for the immunodetection and identification of tumor cells in all subtypes of Hodgkin disease. As many as 100% of Hodgkin disease cases display positivity for CD40, irrespective of the antigenic phenotype. In contrast, CD40 was immunodetected in only one-third of anaplastic large-cell lymphomas, whereas almost 85% of B-cell non-Hodgkin lymphomas were positive. In-vitro engagement of CD40 by its soluble ligand CD40L enhanced both clonogenic capacity and colony cell survival of Hodgkin disease cell lines. Recombinant CD40L induced interleukin-8 secretion and enhanced IL-6, TNF, and lymphotoxin-α release from cultured Reed–Sternberg cells. These cytokines play a significant role in the clinical presentation and pathology of Hodgkin disease, a tumor of cytokine-producing cells. CD40L has pleiotropic biologic activities on Reed–Sternberg cells, and the CD40/CD40L interaction might be a critical element in the deregulated cytokine network and cell contact-dependent activation cascade typical of Hodgkin disease.

Other applications of CD40 include the study of ulcerative colitis, in which an upregulation of CD40 has been demonstrated in epithelial cells of the colon both in the active state and in remission. Similarly, increased CD40 expression was found in the B cell, macrophage, and dendritic cell compartments in acute ileitis following oral infection with *Toxoplasma* in mice, suggesting that CD40/CD154 interaction is an essential component for development of inflammation in the experimental model. CD40 is also expressed in neuronal cells of the brain.

Comments

CD40 shows distinctive immunolocalization to the cell membrane and as a paranuclear dot similar to that of CD30 and CD15.

CD40 is expressed on B cells, macrophages, dendritic cells, endothelial cells, fibroblasts, keratinocytes, carcinomas, most B-cell lymphomas, and some B-ALL, and is not expressed on plasma cells.

Selected reference

Carbone A, Gloghini A, Gruss HJ, Pinto A. CD40 ligand is constitutively expressed in a subset of T cell lymphomas and on the microenvironmental reactive T cells of follicular lymphomas and Hodgkin's disease. *American Journal of Pathology* 1995; 147: 912–22.

CD43

Sources/clones

Becton Dickinson (Leu-22), Biodesign (BL-E/G3), Biogenesis (MEM59), Biogenesis/Biosource (WR14), Biogenex (MT1), Caltag Laboratories (BL-TP43), Coulter (DFT1), Cymbus Bioscience (DFT1), Dako (DFT1), Labvision Corp. (BRA7G), Novocastra (polyclonal), Pharmingen (HIS17, S7, 1G10), Sanbio/Accurate (BLEG3), Sanbio/Monosan (MEM-59), Serotec (DFT1, DR-14), Shandon Lipshaw (DFT1).

Fixation/preparation

Generally (especially MT1 and DFT-1) applicable to formalin-fixed paraffin-embedded sections, but requires enzyme (trypsin) pretreatment before immunostaining. HIER enhances immunoreactivity.

Background

MT1 and the identical antibody DFT-1 recognize a sialoantigen present on normal T cells, myeloid cells, and macrophages. Megakaryocytes are variably positive. Both antibodies belong to the CD43 cluster. There is evidence that the antibody MT1, originally thought to belong to CD45, binds to an entirely unrelated molecule. Both MT1 and DFT-1 recognize surface antigens (190, 110, and 100 kDa).

Applications

In a review of several published series, CD43 (MT1) was shown to immunoreact with 30% of low-grade B-cell lymphomas, approximately 90% of T-cell lymphomas, 69% of B-cell and 97% of T-cell lymphoblastic lymphomas, and 44% of anaplastic large-cell lymphomas. However, it should be noted that CD43 also highlights myeloid cells and macrophages and may be employed as a marker of granulocytic tumors (Appendix 2.5). Although normal small B lymphocytes are CD43-negative, most low-grade B-cell lymphomas are CD43-positive. However, hairy cell leukemia, MALT lymphoma, and follicle center cell lymphomas are notable exceptions. Therefore CD43 is not useful for distinguishing between T-cell and B-cell lymphocytic lymphoma. Furthermore, although CD43 is a reliable marker of mantle cell lymphoma (MCL), it cannot immunophenotypically distinguish MCL from T-cell or B-cell lymphoblastic lymphomas. CD43 marks plasmacytoma/myeloma and is more often positive than negative in peripheral T-cell lymphomas.

CD43 is the only antibody that is positive in 100% of extramedullary myeloid tumors, irrespective of the differentiation of the myeloid cells. Furthermore, staining is always intense and widespread.

Comments

CD43 remains behind CD3 and UCHL1 (CD45RO) as a marker of T-cell lymphomas. Nevertheless, in appropriate immunohistochemical panels CD43 does play a role in the identification of low-grade B-cell lymphomas (Appendix 2.1) and myeloid disorders. Normal tonsil is useful as a control since paracortical cells are CD43-positive, while follicle center cells are negative. The expression of CD43 in a large B-cell lymphoma may be an indicator of dedifferentiation from a small-cell lymphoma. There is ample evidence that CD43 is not specific for T cells. Together with CD79a and Tdt, this marker is useful in separating lymphoblastic lymphoma from Ewing's sarcoma, which is consistently negative for these antigens.

CD43 is positive on most T cells, activated B cells, NK cells, granulocytes, monocytes, megakaryocytes, and 90% of T-cell lymphomas. It is co-expressed with CD20 in small lymphocyte lymphoma but not in benign cells, granulocytic sarcomas, acute myeloid leukemia, most acute lymphoblastic leukemia, plasmacytomas, and mast cell disease.

Selected references

Flavell DJ, Flavell SU, Jones DB, Wright DH. Two new monoclonal antibodies recognising T-cells (DF-T1) and B-cells (DF-B1) in formalin fixed paraffin embedded tissue sections. *Journal of Pathology* 1988; 155: 343A.

Poppema S, Hollema H, Visser L, Vos H. Monoclonal antibodies (MT1, MT2, MB1, MB2, MB3) reactive with leukocyte subsets in paraffin-embedded tissue sections. *American Journal of Pathology* 1987; 127: 418–29.

CD44

Sources/clones

CD44

Available from Biodesign (T2.F4, BU52), Cymbus Bioscience (F10–44–2), Dako (DF1485, 2B11), Immunotech (J.173), Oncogene (A3D8, AIG3), Pharmingen (OX-49), RDI (F10–44–2), Sanbio (MEM-85), Sera Lab (A3D8, AIG3), Serotec (F10–44–2), Sigma (A3D8).

CD44v6

Available from R & D Systems (2F10), and various isoforms including v4, v5, v6, v7, and v7-v8 are available from Bender MedS.

Fixation/preparation

The antibodies, particularly A1G3, are effective in formalin-fixed paraffin-embedded tissues, but staining is optimal only after microwave-induced epitope retrieval in citrate buffer at pH 6.0. Enzyme digestion should not be performed, as this has been shown to alter the integrity of the antigen.

Background

The CD44 receptor is also known as phagocytic glycoprotein (Pgp-1), extracellular matrix receptor III (ECM-III), B-cell p80 antigen, lymphocyte homing receptor (Hermes antigen), and hyaluronate cellular adhesion molecule (H-CAM). CD44 shows considerable homology with the cartilage link proteins involved in adhesion between hyaluronate and other proteoglycans in the extracellular matrix including collagen, fibronectin, and ankyrin. Besides this function, CD44 has since been found to have a role in recognition between lymphocytes and endothelial cells and in lymphocyte homing to the reticuloendothelial tissues. This latter function has led to interest in its possible role in the regulation of tumor cell dissemination.

The CD44 family of glycoproteins exists in a number of variant isoforms, the most common being the standard 85–95 kDa or hematopoietic variant (CD44s) that is found in mesodermal cells such as hematopoietic, fibroblastic, and glial cells, and in some carcinoma cell lines. The receptor is coded in five distinct domains located on the short arm of chromosome 11. The heterogeneity in the CD44 molecule may result from post-translational modification of the protein, and/or splicing of up to 10 exons may result in variant isoforms of higher molecular weight (140–160 kDa) which may be expressed individually or in various combinations, with potentially diverse functions. Higher-molecular-weight isoforms have been described in epithelial cells (CD44v) and are thought to function in intercellular adhesion and stromal binding. While the other functions and distributions of the CD44 family have not yet been completely elucidated, they are also known to participate in embryonic development and angiogenesis as well as in other molecular processes associated with specific adhesions, signal transduction, and cell migration. The demonstration of a concordance of the cell proliferation nuclear antigen Ki-67 and CD44 expression in adenomatous polyps, colonic carcinomas, and adjacent mucosa raises the possibility of involvement of CD44 in stimulating cell growth.

Following the discovery that the splice variants, especially exon v4–7, initiated the lymphatic spread of rat pancreatic carcinoma cells, the role of the highly interspecies conserved CD44 in human tumor progression and metastasis has been examined. It appears that the CD44–hyaluronate interaction is central to tumor invasiveness, the receptor allowing the uptake and subsequent degradation of matrical hyaluronate. While many human tumors express CD44, a positive correlation between increased CD44v expression and tumor progression and/or dedifferentiation has been demonstrated in only some. Such tumors include non-Hodgkin lymphoma, hepatocellular carcinoma, breast carcinoma, renal cell carcinoma, colonic carcinoma, some soft tissue tumors, metastatic melanoma, prostatic carcinoma, and gastric cancer. Conversely, CD44v expression is downgraded in other tumors, including neuroblastomas and squamous cell and basal cell carcinomas of the skin.

Applications

The suggestion that there is a positive association between CD44 isoform expression and progression in human tumors has important implications for diagnosis and prognosis. Unfortunately, the situation is not yet clear-cut. Confusion over the complicated exon boundaries, compounded by the different nomenclatures employed by researchers, has added to problems in identifying the true metastasis-associated isoform. Furthermore, stromal cells may contribute to the isoform pattern detected. For example, activated lymphocytes may express the so-called metastasis-associated variant of CD44, emphasizing the importance of immunohistological assessment as a method that allows morphologic discrimination.

Comments

Currently, applications of CD44 still lie in the research domain. While antibodies to specific isoforms are available, some reactive in fixed paraffin-embedded tissues, the antibody to pan-CD44 molecule has been the most widely used in paraffin sections. Microwave epitope retrieval is essential for the demonstration of the antigen. While CD44 is a plasmalemmal determinant, both cytoplasmic and cell membrane staining patterns have been demonstrated in non-neoplastic and neoplastic cells. It has been suggested that exclusive cytoplasmic staining may reflect the overproduction of the protein so that not all of it can be incorporated into the cell membrane. Alternatively, the production of aberrant forms or massive shedding of the CD44 molecule from the cell membrane could account for this pattern of staining.

Selected reference

East JE, Hart IR. CD44 and its role in tumor progression and metastasis. *European Journal of Cancer* 1993; 29A: 1921–2.

CD45 (leukocyte common antigen)

Sources/clones

CD45

Available from a large number of sources including Biodesign (ALB12, J.33, MEM 28, T29/33), Biogenex, Bioprobe (bra 55, ICO-46, LT46), Cymbus Bioscience (MEM 28, RVS-1, F10-89-4), Dako (T29/33, 2B11, PD7/26), GenTrak, Immunotech (J.33, ALB 12), Oncogene (MEM 28, T29/33, J.33), Pharmingen (H130, CT-1, 30F11.1), RDI (F-10-89-4, CLB-T200/1), Sanbio (BL-leuk-45), Sera Lab (F10–89–4), Serotec (YTH54.12, YTH24.5), and Sigma.

CD45R

Available from Accurate/Ancell (351C5), Biodesign (DFB1, F8-11-13, MEM56), Biogenex, Bioprobe (LT45R), Cymbus Bioscience (DFB1), GenTrak, RDI (DFB1), Pharmingen (HIS24, DNL-1.9, 16A, 23G2, RA3-6B2), Sera Lab, Serotec.

CD45RO

Available from Accurate/Ancell (UCHL1), Biodesign (UCHL1), Biotest (UCHL1), Cymbus Bioscience (UCHL1), Dako (UCHL1, OPD4), GenTrak, Immunotech (UCHL1), Sera Lab (UCHL1), Serotec (UCHL1).

CD45RA

Available from Accurate (YTH80.103), Biodesign (ALB11, F8-11-13), Cymbus Bioscience (F8-1-3, MEM 56), Dako (4KB5), GenTrak, Immunotech (ALB11), Pharmingen (14.8), RDI (F8-11-13), Sanbio (MEM-56), Sera Lab, Serotec (B-C15, F8-11-13).

CD45RB

Available from Axcel/Accurate, Cymbus Bioscience, Dako (PD7/26),

CD45RC

Available from Pharmingen (HIS25) and Serotec (YTH80.103).

Fixation/preparation

The CD45 antibodies that are commercially available are mostly effective in paraffin-embedded tissues as well as in frozen sections.

Background

The CD45 cluster of antibodies recognizes a family of proteins known as the leukocyte common antigen (LCA) exclusively expressed on the surface of almost all hematolymphoid cells and their progenitors. The CD45 antibody is one of the most specific antibodies currently available for diagnostic use. Virtually all hematolymphoid cells, including T and B lymphocytes, granulocytes and monocytes, and macrophages, with the exception of maturing erythrocytes and megakaryocytes, express CD45. To date, proteins of the leukocyte common antigen family have not been conclusively shown on any non-hematolymphoid cells.

The CD45 proteins are coded for by a single gene located on chromosome lq31–32. The gene is composed of 33 exons that code for the cDNA sequence as well as both 5′ and 3′ non-translated regions. Differential usage of three exons termed A, B, and C is known to generate eight different mRNAs and at least five proteins in the CD45 protein family. The complete CD45 protein consists of a large cytoplasmic domain of 707 amino acids, a transmembrane region of 22 amino acids, and an external domain of 391–552 amino acids depending on the pattern of exon splicing. By electron microscopy, the CD45 proteins consist of a globular structure of 12 nm, representing the cytoplasmic domain, and a rod-like structure of 18 nm, representing the external domain.

There is high conservation of the cytoplasmic domain among mammals, and it shows homology with placental tyrosine phosphatases. Consistent with this homology, the CD45 protein has intrinsic tyrosine phosphatase activity and belongs to a family of protein tyrosine phosphatases that includes 16 other members, at least seven of which are transmembrane proteins.

The precise function of the CD45 proteins is not known, but they appear to play an important role in early lymphocyte activation. Protein tyrosine phosphatase can counter the actions of protein tyrosine kinases, enzymes known to be induced in early T-cell activation that may represent the primary signaling event initiated by the T-cell receptor. CD45 expression is inversely related to spontaneous tyrosine phosphorylation of multiple proteins, which has a fundamental role in regulating T-cell calcium levels. CD45 is required for both T-cell antigen receptor and CD2-mediated activation of T-lymphocyte protein tyrosine kinase, and CD45 is physically linked to both CD2 and the T-cell receptor on the surface of memory T lymphocytes. The differences in structure among the external domains of the different CD45 proteins probably determine the specific target stimuli for the different cell types expressing CD45. Similarly, CD45 may also be important for B-cell function. Antibodies to CD45 inhibit an early phase in the activation of resting B cells and are able to inhibit *c-myc* induction in B cells.

As a result of post-translocational change of the mRNA of the A, B, and C exons, several isoforms are produced. By strict definition, CD45 antibodies are monoclonal antibodies, which react with all isoforms of CD45 proteins, and there are several subclusters of antibodies that detect different species of CD45 proteins. These have molecular weights of 220 kDa representing the ABC isoform, 205 kDa probably representing distinct AB and BC isoforms, 190 kDa representing the B isoform, and 180 kDa representing the O isoform. The restricted CD45 antibody refers to those that recognize subsets of CD45 proteins but not the entire class, and these CD45R antibodies can be further subdivided into CD45RA, CD45RB, and CD45RO depending on the isoform recognized by the antibody. To date, there are no monoclonal antibodies that specifically recognize the C isoform. CD45RA antibodies generally precipitate the 220 and 205 kDa proteins (ABC and AB isoforms), CD45RB the 220, 205, and 190 kDa proteins (ABC, AB, BC, and B isoforms) and CD45RO the 180 kDa protein (O isoform).

Many of the CD45 antibodies are sensitive to neuraminidase, consistent with the suggestion that these antibodies recognize epitopes that are associated with carbohydrates and, possibly, terminal sialic acids. PD7 is a CD45RB antibody and labels all known CD45 proteins with the exception of the ones lacking exons A, B, and C, whereas 2B11 reacts against AB protein but not others. The combination of PD7 with 2B11 as a CD45–CD45RB cocktail (Dako) allows a reliable method of detecting LCA in hematolymphoid cells. CD45 proteins are major components of the membranes of lymphocytes and form about 10% of the lymphocyte surface, accounting for much of the carbohydrate present on the membrane. The staining with CD45 antibodies is membranous, although there may be some staining of the Golgi. Histiocytes exhibit minimal cell membrane staining, and phagocytic cells show immunolocalization of the antigen to secondary lysosomes.

Applications

The CD45 proteins are the most specific of diagnostic antibodies currently available. A cocktail of PD7-2B11 (CD45–CD45RB) antibodies is a reliable marker of cells fixed in formalin as well as in cryostat sections and fresh cell preparations. It is, therefore, an essential component of the panel to distinguish anaplastic large-cell tumors, which include the entities malignant lymphoma, melanoma, and carcinoma (Appendix 1.10). It is also an essential component of panels to separate small-cell tumors of lymph nodes, skin, bone, and other sites (Appendix 1.6, 1.11, 1.12), in adults as well as in children. The reactivity of anti-LCA antibodies is between 93% and 99% for a cross-spectrum of different subtypes of B- and T-cell lymphomas.

In classic Hodgkin disease, excluding the nodular L&H lymphocyte-predominant subtype, membrane staining for LCA is rare, although cytoplasmic staining may be seen. Cytoplasmic staining may be spurious, as similar cytoplasmic staining can be found in non-hematolymphoid neoplasms. By contrast, the majority of nodular L&H lymphocyte-predominant Hodgkin disease shows positivity for PD7 and/or 2B11, and this subtype is now thought to be distinctly different from classic Hodgkin disease.

Anaplastic large-cell lymphoma may show positivity for LCA in only 50–87% of cases, although this figure may be higher in frozen section material. Furthermore, anaplastic large-cell lymphoma may also show staining for epithelial membrane antigen, making its immunohistochemical differentiation from anaplastic carcinoma difficult. These tumors express CD30 and, in 60% of cases, are of activated T-cell phenotype showing staining for CD45RO and/or CD43 in paraffin sections.

Among other hematolymphoid neoplasms, plasmacytomas show a variable degree of positivity for LCA, ranging from 0% to 20% of cases. Hairy cell leukemia has been found to be uniformly positive for PD7-2B11, and CD45 expression has been found in all cases of acute leukemias of T-cell lineage and in over 80% of cases of B-cell lineage. Failure of expression of CD45 in acute childhood lymphoblastic leukemia appears to be associated with other favorable prognostic features such as lower leukocyte counts and serum lactic dehydrogenase levels and is associated with chromosomal hyperdiploidy. Mast cell disease appears to be positive for PD1–2B11, and polycythemia vera and extramedullary hematopoiesis have been reported as negative although only a few cases were studied. In keeping with the low expression in histiocytes, true histiocytic tumors were found to be negative for PD7–2B11, whereas cases of Langerhans histiocytosis were reported to be positive. The rare cases of interdigitating reticulum cell sarcoma that have been studied have been reported to be positive for PD7, similar to non-neoplastic interdigitating reticulum cells. Cases of CD45-negative, keratin-positive large-cell lymphomas have been reported, but these are exceptionally rare.

While larger series have reported a total absence of staining for LCA in non-hematolymphoid neoplasms, there have been rare case reports of staining examples of primitive sarcoma, probably rhabdomyosarcoma.

CD45RA (4KB5)

The CD45RA group of antibodies recognize the 220 kDa and 205 kDa variants of CD45 encoded by exon A. These isoforms are expressed on the surface of most B cells, as well as post-thymic, naïve T cells and some medullary thymocytes. MT2 is thought to recognize a carbohydrate moiety and is negative in normal germinal centers, unlike antibodies MB1 and KiB3, which appear to bind to the peptide backbone of CD45RA, staining mantle zone and follicular center cells. In the paracortical areas of lymph nodes, there are approximately equal numbers of CD45RO+ and CD45RA+ cells. In paraffin-embedded sections, MB1 and 4KB5 stain over 80% of cases of B-cell lymphomas, while MT2 stains only 57% of such cases. Small lymphocytic lymphoma has the highest rate of positivity, while small non-cleaved cell lymphoma has the lowest. Fifty-seven percent of cases of follicular center lymphoma are positive for MT2, and this pattern of staining has been exploited for diagnostic purposes, as only weak or absent scattered positivity for MT2 is seen in reactive germinal center cells. Neoplastic follicles are labeled by MT2 whereas reactive follicles are not. This difference in staining patterns with MT2 has been postulated to be due to differences in the sialation of the CD45 protein present on these B cells. T-cell lymphoma has a much lower incidence of positivity with CD45RA antibodies, which is seen in about 10% of cases.

CD45RA+ mycosis fungoides is a rare form of the disease with T-helper phenotype (CD3+/CD4+/CD8−/CD45RO+), often with loss of lineage markers.

CD45RO (UCHL1, OPD4)

CD45RO antibodies recognize the 180 kDa (O isoform) variant of CD45. UCHL1 antibody reacts with approximately 90% of cortical thymocytes, 50% of medullary thymocytes, and approximately 50–70% of CD2− and CD3+ peripheral blood and lymph node T cells. It rarely, if ever, reacts with benign B cells. While most mature T cells are CD45RO-positive (Appendix 2.2), some normal T-cell subsets are constitutively CD45RO-negative and CD45RA-positive, and the CD45RO+ cells slowly increase in number to reach the adult level of about 50% by the age 10–20 years. CD45RO− cells include naïve CD4+ T cells which predominate in neonates, and some CD8+ or CD4−/CD8− subsets found in intestinal intraepithelial T cells and enteropathy-associated T-cell lymphoma.

In the differentiation of low-grade B-cell from T-cell lymphomas, the approximated test analysis figures for UCHL1 are as follows: sensitivity 95%, specificity 95%, accuracy 95%. In contrast, in high-grade lymphomas, the same parameters are 80%, 85%, and 83% respectively. Stem cells giving rise to both erythroid and myeloid cells as well as primitive erythroid colony-forming cells express the 180 kDa isoform of the CD45 protein recognized by CD45RO, but more mature erythroid forms lack CD45 expression. Most granulopoietic colony-forming cells are CD45RO-negative, while mature monocytes or macrophages and myeloid cells are generally CD45RO-positive. These latter cells do not stain with the antibody OPD4, the difference in reactivity possibly due to a difference in the carbohydrate structure of the epitope presented on these cells.

Enumeration of CD45RO+ inflammatory cells, together with CD8, neutrophil elastase, CD68, and mast cell tryptase, has been employed in an attempt to distinguish ulcerative colitis and Crohn's disease, but the results require confirmation.

The OPD4 antibody is not, as originally claimed, specific for CD4+ T cells. It reacts very similarly to clone UCHL1 and differs only in having a low sensitivity for T-cell lymphoma and is not reactive with monocytic cells.

CD45 is positive on all hematopoietic cells, and strong expression is seen on lymphocytes. The antigen may not be found on non-hematopoietic cells, lymphoplasmacytic lymphoma, lymphoblastic lymphoma, anaplastic lymphoma, and multiple myeloma. CD45RA is expressed on naïve and activated T cells and medullary thymocytes. CD45RO is expressed on memory and activated T cells, thymocytes, some B cells, and weakly on granulocytes and macrophages. The antigen is expressed on about 75% of T-cell lymphomas, with variable expression in T-cell lymphoblastic lymphoma.

Selected references

Poppema S, Lai R, Visser L. Monoclonal antibody OPD4 is reactive with CD45RO but differs from UCHL1 by the absence of monocyte activity. *American Journal of Pathology* 1991; 139: 725–9.

Weiss LM, Arber DA, Chang KL. CD45: a review. *Applied Immunohistochemistry* 1993; 1: 166–81.

CD54 (ICAM-1)

Sources/clones

Accurate (1304.100.40), Biodesign (84H10, 15.2, MEM-111, MEM-112), Biogenesis (MEM-12), Biogenex (BBIG-1), Biosource (BC14, RR1-1), Caltag Laboratories (MEM111), Coulter (84H10), Dako (6.5B5), Exalpha Co. (D3.6), Immunotech (84H10), Novocastra (15.2), Pharmingen (3E2, HA58), Sanbio/Monosan (MEM-111), Serotec (84H10), Zymed (My13).

Fixation/preparation

Apart from clone My13, which is applicable to both frozen and paraffin-embedded tissue sections, all the antibodies are applicable to frozen sections only. In certain instances acetone fixation is recommended.

Background

Cell-to-cell adhesion is critical in the generation of effective immune responses and is dependent upon the generation of a variety of cell surface receptors. Intercellular adhesion molecule-1 (ICAM-1, CD54) is an inducible cell surface glycoprotein expressed at a low level on a subpopulation of hematopoietic cells, vascular endothelium, fibroblasts, and certain epithelial cells. However, its expression is dramatically increased at sites of inflammation, providing important means of regulating cell–cell interactions and hence inflammatory responses. ICAM-1 is induced by proinflammatory cytokines such as interleukin-1, tumor necrosis factor-α, or interferon-γ.

The CD54 antigen (ICAM-1) is a 90 kDa integral membrane glycoprotein with seven potential N-linked glycosylation sites.

Applications

The CD54 antigen is expressed on monocytes and endothelial cells. It is also a lymphokine-inducible molecule and has been shown to be a ligand for LFA-1-mediated adhesion. Expression of the antigen can be induced or upregulated on many cell types including B and T lymphocytes, thymocytes, fibroblasts, keratinocytes, and epithelial cells. In its function of mediating immune and inflammatory responses, CD54 antigen mediates adhesion of T cells with antigen-presenting cells and is involved in T-cell to T-cell and T-cell to B-cell interactions. Mice bearing a null mutation of CD54 have been found to display no inflammatory cell infiltrate in the lung following thoracic irradiation, suggesting that agents that block CD54 function may prevent radiation-induced pulmonary fibrosis.

Increased expression of ICAM-1 has been associated with many types of atherosclerotic lesions. In rejecting kidneys the antibody highlights all infiltrating cells strongly as well as glomerulus epithelium, endothelium on capillaries, vessels, and mesangium.

Comments

CD54 is expressed in both B and T cells, monocytes, endothelial cells, and a variety of epithelial cells and thus has low specificity. CD54 may be strongly positive on mantle cell lymphomas of the spleen.

Selected reference

Ohh M, Takei F. New insights into the regulation of ICAM-1 gene expression. *Leukemia and Lymphoma* 1996; 20: 223–8.

NOTES

CD56 (neural cell adhesion molecule)

Sources/clones

Dako (MOC-1, T199), Monosan (123C3), Research Diagnostics (ERIC-1), Zymed (123C3).

Fixation/preparation

Applicable to formalin-fixed paraffin sections. Requires pretreatment with microwave or pressure cooker antigen/epitope retrieval in citrate buffer. Enzymatic pretreatment has been shown to markedly decrease reactivity. The antibody to CD56 may also be applied to frozen sections or cell smears.

Background

CD56, the neural cell adhesion molecule (NCAM), was discovered in a search for cell surface molecules that contribute to cell–cell interactions during neural development. Human peripheral cells capable of non-MHC-restricted cytotoxicity express the CD56 antigen. NCAM has at least three isoforms, generated by differential splicing of the RNA transcript from a single gene located on chromosome 11. The core polypeptide of CD56 appears to be the 140 kDa isoform, which is variably glycosylated and sialylated to produce mature species with molecular weights ranging from 175 to 220 kDa. The CD56 antigen itself appears not to participate directly in the cytolytic activity of NK cells. Subsequent immunohistochemical studies have shown that NCAM is widely expressed in neural and neuroendocrine tissues. Antibody clone 123C3 recognizes a heterodimeric glycoprotein with the 145 and 185 kDa isoforms of NCAM, while clone ERIC-1 has been reported with two human isoforms of NCAM, 145 and 180 kDa. T199 is a 135/220 kDa single chain glycosylated and sialylated protein expressed on CD2+/CD3−/CD16+ natural killer (NK) cells and neuroectodermal cells. Autopsy tissue has been used to demonstrate strong CD56 immunoreaction in peripheral nerve, adrenal zona glomerulosa and medulla, and synapses in cerebral cortex. CD56 also marks thyroid follicular epithelium, proximal renal tubules, hepatocytes, gastric parietal cells, and pancreatic islet cells.

Applications

Merkel cell carcinoma, neuroblastoma, ganglioglioma, oligodendroglioma, glioblastoma multiforme, pheochromocytoma, retinoblastoma, laryngeal and pulmonary squamous cell carcinoma, pulmonary and intestinal carcinoid, pulmonary small-cell undifferentiated carcinoma, pancreatic neuroendocrine tumors, hepatocellular carcinoma, renal cell carcinoma, and follicular and papillary thyroid carcinoma mark positively with CD56 antibodies. For neuroendocrine tumors, CD56 should be used in conjunction with chromogranin A and synaptophysin. CD56 has been found to be negative in Ewing's sarcoma, nasopharyngeal carcinoma, colonic adenocarcinoma, melanoma, meningioma, follicular center cell lymphoma, hairy cell leukemia, and multiple myeloma. However, the current major application of CD56 in paraffin sections is in the diagnosis of NK and NK-like T-cell lymphoma, i.e., CD56 being a marker for natural killer cells (Appendix 2.6). CD56+ lymphomas are heterogeneous, encompassing several entities: nasal/nasopharyngeal NK/T-cell lymphoma, nasal type (extranasal) NK/T cell lymphoma, aggressive NK-cell leukemia/lymphoma, and the newly described blastoid NK-cell lymphoma. The nasal form represents the prototype of this group and is referred to as angiocentric lymphoma in the REAL classification. Besides co-expression of CD3, such tumors are often labeled by EBER-1 so that therapeutic measures directed against the EB virus should be researched. Since CD56-positive lymphomas do not always show angiocentricity, and angiocentricity may occur in other lymphoma types, the term NK/T-cell lymphoma or T/NK-cell lymphoma appears to be more appropriate. Two other types of T-cell lymphoma show a particularly high frequency of CD56 expression: hepatosplenic δ/γ-T-cell lymphoma (63% CD56+) and S100 protein-positive T-cell lymphoma.

Microvillous lymphomas are a group of B-cell lymphomas that frequently express CD56. These rare, poorly defined transformed cell lymphomas are characterized by a cohesive sinus growth pattern and ultrastructural cytoplasmic processes. They have been compared to transformed follicle center cells and follicular dendritic cells; they show clonal heavy chain immunoglobulin rearrangement, and mark with CD74, CDw75, and CD20 but not DBA.44, CD21, or CD35. About half of such tumors express CD56, suggesting a role for adhesion molecules in the distribution of these lymphomas.

An unusual cutaneous blastic tumor co-expresses CD56 and terminal deoxynucleatidyl transferase (TdT) and has been termed blastic natural killer cell lymphoma. These tumors are likely to be of primitive/undifferentiated hematopoietic origin and may progressively develop bone marrow involvement by blast cells with myeloid immunophenotype that are negative for CD56 and TdT.

CD56 expression may predict occurrence of CNS disease in acute lymphoblastic leukemia, and the expression of this antigen in multiple myeloma correlates with the presence of lytic bone lesions and distinguishes myeloma from lymphomas with plasmacytoid differentiation and from monoclonal gammopathy of undetermined significance. CD56 is expressed by both myeloma cells and osteoblasts, the expression of CD56 perhaps contributing to bone lysis by causing a decrease in osteoid formation.

Another rare malignancy with CD56+/CD4+ immunophenotype has been shown to correspond to the so-called type 2 dendritic cell or plasmacytoid dendritic cell. Such tumors typically present with cutaneous nodules associated with lymphadenopathy or splenic enlargement, or both, and massive bone marrow infiltration. The disease is rapidly fatal, but there is a purely cutaneous form that is indolent.

Comments

Clearly CD56 antibodies are essential for the diagnosis of NK/T-cell lymphomas, which show a predilection for the upper aerodigestive tract, skin, testes, skeletal muscle, gastrointestinal tract, and other extranodal sites and pursue an aggressive clinical course. Furthermore, this antibody may be used to detect residual disease in CD56+ NK/T-cell lymphoma in which the neoplastic lymphoid cells are small and show minimal atypia, especially in small biopsies.

CD56 is expressed in NK cells, activated T cells, cerebellum, brain, neuromuscular junctions, normal and neoplastic neuroendocrine tissues, myeloma, and myeloid leukemia.

Selected reference

Chan JKC. CD56-positive putative natural killer (NK) cell lymphomas: nasal, nasal-type, blastoid, and leukemic forms. *Advances in Anatomic Pathology* 1997; 4: 163–72.

CD57

Sources/clones

Becton Dickinson (Leu-7), Biodesign (NCI), GenTrak, Immunotech (NCI), Sanbio (6-13-19-1), Serotec (NC-1).

Fixation/preparation

Most antibodies are reactive in fixed paraffin-embedded tissues, and immunoreactivity is enhanced by HIER.

Background

CD57 antibodies detect a HokDa protein encoded by a gene on chromosome 11. The protein is present on some peripheral lymphocytes but not in monocytes, granulocytes, platelets, or erythrocytes. CD57+ lymphocytes increase with age and represent 10–20% of lymphocytes in most adults. They mostly include a subset of CD8+ T lymphocytes as well as natural killer (NK) cells. A subpopulation of peripheral lymphocytes that reacts with this marker includes large granular lymphocytes. This antibody also reacts with both CD3+ and CD3– non-B lymphocytes. The CD3– lymphocytes demonstrate NK cell activity and have large cytoplasmic granules that are not seen in the CD3+ cells. CD3+/CD57+ T cells are primarily suppressor lymphocytes with CD8 expression, though CD4+/CD8–/CD57+ T cells have been described, and CD8+ CD57+ HLA-DR+ T cells have also been identified. CD3+/CD8+/CD57+ lymphocytes are positive for CD45RA but not CD45RO. While this phenotype is characteristic of naïve T lymphocytes, the CD57+ cells differ from other naïve T cells by failing to lose the CD45RA antigen when stimulated with alloantigens. These cells also differ from other T lymphocytes by their increased ability to acquire the HLA-DR antigen in the absence of antigen-specific cytotoxic activity against allogeneic target cells.

The frequency of CD57+ lymphocytes in solid tissues varies according to site. CD57+ lymphocytes are increased in term placental tissue, but not in decidua of early pregnancy. CD57+ lymphocytes are decreased in bronchoalveolar lavage specimens compared with peripheral blood in the same patient, and they represent less than 2% of all nasal mucosal lymphocytes. CD57+ lymphocytes are rare in both the endometrium and the uterine cervix. They are also rare in the thymus and in the bone marrow, where they constitute no more than 1% of all nucleated cells.

CD57+ lymphocytes have a different distribution to that of CD8+ cells in the tonsils and lymph nodes, with the CD57+ cells located primarily within the germinal centers. These germinal center cells are CD3+ T cells, which also express the CD4 antigen. Similar to the CD57+/CD4+ T cells in cytomegalovirus (CMV) carriers, the CD4+ germinal center cells do not display the usual helper activity of classic CD4+ lymphocytes.

CD57+ cells in the spleen are seen mostly in the germinal centers of the white pulp, or as a rim of cells around the central white pulp.

The HNK-1/Leu-7 antibody also reacts with cells other than lymphocytes. CD57 antibodies react with an antigen present in the central and peripheral nervous system myelin and oligodendroglia and Schwann cells. Some neural adhesion molecules also contain a carbohydrate epitope that is recognized by CD57 antibodies. The reactivity is due to part of the myelin-associated glycoprotein having a similar molecular weight (110 kDa) to the CD57 lymphocyte antigen.

Besides neural-associated cells, CD57 antibodies immunoreact with prostatic epithelium, pancreatic islets, adrenal medulla, renal loops of Henle and proximal tubules, chromaffin cells of the gut, gastric chief cells, epithelial cells of the outer thymic cortex, and some cells in the fetal bronchus. They are also detected in the prostatic seminal fluid.

Applications

CD57+ lymphocytes are increased in patients following bone marrow transplantation. This increase often persists for years after the procedure. The majority of these cells are CD57−/CD8+ T lymphocytes, which form up to two-thirds of the peripheral blood T lymphocytes, with a small expansion in CD57+/CD4+ cells.

The relationship of this increase in CD57+ cells to graft-versus-host disease is controversial, some workers finding a correlation between the increase in CD57+ cells and the onset of disease while others have not. Some investigators have noted the expansion of the CD57+ population with reactivation of CMV after transplantation, similar to the increase in CD57+ cells seen in healthy carriers of CMV.

CD57+ cells are also elevated in the peripheral blood in some solid organ transplant patients. Up to 20% of renal allograft, 66% of cardiac allograft, and 44% of liver allograft recipients had more than 20% peripheral blood CD57+ CD3+ lymphocytes, the majority of these cells also being CD8+. As with bone marrow transplantation, the elevation of CD57+ correlated with a rise in CMV titers and may show poorer graft survival.

CD57+ cells are also elevated in human immunodeficiency virus (HIV) infections. CD57+ CD8+ lymphocytes are increased through the clinical progression of the infection, while CD57+ and CD57− NK cells remain normal.

Peripheral blood CD57+ cells may be increased in patients with adult-onset cyclic neutropenia, whereas no elevation is seen in childhood-onset cases. The adult-onset variant of cyclic neutropenia has been found to be steroid-responsive.

Circulating CD57− lymphocytes are elevated in patients with Crohn's disease, with many of these cells being CD8-positive, corresponding to the increase in suppressor cell function found in such patients. Elevations in peripheral blood CD57+ cells may also be seen in rheumatoid arthritis.

Large granular lymphocytosis (LGL) is by far the most common CD57+ lymphoproliferative disorder. LGL cells are usually CD2-positive and may be divided into T-cell and NK-cell types based on CD3 expression. CD3+ cases are generally associated with clonal T-cell gene rearrangement. The T-cell cases are usually CD57-negative and CD8-positive, and may be further typed according to the presence (type 1) or absence (type 2) of the NK-associated antigen CD16. Immunostaining of the spleen may be useful in the evaluation of resected spleens in LGL patients. CD57+ lymphocytes are found in the splenic red pulp, while the expanded pulp nodules are usually not involved.

Elevations of peripheral blood CD57+ lymphocytes may be associated with non-neoplastic states such as in CMV carriers, possibly in chronic hepatitis, in ankylosing spondylitis, and more frequently in rheumatoid arthritis and Felty's syndrome. Synovial fluid CD57+ cells may also be elevated in rheumatoid arthritis. Clonal T-cell receptor gene rearrangement has been demonstrated in some cases of rheumatoid arthritis, especially those with Felty's syndrome.

NK/T-cell lymphomas frequently affect the nasal and extranasal sites and show similarities to LGL. The lymphoma cells display large cytoplasmic granules with either a T-cell or an NK-cell phenotype. They are also mostly positive for the Epstein–Barr virus and display an angiocentric pattern of infiltration with necrosis and an aggressive clinical course. Unlike LGL, NK/T-cell lymphomas are CD57-positive in less than 10% of cases, with most cases being CD56-positive, so CD57 antibodies alone are unreliable NK cell markers of such lymphomas.

CD57 expression is seen in just over 20% of T-lymphoblastic lymphomas, but the expression of CD57 does not correlate with NK activity in these cases, and the significance of the expression of this antigen is unknown. Less than 2% of other types of T-cell lymphoma are CD57-positive, and the antigen does not appear to be expressed in B-cell lymphomas, monocytic leukemia, or Langerhans histiocytosis. Increases in presumably non-neoplastic CD57+ cells may be seen in the neoplastic follicles of follicular lymphomas, especially of the small cleaved cell type, and in cases of nodular L&H Hodgkin disease where the CD57+ cells often rosette around CD20+ L&H cells, providing a useful pointer to the diagnosis. The CD57+ cells in the latter condition are also CD4-positive and can be seen in about 25–30% of cases of nodular lymphocyte-predominant Hodgkin disease. Interestingly, a variant of classic Hodgkin disease that produces follicles with small, eccentric germinal centers and expanded mantle zones containing classic Reed–Sternberg cells shows similar CD57+ resetting of the latter cells, mimicking nodular L&H Hodgkin disease. Similar distribution and increases in CD57+ cells were not found in nodular sclerosing Hodgkin disease, T-cell-rich B-cell lymphoma, or follicular lymphoma.

CD57 expression may be observed in a variety of solid tumors, the most common of which are lung tumors. Almost half of small-cell lung carcinomas and about 85% of carcinoid tumors are CD57-positive. In non-small-cell lung carcinoma the identification of neuroendocrine-associated antigens such as CD57 has been shown to be predictive of response to chemotherapy. The expression of CD57 antigen in small-cell carcinoma and carcinoid is generally widespread in the tumor but only focal in non-small-cell lung carcinomas. Sampling errors should be taken into consideration in the assessment and, because of the low sensitivity and specificity of CD57 antibodies, other neuroendocrine-associated markers such as chromogranin, synaptophysin, and neuron-specific enolase should be employed.

Other non-hematopoietic neoplasms that express CD57 include the majority of thyroid carcinomas, especially papillary carcinoma, while CD57 expression is present in only 30% of benign thyroid proliferations. CD57 may be used to separate medullary carcinomas from other thyroid carcinomas, although there have been some reported examples of positivity in medullary carcinomas. Strong CD57 staining of the majority of the tumor cells is indicative of papillary or follicular carcinoma and uncommon in benign thyroid proliferations and medullary carcinoma.

The CD57 antigen is expressed in prostatic epithelium, but the marker does not discriminate between benign and neoplastic cells. Metanephric adenomas are strongly and diffusely positive for CD57 and WT1, with focal staining for CK7 but no staining for CD56 and desmin. While Wilms tumor was also strongly positive for WT1 in the blastema and epithelial components, there was no staining for CD57 in these components, and some cases were diffusely positive for CD56.

Epithelial cells of thymomas are usually CD57-positive, while only some thymic carcinomas express the antigen. Over half of malignant mesotheliomas are reported to express CD57, although they generally do not react with other neuroendocrine markers. Among the soft tissue tumors, the majority of neural tumors, especially neuromas, schwannomas, and neurofibromas, react with CD57 antibodies. Most malignant peripheral nerve sheath tumors are CD57, but the antigen may also be expressed by other sarcomas such as synovial sarcoma and leiomyosarcoma. Therefore the marker on its own is not a useful diagnostic discriminant and should be used in an appropriate panel of antibodies in order to separate the various spindled and pleomorphic soft tissue tumors. Similarly, because CD57 may be expressed by a variety of small round cell tumors including neuroblastomas, it is not a useful diagnostic discriminant for this group of poorly differentiated tumors.

In the central nervous system, CD57 expression may be seen in normal oligodendroglia and other nervous system cells as well as in their corresponding tumors. Oligodendrogliomas perhaps show the most extensive degree of CD57 positivity compared to astrocytomas and glioblastomas, which demonstrate fewer positive cells. Among skin tumors, the expression of CD57 closely parallels that of S100 protein, although the two are not identical. Neither was found to be useful in the distinction of eccrine from apocrine tumors. Melanocytic proliferations and melanomas may show variable positivity for CD57, whereas reports of the expression of this antigen in Merkel cell carcinoma are conflicting, the antigen being absent in some series and positive in half the tumors in another study. CD57 positivity is also seen in other tumors, including a large proportion of granular cell tumors, paragangliomas, and pheochromocytomas. Embryonal carcinomas and dysgerminomas are also reported to be positive for CD57 in most cases.

Comments

The CD57 antigen is most useful in the identification of large granular lymphocyte disorders (Appendix 2.6) and assists in the identification of L&H cells of lymphocyte-predominant Hodgkin disease. The CD57+ cells that are CD4+ T cells form rosettes around CD20+ L&H cells. Elevation of peripheral blood CD57+ lymphocytes may be seen following some viral infections such as CMV, in patients following bone marrow or solid organ transplantation. CD57 should not be used alone as a marker of NK cells, neuroendocrine cells, or neural cells and must be employed in combination with other antibodies in a panel, particularly if used for diagnostic purposes. The antibody is immunoreactive in fixed paraffin-embedded tissues, especially following heat-induced epitope retrieval (HIER).

CD57 is expressed on an NK-cell subset, T-cell subset, brain, neuroectodermal tumors, small-cell lung carcinoma, prostatic epithelium and tumors, nerve sheath tissues, and tumors.

Selected reference

Arber DA, Weiss LM. CD57. A review. *Applied Immunohistochemistry* 1995; 3: 137–52.

NOTES

CD68

Sources/clones

Accurate (EVM11), Biodesign (BL-M68), Caltag Laboratories (BL-M68), Dako (KP1, PG-M1, EVM11), Sanbio/Monosan/Accurate (BLAD8), Serotech (KiM6).

Fixation/preparation

EVM11 is applicable only to frozen sections, but KP1 and PG-M1 monoclonal antibodies are applicable to formalin-fixed paraffin sections, acetone-fixed cryostat sections, and fixed cell smears. Anti-macrophage reagents recognizing formalin-resistant epitopes require microwave or enzyme pretreatment with trypsin or pronase before immunostaining to reduce background staining.

Background

The best macrophage reagents produced to date are those recognizing the CD68 antigen. This 110 kDa antigen belongs to a family of acidic, highly glycosylated lysosomal glycoproteins that include the lamp-1 and lamp-2 molecules. CD68 is the human homolog of the murine macrosialin antigen and is present in the cytoplasmic granules of monocytes, macrophages, neutrophils, basophils, and large lymphocytes. This antigen is also expressed to some degree in the cytoplasm of some non-hematopoietic tissue. However, the function of the molecule is to date unknown.

The monoclonal antibody KP1 (IgG1κ) was raised against lysosomal granules prepared from lung macrophages and recognizes the 110 kDa CD68 antigen. This antibody labels monocytes and macrophages in a wide range of tissues, e.g., lung macrophages, germinal center macrophages, and Kupffer cells. Osteoclasts and myeloid precursors in bone marrow are also strongly labeled. In frozen sections, KP1 stains endothelium and hepatocytes weakly. Strong labeling of blood monocytes (granular/cytoplasmic), neutrophils, and basophils is also demonstrated with KP1. KP1 antigen is expressed as an intracytoplasmic molecule, associated with lysosomal granules.

The murine PG-M1 monoclonal antibody (IgG3κ) was raised against spleen cells of Gaucher's disease. Reactivity with cells transfected with a human cDNA encoding for the CD68 antigen confirms PG-M1 as a member of the CD68 cluster. In normal tissue, PG-M1 is comparable to KP1; however, in bone marrow paraffin sections, PG-M1 strongly stains macrophages but not granulocytes and myeloid precursors. PG-M1 also shows immunopositivity with mast cells and synovial cells.

Applications

Malignant histiocytosis and true histiocytic lymphoma express the CD68 macrophage marker. These tumors should be CD68-positive, but unlabeled with antibodies to CD30, T-cell and B-cell antigens, and cytokeratins. Acute myeloid leukemias (AMLs) are identified by the presence of CD68 antigen. While KP1 recognizes M1–M5 types, PG-M1 immunoreaction is confined to M4 (myelomonocytic) and M5 (monocytic) types of AML. The CD68 antibodies are also able to distinguish between monocyte/macrophage and lymphoid leukemias (Appendix 2.4). While this is useful in identifying granulocytic sarcoma (Appendix 2.5), some B-cell neoplasms (notably small lymphocytic lymphoma and hairy cell leukemia) show weak cytoplasmic staining in the form of a few scattered granules. Mast cell proliferations and "plasmacytoid monocytes" are usually stained by both the KP1 and PG-M1 antibodies. The CD68 antigen is also expressed to varying degrees in Langerhans and interdigitating reticulum cell sarcomas, as well as Langerhans cell histiocytosis. Other accessory cell tumors such as follicular dendritic cell sarcomas may be positive for CD68. CD68 is a good marker for Gaucher cells, with accentuation of the striations in the characteristic cells.

Macrophages may be present either as rare scattered cells or as large cellular infiltrates in some T-cell and B-cell lymphomas, leading to erroneous diagnoses of histiocytic malignancies. Dual immunocytochemical labeling with CD68 antigen and T/B-cell antigen is useful in delineating the two populations. The identification of macrophages is also crucial in the diagnosis of granulomatous diseases, storage diseases, and certain types of lymphadenitis, e.g., Kikuchi's lymphadenitis. In the latter condition macrophages phagocytosing apoptotic bodies and cells known as "plasmacytoid monocytes" and "crescentic histiocytes" are easily recognized with antibodies against CD68, avoiding a misdiagnosis of a high-grade lymphoma.

Comments

Caution is advised in the immunophenotypic interpretation of histiocytes, since the distinction between "uptake" and "synthetic" patterns should be borne in mind. KP1 would appear to be superior to PG-M1, particularly with respect to the wider recognition of AML. The latter antibody also carries the distinct disadvantage of being demonstrated in about 10% of melanomas. Tissue rich in macrophages is suitable as a positive control.

CD68 is expressed on macrophages/monocytes, basophils, neutrophils, mast cells, dendritic cells, myeloid and CD34+ progenitor cells, B and T cells, 50% of acute myeloid leukemias, some B-cell lymphomas, hairy cell leukemia, Langerhans cell histiocytosis, mastocytosis, and some melanomas.

Selected references

Pulford KAF, Rigney EM, Micklem KJ, et al. KP1: a new monoclonal antibody that detects a monocyte/macrophage associated antigen in routinely processed tissue sections. *Journal of Clinical Pathology* 1989; 42: 414–21.

Pulford KAF, Sipos A, Cordell JL, Stross WP, Mason DY. Distribution of the CD68 macrophage/myeloid associated antigen. *Immunology* 1990; 2: 973–80.

CD71

Sources/clones

Thermal Scientific (10F11, mouse monoclonal IgG2b).

Fixation/preparation

The antigen is preserved in formalin-fixed paraffin-embedded (FFPE) tissues.

Background

CD71, also known as the transferrin receptor, represents a major cellular receptor for iron. CD71 is expressed in all proliferating cells, often at high levels, because of their metabolic need for iron. Among specific cell lineages, CD71 is most highly expressed by erythroid precursors, whose great need for iron is necessitated by heme synthesis and differentiation, rather than proliferation. In iron-replete non-erythroid cells, CD71 is downregulated to prevent excessive iron intake, which can be toxic to the cell.

Applications

In the immunohistochemistry lab, where other markers of cellular proliferation are more standard than CD71 (e.g., Ki-67), CD71 is of greatest utility in identifying erythroid precursors in bone marrow specimens. The very high-level expressed CD71 on the surface of erythroid precursors (it stains in a membranous pattern), makes it the best marker of this cell population in our experience. The disparity in expression levels between non-erythroid and erythroid cells leads to minimal background staining of non-erythroid tissues. Importantly, because of the very high level of CD71 expression in erythroid precursors, the antibody works well on virtually all decalcified bone marrow biopsies in our experience, in addition to outstanding performance in non-decalcified bone marrow clots and particle preparations.

CD71 expression is turned on at high levels as soon as a myeloid progenitor commits to the erythroid lineage, and is significantly downregulated when erythroid precursors extrude their nuclei and become mature erythrocytes. CD71 identifies the full spectrum of nucleated erythroid precursors in the marrow, from proerythroblasts up through orthochromatic erythroblasts. Because it marks the entirety of nucleate erythroid differentiation, CD71 may be used with a pan-myeloid marker such as CD15 or CD33 to determine the myeloid:erythroid ratio by immunohistochemistry in bone marrow FFPE.

When combined with antibodies to E-cadherin (a proerythroblast marker) and glycophorin-A (a marker of post-proerythroblast cells), this combination of antibodies can yield valuable insight about the extent to which the erythroid maturation is "left shifted" to immaturity.

There is some literature associating increased CD71 expression with adverse prognosis in solid tumors such as carcinoma, but CD71 immunohistochemistry does not appear to be used routinely for this purpose.

Selected references

Dong HY, Wilkes S, Yang H. CD71 is selectively and ubiquitously expressed at high levels in erythroid precursors of all maturation stages: a comparative immunochemical study with glycophorin A and hemoglobin A. *American Journal of Surgical Pathology* 2011; 35: 723–32.

Habashy HO, Powe DG, Staka CM, et al. Transferrin receptor (CD71) is a marker of poor prognosis in breast cancer and can predict response to tamoxifen. *Breast Cancer Research and Treatment* 2010; 119: 283–93.

Marsee DK, Pinkus GS, Yu H. CD71 (transferrin receptor): an effective marker for erythroid precursors in bone marrow biopsy specimens. *American Journal of Clinical Pathology* 2010; 134: 429–35.

NOTES

CD74 (LN-2)

Sources/clones

American Research Products (MB3), Ancell/Pharmingen (MB741), Biodesign (BU43, BU45), Biogenex (LN-2), Cymbus Bioscience (BU45), Dako (LN-2), Harlan Sera Lab/Accurate (2G5), ICN Biomedicals (LN-2), Immunotech (LN-2), Novocastra (LN-2), Pharmingen (LN-2), RDI (BU45, LN-2), Serotec (BU 45), Sigma Chemical (LN-2), Zymed (LN-2).

Fixation/preparation

This antibody is applicable to formalin-fixed paraffin-embedded tissue sections, frozen sections, and cytological preparations. Immunoreaction may be improved with microwave antigen retrieval in citrate buffer.

Background

The CD74 antigen represents a membrane-bound subunit of the MHC class II-associated invariant chain that is encoded by the gene located on chromosome 5 region q31–q33. The monoclonal antibody LN-2 recognizes nuclear and cytoplasmic antigens of molecular weights 35 kDa and 31 kDa respectively in routinely processed tissues. MB3, another mononuclear antibody, is thought to be identical to LN-2. LN-2 reacts with about 50% and 75% of activated and resting L20+ B cells in the peripheral blood and tonsils respectively. LN-2 is positive in less than 3% of CD3+ T cells. Very weak staining may be seen on circulating monocytes, and granulocytes are negative.

In lymph nodes, LN-2 positivity is seen primarily in germinal center and mantle cells. Staining is strongest in small germinal center cells and in mantle cells. Plasma cells are not labeled. The vast majority of cells in the interfollicular areas are negative, except for interdigitating dendritic reticular cells, which are often strongly positive. Besides distinct staining of the nuclear membrane there may be diffuse or paranuclear cytoplasmic staining, the pattern of staining being similar in both fixed and frozen tissue sections.

Thymocytes are negative for LN-2 but thymic dendritic cells may often be positive. Other cells that may be positive for LN-2 include sinusoidal histiocytes, epithelioid histiocytes, splenic red pulp histiocytes and Langerhans-type giant cells. In addition, some epithelial cells and corresponding carcinomas may be positive, but the staining of LN-2 in these cells is often diffuse in the cytoplasm and the distinctive nuclear membrane staining is not observed.

Applications

The LN-2 antibody stains about 90% and 20% of low-grade B-cell and T-cell lymphomas respectively. In high-grade lymphomas, the corresponding figures are 85% and 75%, so its value as a discriminator is less in large-cell lymphomas. The pattern of labeling is also different. In small lymphocytic lymphoma, LN-2 shows either nuclear membrane or dot-like cytoplasmic positivity, whereas in small cleaved cells nuclear membrane staining is the predominant pattern. In the mixed cell lymphomas and large-cell lymphomas, LN-2 stains the nuclear membranes of the small cleaved cells but only some of the larger cells exhibit cytoplasmic staining, the minority displaying bright cytoplasmic globules.

Reed–Sternberg cells also stain with LN-2, exhibiting cytoplasmic, cytoplasmic membrane, and nuclear membrane staining in about two-thirds of cases. The antigen is expressed in about 60% of precursor B-cell ALLs/LBLs, about 50% of AMLs (excluding FAB M6 AML), most cases of CML, granulocytic sarcomas, and true histiocytic sarcomas.

LN-2 antigen is strongly expressed by cells of malignant fibrous histiocytoma (MFH) but not atypical fibroxanthoma (AFX). LN-2 immunoreactivity appears to distinguish between these two histologically similar yet biologically distinct tumors with a high degree of statistical significance. The antigen was not expressed or only weakly expressed on dermatofibroma and dermatofibrosarcoma protuberans. LN2 has also been observed to label some epithelial tumors, including adenocarcinoma of the uterus, squamous cell carcinoma of the lung, transitional cell carcinoma of the bladder, and renal cell carcinoma.

Comments

LN-2 is immunoreactive in formalin-fixed paraffin-embedded tissue sections. It is only poorly reactive in ethanol-fixed tissues, and B5 fixation produces reduced positivity and a high background staining. The staining in B5-fixed tissues tends to be of the nuclear membranes and the perinuclear cytoplasm of B cells, whereas in formalin-fixed tissues, paranuclear dot-like globules are more common. Trypsinization destroys LN-2 reactivity, and neuraminidase treatment does not affect it. Given the contrasting immunoreactivity of LN-2, it is possible that other applications of LN-2 are yet to be discovered. Benign or neoplastic B-cell tissue is recommended for optimization of this antibody.

CD74 is expressed on B cells, activated T cells, macrophages, endothelial cells, and a variety of epithelial cells and corresponding tumors.

Selected reference

Lazova R, Moynes R, May D, Scott G. LN-2 (CD74): a marker to distinguish atypical fibroxanthoma from malignant fibrous histiocytoma. *Cancer* 1997; 79: 2115–24.

CDw75 (LN-1)

Sources/clones

Biogenex (LN-1), Dako (LN-1), Immunotech (LN-1), Novocastra, Sigma Chemical (LN-1), Zymed (LN-1).

Fixation/preparation

Enzyme or heat pretreatment before immunostaining improves immunodetection.

Background

The CDw75 epitope is a sialylated carbohydrate determinant generated by the β-galactosyl α-2,6 sialyltransferase, and it has a molecular weight of 53 kDa. Sialyltransferase catalyzes the incorporation of sialic acid to the carbohydrate group of glycoconjugates. Alterations on the cell surface of the oligosaccharide portion of glycoproteins and glycolipids are thought to play a role in tumorigenesis. Sialyltransferase has been found elevated in different tumor tissues and in serum of cancer patients. Further, the amount of sialic acid correlates with the invasiveness and metastasizing potential of several human tumors. Therefore the CDw75 epitope can be viewed as a target for identifying biologically aggressive tumors.

LN1 belongs to the CDw75 group of antibodies and recognizes a sialo antigen (45–85 kDa). LN1 stains B lymphocytes in the germinal center with no reaction with T cells. It also reacts with a variety of epithelial cells including distal renal tubules, mammary glands, bronchus, and prostate.

Applications

CDw75 antigen expression has been examined in breast lesions. Duct carcinoma showed diffuse cytoplasmic staining in 21% of in-situ and 35% of invasive carcinomas respectively. No correlation was demonstrated between immunoreactivity for CDw75 in breast carcinoma and their metastatic potential. However, CDw75 was more frequently expressed in high-grade carcinomas. A positive immunoreaction was demonstrated in benign proliferating lesions: intraductal papillomas (2/3) and epitheliosis in fibrocystic disease (10/14). This high frequency of immunoreactivity among the benign breast lesions was ascribed to activation of epithelial cells.

CDw75 epitope expression has also been examined in gastric carcinomas and their metastases. About 50% were immunopositive for CDw75 antigen in the primary tumors or metastases. In contrast to breast carcinomas, a close relationship was found between antigen in primary tumors and their respective metastases. In addition, antigen expression correlated with an infiltrative growth pattern, lymphatic invasiveness, and aneuploidy, while no correlation was found with gastric carcinoma morphology, lymphoid infiltrate, vascular invasion, or gastric wall penetration. Hence, CDw75 expression appears to be a good indicator of biologic aggressiveness of gastric carcinoma. In view of the contrasting results between breast and gastric carcinoma, further studies examining CDw75 expression in these and other cancers are awaited.

LN1 is an excellent marker for B-cell lymphomas, especially follicular-derived lymphomas (Appendix 2.1). In B cells, the LN1 antibody produces a typical membrane and cytoplasmic (paranuclear "dot-like" or Golgi) staining pattern. No immunoreaction is present with small lymphocytic lymphomas and T-cell lymphomas. LN1 also reacts with L& H cells in nodular lymphocyte-predominant Hodgkin disease. In a study of CD10, Bcl-6, and CDw75 as markers of follicle center cell lymphomas, it was found that CDw75 was the most sensitive (97%), closely followed by Bcl-6 (90%), with CD10 being the least sensitive (80%). A combination of all three markers has been shown to produce a sensitivity of 100%.

Comments

Follicular lymphomas or epitheliosis of the breast or gastric carcinoma is most suitable for use as positive control tissue.

Selected reference

Dunphy CH, Polski JM, Lance Evans H, Gardner IJ. Paraffin immunoreactivity of CD10, CDw75, and Bcl-6 in follicle center cell lymphoma. *Leukemia and Lymphoma* 2001; 41: 585–92.

CD79a

Sources/clones

Becton Dickinson (HM47), Dako (JCB117, HM57), Immunotech (HM47), Novocastra (11E3, 11D10, HM47/A9).

Fixation/preparation

This antibody is applicable to paraffin-embedded tissue sections. Heat pretreatment in citrate buffer is necessary for antigen retrieval to improve staining pattern. CD79a may also be applied to acetone-fixed cryostat sections and fixed cell smears.

Background

Membrane-bound immunoglobulin (mIg) on human B lymphocytes is non-covalently associated with a disulfide-linked heterodimer, which consists of two phosphoproteins of 47 kDa and 37 kDa, encoded by the *mb-1* and *B29* genes respectively. Association of IgM with the mb-1 protein is necessary for membrane expression of the B-cell antigen receptor complex. When antigen is bound to this B-cell complex, a signal transduction is transmitted to the interior of the cell, accompanied by phosphorylation of several components following induction of tyrosine kinase activity. The mb-l/B29 dimer seems to be analogous to the association of the T-cell receptor with the CD3 components.

Studies have shown that mb-1 is present throughout B-cell differentiation and is B-cell-specific. Its high degree of specificity is probably a reflection of its crucial role in signal transduction after antigen binding to the B-cell antigen receptor complex. The mb-1 and B29 proteins were designated CD79a and CD79b at the Fifth International Workshop on Human Leucocyte Differentiation Antigens in 1993. JCB117 was raised against the recombinant protein-containing part of the extracellular portion of the CD79a (mb-1) polypeptide. Clone HM57 was raised against a synthetic peptide sequence comprising amino acids 202–216 of mb-1 protein. This oligopeptide represents the intracytoplasmic C-terminal part of the mb-1 protein.

Applications

The mb-1 (CD79a) chain appears before the pre-B-cell stage and is still present at the plasma cell stage. JCB117 reacts with human B cells in paraffin-embedded tissue sections including decalcified bone marrow trephines. When applied to paraffin-embedded tissue biopsies, it reacted with the majority (97%) of B-cell neoplasms. This covered the full range of B-cell maturation including 10/20 cases of myeloma/plasmacytoma. This antibody also labeled precursor B-cell acute lymphoblastic leukemia (ALL), making it the most reliable B-cell marker detectable on paraffin-embedded specimens. T-cell and non-lymphoid neoplasms were negative, indicating that JCB117 may be of value in the identification of B-cell neoplasms.

The mb-1 protein has also been detected in nodular lymphocyte-predominant Hodgkin disease using monoclonal antibody JCB117; however, only 20% of non-lymphocyte-predominant cases expressed mb-1. A rare phenotypic characterization has been demonstrated in mediastinal large B-cell lymphomas, with the majority being mb-1-positive/Ig-negative.

Comments

We have found JCB117 to be superior to HM57, the latter demonstrating cross-reactivity with smooth muscle in paraffin sections.

CD79a is a marker of precursor B cells, expressed early in B-cell differentiation and often positive when other mature B-cell markers are negative (Appendix 2.1). It is expressed on megakaryocytes. CD79a has been shown on pre-T-acute lymphoblastic leukemia and rarely in peripheral T-cell lymphomas, normal T cells being negative for the antigen. As CD79a is only weakly positive in some B-cell lymphomas, it is preferable to use CD20 as the first-line marker of mature B-cell lymphomas.

Selected references

Chu PG, Arber DA. CD79: a review. *Applied Immunohistochemistry and Molecular Morphology* 2001; 9: 97–106.

Mason DY, Cordell JL, Brown MH, *et al*. CD79a: a novel marker for B cell neoplasms in routinely processed tissue samples. *Blood* 1995; 86: 1453–9.

CD99 (p30/32^{MIC2})

Sources/clones

Dako (12E7), Pharmingen (MIC2), Signet (013).

Fixation/preparation

All three clones of antibodies show enhanced immunoreactivity following HIER.

Background

The p30/32^{MIC2} antigen, also referred to as CD99 or the *MIC2* gene product, is a cell-surface glycoprotein of relative molecular weight of 30–32 kDa that appears to be involved in cell adhesion processes. It is recognized by a number of monoclonal antibodies including RFB-1, 12E7, HBA71, and 013, although there is some demonstrable difference in sensitivity and perhaps specificity.

CD99 was first described as a polypeptide expressed in T-cell acute lymphoblastic leukemia (T-ALL) and T-ALL-derived cell lines, as well as in a subset of cortical thymocytes. CD99 was also found on a group of hematopoietic precursor cells in the human bone marrow including terminal deoxynucleotidyl transferase-positive cells and myelo-monocyte progenitors, the expression decreasing with maturation of cells in the latter series. The *MIC2* gene has been mapped to the terminal region of the short arm of the X chromosome (Xp22.32-pter) and the euchromatin region of the Y chromosome (Yq11-pter). The gene is expressed in both sexes and escapes X inactivation, making it the first described pseudo-autosomal gene in humans.

The main application of this antigen has been for the differentiation of the group of small round cell tumors in childhood, as the marker is strongly expressed in Ewing's sarcoma (ES) and the closely related peripheral/primitive neuroectodermal tumors (PNETs). Both show strong membrane and cytoplasmic staining with clones 12E7, HBA71, and 013. There is positive staining in acute lymphoblastic lymphoma and related leukemias, and in rhabdomyosarcoma, although to a much lesser degree. More recently, immunoreactivity for this marker has been shown in a much wider spectrum of normal tissues and ependymal cells, pancreatic islet cells, urothelium, some squamous cells, columnar epithelial cells, fibroblasts, endothelial cells, and granulosa/Sertoli cells. Among the spindle cell neoplastic tissues which show variable positivity for CD99 are synovial sarcomas, meningiomas, solitary fibrous tumors, and only very rarely mesotheliomas. Epithelial tumors expressing CD99 include neuroendocrine tumors such as islet cell tumors, carcinoid tumors, and pulmonary oat cell carcinomas, but apparently not Merkel cell carcinomas of the skin. Granulocytic sarcomas have been shown to stain for CD99.

Applications

CD99 antibodies have proven usefulness for the separation of Ewing's sarcoma and PNETs from the other small round cell tumors in childhood (Appendix 1.3, 1.11). In addition, this marker can be employed as a diagnostic discriminator for the identification of thymic cortical T cells associated with thymic neoplasms (Appendix 1.12), and in the differential diagnosis of spindle cell tumors (Appendix 1.23). The latter include synovial sarcoma, hemangiopericytoma, meningioma, and solitary fibrous tumors, all of which show variable extents of positivity. The demonstration of CD99 in mesenchymal chondrosarcoma emphasizes the need for caution if this marker is to be employed as a diagnostic discriminator for small round cell tumors. Furthermore, the immunoexpression of CD99, while most common in ES/PNET (100%), may also be seen in rhabdomyosarcoma, non-Hodgkin lymphoma, and synovial sarcoma and needs to be used in combination with antibodies to Fli-1 and Tdt to increase the diagnostic yield. CD99 expression in retinoblastoma is much less common than in PNET.

Ependydomas express CD99 strongly in a membranous pattern with intracytoplasmic or intercellular dots. B-cell lymphoblastic lymphoma has also been shown to immunoexpress CD99. Benign spindle stromal tumors of the breast, which encompass spindle cell lipoma-like tumor, solitary fibrous tumor, and myofibroblastoma, share the common immunophenotype of vimentin+/CD34+/Bcl-2+/CD99+ and may have a common histiogenesis. CD99 has also been described on a number of other tumors including superficial acral fibromyxoma, proximal epithelioid sarcoma, spindle cell epithelioma of the vagina, neuroepithelial tumors of the kidney, and tumors of sex cord–stromal differentiation. Dot-like positivity with CD99 has been seen in pancreatic neuroendocrine tumors.

Comments

Initial enthusiasm for the specificity of CD99 has been tempered by the realization of the wide spectrum of tumors that may express the antigen. Immunoreactivity is enhanced following heat-induced epitope retrieval (HIER). Both 013 and 12E7 have been very effective in our hands but it should be noted that they show different sensitivities, perhaps reflecting different specificities. Positive staining for CD99 occurs as strong membrane immunolocalization, whereas variable heterogeneous staining may be seen in some cases of non-Hodgkin lymphoma and in occasional Reed–Sternberg cells and their variants.

CD99 is expressed on a variety of cells and tumors that include Ewing's sarcoma/PNET, T-cell lymphoblastic lymphoma, synovial sarcoma, rhabdomyosarcoma, some cases of Wilms tumor, ovarian granulosa cells, pancreatic islets, and infant thymus.

Selected references

Stevenson AJ, Chatten J, Bertoni F, Miettinen M. CD99 (p30/32MIC2) neuroectodermal/Ewing's sarcoma antigen as an immunohistochemical marker. Review of more than 600 tumors and the literature experience. *Applied Immunohistochemistry* 1994; 2: 231–40.

Vartanian RK, Sudilovsky D, Weidner N. Immunostaining of monoclonal antibody 013 (anti MIC2 gene product) (CD99) in lymphomas. Impact of heat-induced epitope retrieval. *Applied Immunohistochemistry* 1996; 4: 43–55.

Weidner N, Tjoe J. Immunohistochemical profile of monoclonal antibody 013: antibody that recognizes glycoprotein p30/32MIC2 and is useful in diagnosing Ewing's sarcoma and peripheral neuroepithelioma. *American Journal of Surgical Pathology* 1994; 18: 486–94.

CD103

Sources/clones

Biogenex (2G5), Coulter (2G5), Dako (Ber-ACT8), Immunotech (2G5), Serotec (295.1).

Fixation/preparation

The antibodies are mainly immunoreactive in cryostat sections of fresh frozen tissue. Immunoreactivity in fixed paraffin-embedded sections has not been reported.

Background

The antibody to CD103, also known as anti-human mucosal lymphocyte 1 antigen (HML-1) and integrin α-E chain, recognizes a T-cell-associated trimeric protein of 150, 125, and 105 kDa, which is expressed on 95% of intraepithelial lymphocytes and only on 1–2% of peripheral blood lymphocytes. CD103 (α-E integrin) antigen is part of the family of β7 integrins on human mucosal lymphocytes which play a specific role in mucosal localization or adhesion. CD103 is a receptor for the epithelial cell-specific ligand E-cadherin and is expressed by a major subset of CD3+, CD8+, CD4− lymphocytes present in the intestinal mucosa. About 40% of isolated intestinal lamina propria lymphocytes (LPLs) have been shown to express HML-1, the majority being CD8-positive. Virtually all LPL expressed CD45RO, whereas only about 50% were CD29-positive, a percentage similar to that in peripheral blood lymphocytes. HML-1+ cells were almost exclusively CD45RA-negative, and the in-vitro expression of HML-1 was inducible on T cells by mitogen. CD103+/CD8+ T lymphocytes have also been demonstrated in the bladder urothelium and their corresponding tumors, the epidermis in inflammatory skin disorders, pancreas in chronic pancreatisis, and graft epithelium during renal allograft rejection.

Applications

Antibodies to CD103 are used for the diagnosis of intestinal T-cell lymphoma. CD103 has been found to be a useful marker of B-cell hairy cell leukemia, which shows strong reactivity for CD22, CD25, CD103, DBA.44 as well as immunoglobulin light chain restriction. The abnormal co-expression of CD103, CD25, and intense CD11c and CD20 on monomorphic, slightly large B lymphocytes has been shown to be highly characteristic of hairy cell leukemia. The antigen may be occasionally expressed by some B-cell lymphomas. The antigen has also been demonstrated in T-cell lymphoblastic lymphoma.

Comments

Current diagnostic applications of antibodies to CD103 are restricted by their immunoreactivity only in fresh cell preparations and cryostat sections. CD103 may be employed as a marker of intraepithelial lymphocytes and activated lymphocytes. It is positive in B-cell hairy cell leukemia, acute myeloid leukemia, enteropathy-associated T-cell lymphoma, and adult HTLV-1-associated T-cell leukemia.

Selected references

Ebert MP, Ademmer K, Muller-Ostermeyer F, et al. CD8+CD103+ T cells analogous to intestinal intraepithelial lymphocytes infiltrate the pancreas in chronic pancreatitis. *American Journal of Gastroenterology* 1998; 93: 2141–7.

Pauls K, Schon M, Kubitza RC, et al. Role of integrin αE(CD103)β7 for tissue-specific epidermal localization of CD8+ T lymphocytes. *Journal of Investigative Dermatology* 2001; 117: 569–75.

NOTES

CD117 (KIT)

Sources/clones

Dako (C-KIT/CD117, polyclonal rabbit).

Fixation/preparation

The antibody can be used on formalin-fixed paraffin-embedded tissue sections without antigen retrieval, but heat pretreatment provides the best staining. Proteolytic enzyme treatment should be avoided.

Background

Tyrosine kinase growth factor receptors are a family of membrane-bound proteins essential for the regulation of cell growth and maintenance of the cells. C-*kit* is a proto-oncogene that encodes for one such growth factor receptor protein, KIT (CD117). C-*kit* maps to chromosome 4 (4q11–12). The gene product KIT is the receptor for stem cell factor (SCF), also known as mast cell growth factor. As a transmembrane type III tyrosine kinase receptor, KIT is phosphorylated as a result of binding with SCF and begins a cascade of intracytoplasmic signals, which are important to the regulation of cell development and growth. Many investigators have shown that c-*kit* expression is essential for the proper development of certain hematopoietic cells, mast cells, melanocytes, and germ cells.

KIT (CD117) is a 145–160 kDa protein, which is structurally related to platelet-derived growth factor. It was originally described in the late 1980s as a cellular homolog of the feline sarcoma retrovirus HZ4-FeSV transforming gene. Since that time, several authors have shown that the KIT protein is constitutively expressed in hematopoietic stem cells, tissue mast cells, basal cells of the skin, epithelial cells of the breast, melanocytes, germ cells, and interstitial cells of Cajal. KIT is not expressed in normal squamous epithelium. The central nervous system shows distinct immunopositivity in certain regions, which is absent in peripheral nerves.

Several publications have extensively demonstrated the utility of KIT staining in the identification and diagnosis of gastrointestinal stromal tumors (GISTs). Moreover, the study of this property of GISTs has led to the development of new treatment modalities targeting the KIT protein as a tyrosine kinase receptor, which is activated in the majority of GISTs. The KIT protein is selectively and competitively bound by STI-571, resulting in inhibition of tyrosine phosphorylation. The effect thereof is to shut down the transcriptional activity in the cell, resulting in growth arrest.

The interstitial cells of Cajal, the proposed pacemaker cells of the GI tract, are believed to represent the cell of origin for GISTs because of their similar immunohistochemical profile, electron microscopic features, and location within the GI tract. Gastrointestinal autonomic nerve tumors (GANTs) have features that overlap with GISTs, including immunoreactivity with KIT, and are viewed by some as a variant of GISTs.

Depending on the study design, 72–100% of GIST tumors are immunopositive with the CD117 antibody. The staining pattern is typically a diffuse cytoplasmic granular staining with membrane accentuation, with occasional cases showing focal perinuclear staining. The panel including CD117, CD34, as well as S100, desmin, and smooth muscle actin (SMA), can effectively differentiate between GISTs, true smooth muscle tumors, and neural tumors (Appendix 1.29), since GISTs do not typically express desmin or S100, but demonstrate immunopositivity for CD117 and/or CD34 and occasionally SMA. Occasional tumors with S100 and desmin positivity may also be classified as GISTs. C-*kit* mutations appear to occur preferentially in the spindle rather than in the epithelioid variant of GIST.

Mast cells are well known to show distinctive membranous and cytoplasmic staining for KIT. Furthermore, similar staining is seen in mast cell disorders and can be used to identify neoplasms of mast cells in bone marrow, skin, lymph nodes, and solid organs. Germ cells and germ cell neoplasms have been the subject of numerous studies looking at c-*kit* mutations and KIT protein expression. Studies have shown membranous staining of malignant germ cells in intratubular germ cell neoplasia (ITGCN) and seminomas, in contrast to cytoplasmic staining in non-seminomatous germ cell neoplasms. The combination of CD30 and CD117 is useful for distinguishing seminomas from embryonal carcinomas (Appendix 1.5): seminomas are CD117+/CD30−, none being CD117−/CD30+, whereas embryonal carcinomas are CD30+/CD117−, none being CD30−/CD117+.

Other tumors have been shown to have KIT immunoreactivity, predominantly with weak to moderate cytoplasmic staining intensity. These include small-cell carcinomas of the lung, ovarian epithelial neoplasms, endometrial carcinomas, thyroid carcinomas, melanomas, certain salivary gland neoplasms, angiosarcomas, breast carcinomas and malignant phyllodes tumors, and acute myeloid leukemia (AML). The deep dermal or nodular components of melanomas tend to show loss of staining for KIT, while the in-situ component stains strongly. Angiomyolipomas generally show strong immunostaining for CD117 in the epithelioid, spindle, and intermediate small round cell components in a frequency slightly higher than Melan-A and HMB-45. Other more recent additions to the CD117+ list include pediatric solid tumors such as osteosarcomas, Ewing's sarcoma, and synovial sarcomas, and, less frequently, neuroblastomas, Wilms, and rhabdomyosarcoma. In addition, occasional immunoreactivity has been encountered in extraskeletal myxoid chondrosarcoma, melanotic schwannoma, metastatic melanoma, and angiosarcoma.

Applications

The potential uses of the KIT (CD117) antibody include the diagnosis of GISTs, mast cell disorders, and seminomatous germ cell neoplasms (Appendix 1.5). As with most antibodies in immunohistochemistry, CD117 should be used in conjunction with others in a panel targeted towards the differential diagnosis. Within the spectrum of mesenchymal neoplasms of the GI tract, CD117, CD34, desmin, S100, and SMA should be the primary panel of choice for most circumstances (Appendix 1.29). In the case of mast cell disorders, care must be taken to include antibodies to B cells, T cells, myeloid markers (since CD117 can stain AML), and histiocytic markers. Despite its expression in diverse tumors, selective application with attention to specific staining patterns makes it a useful marker for tumor diagnosis.

CD117 is expressed on hematopoietic progenitor cells, melanocytes, embryonic/fetal brain, endothelium, gonads, gastrointestinal stromal tumors (GISTs), gastrointestinal autonomic nerve tumors, omental mesenchymal tumors, acute myeloid leukemia, granulocytic sarcoma, small-cell carcinoma of the lung, mast cell disease, some Reed–Sternberg cells, and synovial sarcoma.

Selected references

Arber DA, Tamayo R, Weiss LM. Paraffin section detection of c-kit gene product (CD117) in human tissues: value in the diagnosis of mast cell disorders. *Human Pathology* 1998; 29: 498–504.

Ashman LK. The biology of stem cell factor and its receptor c-kit. *International Journal of Biochemistry and Cell Biology* 1999; 31: 1037–51.

Gibson PC, Cooper K. GD117 (KIT): a diverse protein with selective applications in surgical pathology. *Advances in Anatomic Pathology* 2002; 9: 65–9.

CD123

Sources/clones

Novocastra (Br4 MS Mouse monoclonal IgG2b).

Fixation/preparation

Antigen is preserved in formalin-fixed paraffin-embedded tissue.

Background

The CD123 antigen is a transmembrane protein and the α-chain of the interleukin-3 receptor (IL3R-α). Among normal hematopoietic cells, CD123 is most highly expressed on basophils and plasmacytoid dendritic cells and may be expressed at lower level on monocytes, macrophages, and hematopoietic progenitor cells. Among non-hematopoietic cells that one may see in hematolymphoid tissues, CD123 tends to be highly expressed on vascular high endothelium, and may also be expressed on stromal progenitor cells. Note that the common β-chain that CD123 interacts with to form the high-affinity IL-3 receptor is CDw131; while an IL-3-specific β-subunit has been described in the mouse, no such subunit appears present in humans.

Applications

In non-neoplastic lymphoid tissue, such as lymph node or tonsil, CD123 will uniformly identify high endothelium in a characteristic membranous pattern. Smaller numbers of non-endothelial cells identified in the nodal parenchyma will be largely plasmacytoid dendritic cells (pDCs). In normal bone marrow, the scattered strongly CD123+ cells are likely to be pDCs, while less positive hematolymphoid cells are likely to be basophils. Again, CD123 will identify a subset of vascular endothelial cells. CD123 is expressed in the following hematolymphoid malignancies: (1) blastic plasmacytoid dendritic cell neoplasm (BPDCN), in which CD123 is one of the important lineage-defining antigens for this entity, along with CD4, TCL1, and aberrantly expressed CD56; (2) neoplastic myeloid progenitors in a variety of myeloid neoplasms, including acute myeloid leukemia (AML) bearing the FLT3 internal tandem duplication; (3) the abnormal basophils in chronic myeloid leukemia (CML); (4) the neoplastic B cells in hairy cell leukemia (HCL), but not in potential HCL mimics such as HCL-variant and splenic marginal zone lymphoma with villous lymphocytes.

Selected references

Del Giudice I, Matutes E, Morilla R, *et al.* The diagnostic value of CD123 in B-cell disorders with hairy or villous lymphocytes. *Haematologica* 2004; 89: 303–8.

Julia F, Dalle S, Duru G, *et al.* Blastic plasmacytoid dendritic cell neoplasms: clinico-immunohistochemical correlations in a series of 91 patients. *American Journal of Surgical Pathology* 2014; 38: 673–80.

Kussick, SJ, Stirewalt DL, Yi HS, *et al.* A distinctive nuclear morphology in acute myeloid leukemia is strongly associated with loss of HLA-DR expression and FLT3 internal tandem duplication. *Leukemia* 2004; 18: 1591–8.

NOTES

CD138

Sources/clones

Beckman Coulter (clone B-A38, mouse monoclonal IgG1), Biocare Medical (clone B-A38, mouse monoclonal IgG1).

Fixation/preparation

The antigen is preserved in formalin-fixed paraffin-embedded tissue.

Background

CD138, or syndecan-1, is a transmembrane and surface heparan sulfate proteoglycan implicated in a broad range of physiological functions. CD138 binds to many different growth factors by its heparan sulfate chains and mediates a variety of intracellular functions, including cell-to-cell adhesion, cell signaling, and cytoskeletal reorganization. It is thought that a binding site within the N-terminal region of CD138 is exposed to extracellular factors following cleavage of heparan sulfate by an epithelial heparanase. CD138 binds to extracellular matrix proteins such as collagen and fibronectin, allowing for cellular adhesion. In addition, CD138 has been implicated in growth factor receptor activation for many growth factors including fibroblast growth factor 2 (FGF2) and hepatocyte growth factor (HGF). CD138 has also been shown to be a mediator of HIV adsorption to immune cells by binding to HIV gp120.

Applications

In mammalian cells, CD138 is expressed by two major cell types: (1) in plasma cells, CD138 is uniformly expressed; and (2) CD138 is expressed in a large majority of epithelia, but not all. Just as it is expressed in normal plasma cells, the great majority of neoplasms containing plasmacytic components, including true plasma cell neoplasms/myeloma and B-cell lymphomas with plasmacytic differentiation (i.e., lymphoplasmacytic lymphoma and marginal zone lymphoma), also express CD138. B-lymphoid neoplasms lacking significant plasmacytic differentiation are invariably CD138-negative (e.g., Hodgkin lymphoma).

CD138 immunohistochemistry using clone B-A38 is sensitive to fixation conditions of the tissue, such that plasma cells located centrally in suboptimally fixed tissue show diminished or even absent CD138 expression. Therefore, the laboratory that diagnoses plasmacytic neoplasms should consider having an alternative marker of plasma cells, such as CD38, as a backup antibody. Moreover, because of the prominent CD138 expression on the majority of epithelia, any evaluation of plasma cells adjacent to epithelia (e.g., gastrointestinal tract) should also seriously consider using an alternative plasma cell marker. CD138 immunostaining outside of hematolymphoid lesions should be interpreted with caution, given its widespread expression in normal and neoplastic epithelium.

Note that double-labeling experiments with CD138 and antibodies to immunoglobulin light chains or heavy chains can be used to formally document light chain restriction or heavy chain restriction in plasma cells. Similarly, microbeads containing bound CD138 antibody can be used to purify plasma cells from a complex mixture of other cell populations, such as bone marrow.

Selected references

Bobardt MD, Saphire ACS, Hung HC, et al. Syndecan captures, protects, and transmits HIV to T lymphocytes. *Immunity* 2003; 18: 27–39.

Kambham N, Kong C, Longacre TA, Natkunam Y. Utility of syndecan-1 (CD138) expression in the diagnosis of undifferentiated malignant neoplasms: a tissue microarray study of 1,754 cases. *Applied Immunohistochemistry and Molecular Morphology* 2005; 13: 304–10.

Kato M, Wang H, Kainulainen V, *et al.* Physiological degradation converts the soluble syndecan-1 ectodomain from an inhibitor to a potent activator of FGF-2. *Nature Medicine* 1998; 4: 691–7.

O'Connell FP, Pinkus JL, Pinkus GS. CD138 (syndecan-1), a plasma cell marker immunohistochemical profile in hematopoietic and nonhematopoietic neoplasms. *American Journal of Clinical Pathology* 2004; 121: 254–63.

CD163

Sources/clones
Leica (10D6, mouse monoclonal IgG1).

Fixation/preparation
The antigen is preserved in formalin-fixed paraffin-embedded tissue.

Background
CD163 is a macrophage-associated antigen that functions as a scavenger receptor for the hemoglobin–haptoglobin complex, participating in the elimination of products from erythrocyte hemolysis. While immunohistochemistry detects the membranous and cytoplasmic expression of CD163 on macrophages, note that the extracellular domain of the antigen may be shed into plasma; therefore, soluble CD163 (sCD163) can be measured in serum, and is associated with a variety of inflammatory conditions, including macrophage activation/hemophagocytic syndrome, Gaucher's disease, sepsis, cirrhosis, and HIV infection. In contrast to pan-macrophage markers such as CD68, lysozyme, and CD4, CD163 is only expressed in a subset of macrophages, the so-called M2 form, which represents a unique subset of activated macrophages.

Applications
CD163 is a highly specific marker of M2 macrophages. Interestingly, in reactive lymphoid tissues, CD163 is relatively underexpressed on tingible body macrophages in germinal centers, presumably because these have an M1 activation state. In contrast, interfollicular macrophages typically do express CD163. Because of CD163's strong membranous and cytoplasmic expression in macrophages, it identifies almost the entirety of the macrophage, in contrast to the more centrally located CD68 reactivity. As a result, if one compares CD163 and CD68 immunohistochemistry in a bone marrow or other macrophage-rich tissue, CD163 immunoreactivity often occupies a significantly greater area than CD68 reactivity.

CD163 has a significant utility in identifying benign macrophages in a variety of situations. For example, the abnormal macrophages of Rosai–Dorfman (sinus histiocytosis with massive lymphadenopathy) express CD163 in the majority of cases; intracellular defects in CD163 positivity in the abnormal macrophages can help identify the phenomenon of emperipolesis, in which lymphocytes or other inflammatory cells migrate through the macrophage cytoplasm, a characteristic finding of Rosai–Dorfman disease. Similar defects in cytoplasmic CD163 reactivity can help identify engulfed hematopoietic cells in macrophage activation/hemophagocytic syndromes, in which such changes can be subtle by routine bone marrow morphology. In epithelioid cellular collections in bone marrow or other tissues, CD163 immunohistochemistry is useful to confirm macrophage collections or granulomata, and exclude other potential benign and neoplastic mimics, including metastatic carcinoma or melanoma.

Finally, there has been a lot of interest in the association between the activation state of tumor-infiltrating macrophages in a variety of neoplasms; this relationship has been particularly well studied in Hodgkin lymphoma, in which it was initially observed that high numbers of tumor-infiltrating macrophages were associated with an adverse prognosis. Subsequent work in this area has suggested that rather than the absolute number of macrophages, the ratio of CD163+ M2 macrophages to total CD68+ macrophages may be the key prognostic factor, in that increases in this ratio are associated with worse prognosis in classic Hodgkin lymphoma (CHL). Note that increased numbers of intrafollicular M2 macrophages have been associated with adverse prognoses in follicular lymphomas as well.

In addition to identifying diagnostically or prognostically significant benign macrophage populations, CD163 can be used to identify neoplastic macrophages/monocytes in a variety of processes. Histiocytic sarcoma, a rare pleomorphic neoplasm of macrophages, typically expresses CD163, while other histiocytic and dendritic malignancies typically do not (Langerhans cell histiocytosis, indeterminate cell histiocytosis, plasmacytoid dendritic cell neoplasms, etc.).

Selected references

Lau SK, Chu PG, Weiss LM. CD163: a specific marker of macrophages in paraffin-embedded tissue samples. *American Journal of Clinical Pathology* 2004; 122: 794–801.

Klein JL, Nguyen TT, Bien-Willner GA, *et al.* CD163 immunohistochemistry is superior to CD68 in predicting outcome in classical Hodgkin lymphoma. *American Journal of Clinical Pathology* 2014; 141: 381–7.

Kridel R, Xerri L, Gelas-Dore B, *et al.* The prognostic impact of CD163-positive macrophages in follicular lymphoma: a study from the BC Cancer Agency and the Lumphoma Study Association. *Clinical Cancer Research* 2015; 21: 3428–35.

Nguyen TT, Schwartz EJ, West RB, *et al.* Expression of CD163 (hemoglobin scavenger receptor) in normal tissues, lymphomas, carcinomas and sarcomas is largely restricted to the monocyte/macrophage lineage. *American Journal of Surgical Pathology* 2005; 29: 617–24.

CDK4

Sources/clones

Abbiotec (IML-4, polyclonal), Abcam (polyclonal), Abgent (polyclonal), Abnova (polyclonal), Acris (DCS-31.2, DCS156, polyclonal), Aviva Systems Biology (IML-4, RB15490, polyclonal), Biolegend (polyclonal), Biologo (polyclonal), Biorbyt (polyclonal), Bioss (polyclonal), Cloud-Clone Corp (MAB233Hu22, polyclonal), Creative Biomart (CABT-37824MH), Fitzgerald (DCS-156), Gene Tex (GTX63389, GTX75694, polyclonal), LifeSpan BioSciences (EPR4513, DCS-156, polyclonal), Life Technologies (AHZ0202), MBL International (DCS-156), Merck Millipore (DCS-35), NovaTeinBio (polyclonal), Novus Biologicals (polyclonal), Origene (polyclonal), Progen Biotechnik GmbH (DCS-156), Proteintech (polyclonal), Santa Cruz Biotechnology (polyclonal), Thermo Fisher Scientific (polyclonal), United States Biological (5F180).

Fixation/preparation

Several of the antibody clones/polyclonal antibodies to CDK4 are immunoreactive in fixed paraffin-embedded sections. HIER at 120 °C enhances labeling.

Background

Cyclin-dependent kinase 4 (CDK4) regulates the cell cycle by inhibiting retinoblastoma 1. The *CDK4* gene is located at chromosome 12q13. Aberrent cytogenetic karyotypes containing 12q13–15 within supernumerary ring chromosomes or giant rod chromosomes including amplified copies of the *CDK4* and *MDM2* genes are characteristic of most cases of atypical lipomatous tumors/well-differentiated liposarcoma (ALT/WDLPS) and dedifferentiated liposarcoma (DDLPS). Amplification of chromosome 12q13–15 has been observed in well-differentiated osteosarcoma.

Applications

CDK4 is overexpressed in nearly all well-differentiated and dedifferentiated liposarcomas, most often in concert with MDM-2. This phenomenon reflects the common presence of ring or giant marker chromosomes that contain amplified copies of the *CDK4* and *MDM2* genes. Diagnostic application of CDK4 or MDM-2 immunohistochemistry can be used to diagnose DDLPS, as opposed to other high-grade sarcomas, and in the distinction between benign lipocytic neoplasms and ALT/WDLPS, when the latter show very minimal atypical histologic features. CDK4 also can be used to differentiate retroperitoneal liposarcoma with myxoid differentiation from myxoid/round cell liposarcoma.

Analogous to liposarcoma, 12q13–15 chromosome amplification has been shown to correlate with CDK4 immunoreactivity in well-differentiated osteosarcoma. This CDK4 reactivity can be useful to distinguish low-grade osteosarcoma from morphologic stimulants. Acidic decalcifying solution has been reported to minimally decrease CDK4 staining intensity. Differences in CDK4 immunoreactivity in intermediate- and high-grade osteosarcoma have been reported in the literature.

CDK4 reactivity has been described in other types of sarcoma, including chondrosarcoma of the jaw, leiomyosarcoma, malignant peripheral nerve sheath tumor, myxofibrosarcoma, embryonal rhabdomyosarcoma, alveolar rhabdomyosarcoma, undifferentiated pleomorphic sarcoma, and myxoid/round cell liposarcoma.

Comments

Depending on the reference, immunoreactivity may be enhanced following retrieval at 120 °C in citrate buffer at pH 6.0.

Selected references

Binh MB, Sastre-Garau X, Guillou L, *et al.* MDM2 and CDK4 immunostainings are useful adjuncts in diagnosing well-differentiated and dedifferentiated liposarcoma subtypes: a comparative analysis of 559 soft tissue neoplasms with genetic data. *American Journal of Surgical Pathology* 2005; 29: 1340–7.

Coindre JM, Hostein I, Maire G, *et al.* Inflammatory malignant fibrous histiocytomas and dedifferentiated liposarcomas: histological review, genomic profile, and MDM2 and CDK4 status favour a single entity. *Journal of Pathology* 2004; 203: 822–30.

Dei Tos AP, Doglioni C, Piccinin S, *et al.* Coordinated expression and amplification of the MDM2, CDK4, and HMGI-C genes in atypical lipomatous tumours. *Journal of Pathology* 2000; 190: 531–6.

Dujardin F, Binh MB, Bouvier C, *et al.* MDM2 and CDK4 immunohistochemistry is a valuable tool in the differential diagnosis of low-grade osteosarcomas and other primary fibro-osseous lesions of the bone. *Modern Pathology* 2011; 24: 624–37.

Thway K, Flora R, Shah C, Olmos D, Fisher C. Diagnostic utility of p16, CDK4, and MDM2 as an immunohistochemical panel in distinguishing well-differentiated and dedifferentiated liposarcomas from other adipocytic tumors. *American Journal of Surgical Pathology* 2012; 36: 462–9.

CDX2 (caudal type homeobox 2)

Sources/clones

Abcam (EPR2764Y, AMT28), Cell Signaling Technology (3977), Dako (M3636), Life Technologies (ZC007), Millipore (AB4123), Novocastra (AMT28), Santa Cruz Biotechnology (K-21).

Fixation/preparation

The antibody can be used in formalin-fixed paraffin-embedded tissue. Pretreatment of deparaffinized tissue sections with HIER is required.

Background

Caudal type homeobox transcription factor 2, also known as caudal-related homeobox gene 2 (CDX2), is a homeobox gene that encodes an intestine-specific transcription factor expressed early in development. It is also involved in the regulation of proliferation and differentiation of intestinal epithelial cells, and is expressed in the nuclei of epithelial cells throughout the intestine, from the duodenum to the rectum. While it is not expressed in normal gastric mucosa and the distal-most portions of the intestinal tract (anal canal), CDX2 protein is expressed in primary and metastatic colorectal carcinomas. It is also expressed in intestinal metaplasia of the esophagus and stomach, intestinal-type gastric cancer, small intestinal adenocarcinomas, and mucinous neoplasms of the lung, and in breast, ovary, urinary bladder, and pancreaticobiliary tract.

Applications

CDX2 is a useful marker of intestinal-type differentiation and is expressed in a majority of colorectal adenocarcinomas. Its primary utility lies in determination of the site of origin of metastatic adenocarcinomas of unknown primary sites, both in cytology and in surgical pathology specimens. Though combined expression of CDX2 and cytokeratin 20 with absent cytokeratin 7 expression is useful in the diagnosis of lower intestinal adenocarcinomas, it is not specific and may be seen in intestinal-type adenocarcinomas of the cervix and sinonasal mucosa. Additionally, loss of CDX2 and CK20 is more frequently encountered in mismatch repair-deficient colorectal adenocarcinomas, which should be taken into consideration to differentiate between primary and metastatic colorectal cancer.

CDX2 expression is also frequently noted in primary and metastatic well-differentiated neuroendocrine tumors of the midgut and hindgut.

Comments

Several studies comment on the low sensitivity of CDX2 as an immunohistochemical marker of intestinal origin. The sensitivity of CDX2 and protocols for use must be carefully considered when classifying neoplasms of unknown origin.

Selected references

Bellizzi AM. Assigning site of origin in metastatic neuroendocrine neoplasms: a clinically significant application of diagnostic immunohistochemistry. *Advances in Anatomic Pathology* 2013; 20: 285–314.

da Costa LT, He TC, Yu J, et al. CDX2 is mutated in a colorectal cancer with normal APC/beta-catenin signaling. *Oncogene* 1999; 18: 5010–14.

Freund JN, Domon-Dell C, Kedinger M, et al. The Cdx-1 and Cdx-2 homeobox genes in the intestine. *Biochemistry and Cell Biology* 1998; 76: 957–69.

Jaffee IM, Rahmani M, Singhal MG, et al. Expression of the intestinal transcription factor CDX2 in carcinoid tumors is a marker of midgut origin. *Archives of Pathology and Laboratory Medicine* 2006; 130: 1522–6.

James R, Erler T, Kazenwadel J. Structure of the murine homeobox gene cdx-2. Expression in embryonic and adult intestinal epithelium. *Journal of Biological Chemistry* 1994; 269: 15, 229–37.

Li MK, Folpe AL. CDX-2, a new marker for adenocarcinoma of gastrointestinal origin. *Advances in Anatomic Pathology* 2004; 11: 101–5.

Werling RW, Yaziji H, Bacchi CE, *et al.* CDX2, a highly sensitive and specific marker of adenocarcinomas of intestinal origin: an immunohistochemical survey of 476 primary and metastatic carcinomas. *American Journal of Surgical Pathology* 2003; 27: 303–10.

c-erbB-2 (*HER2, neu*)

Sources/clones

Accurate (CB11, CBE1, polyclonal), Becton Dickinson (3B5), Biogenesis (2G2-91, LY369), Biogenex (EGFR), Coulter (3B5), Dako (polyclonal A0485), Lab Vision (9G6.10, L87, N12, N24, N28.6), Novocastra (CB11, CBE1), Oncogene Science (CNeu), Pharmingen (9G6), Zymed (TAB250).

Fixation/preparation

Most antibodies are immunoreactive in fresh frozen tissue sections as well as in fixed paraffin-embedded sections. HIER enhances immunoreactivity. Enzyme treatment is not necessary.

Background

The c-*erb*B-2 oncogene was discovered in the 1980s by three different avenues of investigation. The *neu* oncogene was detected as a mutated transforming gene in neuroblastomas experimentally induced in fetal rats. The c-*erb*B-2 was a human gene discovered by its homology to the retroviral gene v-*erb*B, and *HER2* was isolated by screening a human genomic DNA library for homology with v-*erb*B. When the DNA sequences were determined subsequently, c-*erb*B-2, *HER2*, and *neu* were found to represent the same gene.

The c-*erb*B-2 gene is located on human chromosome 17q21 and codes for the c-*erb*B-2 mRNA (4.6 kb), which translates to the c-*erb*B-2 protein (pi85). The c-*erb*B-2 oncogene is homologous with, but not identical to, c-*erb*B-1, which is located on chromosome 7 and encodes for the epidermal growth factor receptor. The c-*erb*B-2 protein, a member of the epidermal growth factor receptor family, is a normal cell membrane component of all epithelial cells with extracellular, transmembrane, and intracellular tyrosine kinase activity. Apart from a growth stimulatory function, the molecule plays an important role in the motility of tumor cells. Cell migration depends mainly on actin polymerization and intracellular organization, which is influenced by a vast variety of actin-binding proteins. Second messengers such as phosphoinositides and calcium mediate the regulation of these proteins. Signaling via these second messengers is initiated and regulated by membrane receptors (e.g., receptor tyrosine kinases), and by adhesion molecule interactions (e.g., integrins and selectins) and focal adhesion kinases. As c-*erb*B-2 is a receptor tyrosine kinase, it has a major role in steering second-messenger signaling and thus in actin cytoskeleton reorganization and motility of the cell. The *erb*B-2 is unique among the *erb*B family in that no ligand has yet been identified. Due to this absence, alternative mechanisms are use for *erb*B-2 activation. With overexpression, kinase activation occurs in the absence of ligand because of constitutive homodimerization. At normal expression levels, *erb*B-2 acts as the shared co-receptor for the *erb*B family, and these heterodimeric complexes are activated in response to the partner ligand.

c-*erb*B-2 gene alterations have been reported in diverse human neoplasms and almost exclusively involve amplification of the gene. Amplification involves the repeated duplication of a particular gene sequence, resulting in multiple gene copies within each cell. This results in overexpression of the gene product, as reflected in the levels of mRNA and gene oncoprotein. There is generally good correlation of the c-*erb*B-2 gene amplification with overexpression.

Applications

c-*erb*B-2 has been shown to be amplified in about 20–30% of invasive breast carcinomas, and various studies have correlated the gene amplification or overexpression with other prognostic variables in breast cancer patients. Almost all reported studies have shown a strong correlation with various established adverse factors including large tumor size, unfavorable histologic subtype, high histologic grade, high mitotic index and proliferative activity, positive nodal status, hematogenous spread, and aneuploidy. c-erbB-2 expression has also been shown to be an independent significant prognostic factor in both node-positive and node-negative breast cancer, and the combination of c-erbB-2 positivity and estrogen receptor negativity made it possible to identify a subgroup of patients with the worst clinical outcome.

c-erbB-2 overexpression is more common in invasive ductal and medullary carcinomas than in lobular, colloid, and papillary carcinomas. In intraductal carcinomas, it is almost exclusively seen in large-cell, high nuclear grade, estrogen receptor-negative, and comedo-type intraductal carcinoma (interestingly, a larger percentage of ductal carcinoma in situ than infiltrating ductal carcinoma is positive for c-erbB-2). In-situ lobular carcinoma seldom shows overexpression of the oncoprotein. Overexpression is more common in invasive tumors associated with an intraductal component than in those without, and there is usually concordance between the invasive and intraductal components of an individual tumor. The rates of overexpression and gene amplification do not appear to be different in ductal carcinoma in situ and invasive carcinoma, but appear to be significantly higher in invasive carcinoma with intraductal spread.

Despite the universal observation of a strong correlation with various adverse prognostic factors, conflicting data regarding the prognostic value of c-erbB-2 suggest that overexpression of the oncoprotein may not be a powerful predictor by itself. In any individual patient it should be employed as part of a multivariate approach to guiding treatment and determining prognosis. Overexpression of c-erbB-2 may also serve as a predictor of response to adjuvant treatment, predicting a poor response to chemotherapy and a lack of response to endocrine therapy on relapse, and identifying those patients who are most likely to benefit from high-dose regimens. Furthermore, as c-erbB-2 protein has an extracellular domain and tends to be expressed in more aggressive tumors, it is the target for immunotherapy with the humanized anti-HER2/neu antibody trastuzumab (Herceptin; Genentech, Inc., South San Francisco, CA, USA), particularly for patients with metastatic carcinoma.

Comments

Occasional reports have noted discrepancies between the demonstration of amplification of the c-erbB-2 gene and detection of protein overexpression by immunostaining.

Despite this drawback, immunohistochemistry now appears to be the method of choice in most institutions for assessing c-erbB-2 overexpression. A number of factors account for variability of immunohistochemical results and these include fixation, storage, antigen retrieval, reagent optimization, antibody specificity and its domain, controls, scoring system employed, and interobserver variability. Numerous antibodies to c-erbB-2 are available, including both polyclonal and monoclonal antibodies. In general, monoclonal antibodies are considered more specific. The HercepTest uses a polyclonal antibody (A0485). In general, the Food and Drug Administration (FDA)-approved antibodies detect the internal domain of the c-erbB-2 receptor. Some antibodies such as Zymed TAB250 are against the external domain of the receptor. There is some concern that the external domain of c-erbB-2 may be cleaved so that antibodies to the external domain may not be as sensitive, although this concern has not been substantiated.

Only membrane staining should be accepted as positive staining, and we have found the polyclonal antibody from Dako and monoclonal CNeu to be the most sensitive. HIER-enhanced staining, although producing some increase in cytoplasmic staining, was not a hindrance to interpretation. There is no standardized scoring system for HER2/neu by immunostaining, and disparate systems have been employed; some take into consideration the proportion of positive cells, some only regard the intensity of staining, while others combine the two parameters into one score. The heterogeneity of staining in any section is due to variability of fixation and embedding and probably not to intrinsic tumor properties. The majority of publications score immunostaining of c-erbB-2 in the following manner: $0 =$ no staining; $1+ =$ occasional tumor cells show membranous staining that is fragmented and not circumferential; $2+ =$ scattered tumor cells or small groups of tumor cells show circumferential staining; $3+ =$ strong membrane staining throughout the tumor that may be associated with some cytoplasmic staining. The area of highest intensity of staining is assessed, the area occupying at least 10–20% of the tumor in the section. Successful antigen retrieval will result in normal expression in benign epithelial cells, as the c-erbB-2 is a normal gene. However, such internal controls of benign breast epithelium must not display $>1+$ staining. Data from clinical trials suggest that $3+$ immunoexpression reflects gene amplification and 0 and $1+$ are negative. Scores of $2+$ should proceed to FISH analysis, as a small portion of these cases represent true gene amplification.

Besides fixed paraffin-embedded sections, we have shown that c-erbB-2 immunostaining can also be performed on formalin-fixed cytological preparations; however, scoring of staining in such preparations has not been correlated with gene amplification.

c-*erb*B-2 immunoexpression has been demonstrated in a number of epithelial tumors including carcinomas of the prostate, bile duct, colon and rectum, lung, stomach, head and neck region, and other organs, and may have a role in such tumors.

Selected references

Bobrow LG, Happerfield LC, Millis RR. Comparison of immunohistological staining with different antibodies to the c-*erb*B-2 oncoprotein. *Applied Immunohistochemistry* 1996; 4: 128–34.

DePotter CR. The new-oncogene: more than a prognostic indicator? *Human Pathology* 1994; 25: 1264–8.

NOTES

Chlamydia

Sources/clones

American Research Products (C512F), American Research Products/EY Labs (polyclonal), Biogenex (LM-9, 16-UB), Dako (RR402), Fitzgerald (polyclonal).

C. trachomatis

Accurate (115), Biodesign (168, JDC1), Biogenesis (polyclonal), Pharmingen (CHL888).

C. trachomatis 60 kDa

Biodesign (168), Biogenesis (polyclonal).

C. psittaci

Biogenesis (73–0200, 77–05), Kallestadt Diagnostics, Chaska, MN.

C. pneumoniae

Fitzgerald (M73066).

Fixation/preparation

Most antibodies are applicable to routine formalin-fixed paraffin-embedded tissue.

Background

Genital chlamydial infection is recognized as the world's most common sexually transmitted disease. In the majority of cases the condition is asymptomatic. *C. trachomatis* is associated with various complications of pregnancy and with premature birth and neonatal difficulties. A monoclonal antibody specific for the outer membrane proteins of *C. trachomatis* is available.

C. psittaci is the causative agent of psittacosis. It infects a diverse group of animals, including birds, humans, and other mammals. It is a cause of abortion in sheep, cattle, and goats. Transmission to humans is incidental, with a history of direct contact with contaminated products of conception. The disease is characterized as a mild-to-moderate flu-like illness. However, in pregnancy the human host is especially vulnerable. Gestational psittacosis typically presents as a progressive febrile illness with headaches, complicated by abnormal liver enzymes, low-grade disseminated intravascular coagulapathy, atypical pneumonia, and abnormal renal function. Management includes termination of pregnancy with aggressive antibiotic therapy.

Applications

Diagnosis of gestational psittacosis is dependent on histopathological findings, which consist of an intense acute intervillositis, perivillous fibrin deposition with villous necrosis, and large irregular basophilic intracytoplasmic inclusions within the syncytiotrophoblast. The application of genus-specific monoclonal antichlamydial antibody is useful for rapid confirmation of the diagnosis.

C. trachomatis is a major cause of genital infection. The acquired infection tends to persist and is usually symptom-free. Consequently fetal exposure to chlamydial infection is high, with *C. trachomatis* being demonstrated in the placenta. More often, basophilic intracytoplasmic inclusions are detected in cervical smears, where genus-specific antibody may be applied for diagnostic confirmation. In lymphogranuloma venereum, a small ulcerating primary lesion develops in the genitalia, following by involvement of draining lymph nodes with a suppurative granulomatous inflammation, necrosis, and scarring.

Inclusion bodies may also be demonstrated in lung tissue and secretions in atypical pneumonias caused by *C. trachomatis*. Trachoma/trachoma inclusion conjunctivitis or TRIC infection is common in the tropical zones, being responsible for blindness. The organism initially infects the conjunctival epithelium and it can be demonstrated in smears of these cells by the presence of characteristic intracytoplasmic inclusion bodies.

Chlamydia infection of the cardiovascular system is associated with pericarditis, endocarditis, and myocarditis, and *Chlamydia* particles have also been observed in damaged heart valves and may be associated with lesions of arteriosclerosis and aortic aneurysm. In addition, patients with myocardial infarction show seroconversion against *Chlamydia* lipopolysaccharide. Young patients who died of sudden death showed immunohistochemically detectable *C. pneumoniae* in 53% (17/32) cases of advanced arteriosclerosis of left anterior descending coronary arteries and in 22% (8/37) cases of early lesions. *C. pneumoniae* was found most often in macrophages and less often in smooth muscle cells. The organism has similarly been demonstrated in atherosclerotic plaques in a variety of other vascular sites.

Selected reference

Beatty WL, Morison RP, Byrne GI. Immunoelectron microscopic quantitation of differential levels of chlamydial proteins in cell culture model of persistent *Chlamydia trachomatis* infection. *Infection and Immunity* 1994; 62: 4059–62.

Chromogranin

Sources/clones

Antibodies to chromogranin A are available from Accurate (A3), Biogenesis (A11, LK2H10), Biogenex (A11, LK2H10), Camón (LK2H10), Cymbus Bioscience (LK2H10), Dako (DAK-A3, polyclonal), Enzo (PHE5), Immunotech (LK2H10, C3420), Medac, Milab (CH), RDI (LK2H10), Novocastra (LK2H10), Sanbio (LK2H10), Saxon, Serotec (LK2H10, C3420), Zymed.

Fixation/preparation

The antibodies are immunoreactive in fixed paraffin-embedded sections and frozen sections. HIER does not result in significant enhancement. Fixation in Bouin's or B5 fixative may improve immunogenicity, but background staining is correspondingly increased. Proteolytic digestion does not improve immunostaining.

Background

The chromogranins are a family of soluble acidic proteins of about 68 kDa. They are the major proteins in the peptide-containing dense core (neurosecretory) granules of neuroendocrine cells and sympathetic nerves. Ultrastructural examination has confirmed the localization of chromogranins to the matrix of neurosecretory granules of neuroendocrine cells. While having different molecular weights, the chromogranin subunits are neither identical nor entirely dissimilar and may differ in only two or three amino acid residues, with a minimum homology between any pair of polypeptides of about 33%. The chromogranins in neuroendocrine tissues display both quantitative and qualitative variability. They occur in the highest concentration in the following rank order: adrenal medulla; anterior, intermediate and posterior pituitary; pancreatic islets; small intestine; thyroid C cells; hypothalamus.

The antibody clone LK2H10 to chromogranin of 68 kDa labels most normal neuroendocrine cells and their corresponding neoplasms. The LK2H10 clone was derived from human pheochromocytoma and exhibits cross-reactivity with monkey and pig chromogranins.

Chromogranins are thought to stabilize the soluble portion of neurosecretory granules by interaction with adenosine triphosphate and catecholamines, and are released into the serum after splanchnic stimulation. They have multiple roles in the secretory process of hormones. Intracellularly, they play a role in targeting peptide hormones and neurotransmitters to granules of the regulated pathway by virtue of their ability to aggregate in the low-pH, high-calcium environment of the trans-Golgi network. Extracellular peptides formed as a result of proteolytic processing of chromogranins regulate hormone secretion. The synthesis of chromogranins is regulated by many different factors, including steroid hormones and agents that act through a variety of signaling pathways.

Applications

The major applications of antibodies to the chromogranins are for the identification of neuroepithelial/neuroendocrine differentiation in normal and neoplastic tissues, as well as the neural elements of the brain and gut. Initial experience with clone LK2H10 to chromogranin A revealed less than 100% sensitivity for neuroendocrine cells, especially among those cells and tumors with low concentrations of neurosecretory granules and among tumors such as insulinomas, somatostatinomas, prolactinomas, and corticotropin- and growth-hormone-producing adenomas. However, the rate of positivity has improved with the use of more sensitive immunolabeling procedures.

Chromogranin is the most specific marker for neuroendocrine differentiation and corresponds to the neurosecretory granule, the hallmark of the neuroendocrine cell (Appendix 1.3, 1.4, 1.9, 1.20, 1.29, 1.30, 1.35, 1.37). While it may be used with other neuroendocrine markers such as NSE and PGP 9.5 to improve the diagnostic yield, chromogranin and synaptophysin are the most specific of all neuroendocrine markers.

Comments

As neurosecretory granules tend to be localized beneath the plasma membranes of neuroendocrine cells, their highest density is within the cytoplasmic processes characteristic of such cells. Staining for chromogranin therefore highlights the cytoplasmic processes often not visible in H&E stains; these processes when cut in cross-section show dot-like staining. Aberrant immunoreactivity for chromogranin has been described in normal and neoplastic urothelium, particularly in the umbrella cells, attributed to reactivity with chromogranin-like proteins in the transitional cells.

Chromogranin immunostaining has been employed to resolve the problem of argyrophilia seen in some breast cancers. A subset of such carcinomas (10–20%) have been confirmed to show neuroendocrine differentiation by chromogranin immunolabeling, but the phenomenon appears to have no relationship to established prognostic factors or patient outcome. Histologic grade appears to overcome the phenotype in determining prognosis of neuroendocrine differentiation in breast carcinomas.

Selected reference

Hendy GN, Bevan S, Mattei MG, Mouland AJ. Chromogranin A. *Clinical Investigative Medicine* 1995; 18: 47–65.

c-Myc

Sources/clones

Biogenesis (9E11), Caltag Laboratories (polyclonal), Chemicon, Fitzgerald (polyclonal), Novocastra (polyclonal), Oncogene (9E10, 8, 33), Pharmingen (9E10), Serotec (CT14, polyclonal).

Fixation/preparation

Several clones, including 9E10, are immunoreactive in acetone- or formalin-fixed paraffin-embedded tissue sections.

Background

Myc is the product of the early-response gene *myc*. The *myc* family of oncogenes, c-*myc* and N-*myc*, on chromosome 8, encode three highly related regulatory-cycle-specific nuclear phosphoproteins. Myc protein contains a transcriptional activation domain and a basic helix-loop-helix-leucine zipper DNA-binding and dimerization domain. As a heterodimer with a structurally related protein, Max, Myc can bind DNA in a sequence-specific manner, suggesting that the Myc/Max heterodimer functions as a transcriptional activator of genes that are critical for the regulation of cell growth. When overexpressed or hyperactivated as a result of mutation in certain types of cells, *myc* can cause uncontrolled proliferation. There is evidence that *myc* may have a critical role in the normal control of cell proliferation, and cells in which *myc* expression is specifically prevented in vitro will not divide even in the presence of growth factors. Conversely, cells in which *myc* expression is specifically switched on independently of growth factors cannot enter G_0. If the cells are in G_0 when Myc protein is provided, they will leave G_0 and begin to divide even in the absence of growth factors, a behavior that ultimately causes them to undergo programmed cell death or apoptosis.

The presence of a single oncogene is not usually sufficient to turn a normal cell into a cancer cell. In transgenic mice that are endowed with *myc* oncogene, some of the tissues that express the oncogene grow to an exaggerated size, and with the passage of time some cells undergo further changes and give rise to cancers. However, the vast majority of cells in the transgenic mouse that express the *myc* oncogene do not give rise to cancers, showing that the presence of a single oncogene is not enough to cause neoplastic transformation. Nonetheless, *myc* expression produces an increased risk, as the presence of another oncogene such as *ras* results in a synergistic effect known as oncogene collaboration. The synergism increases the incidence of cancers in the transgenic mouse to a much higher rate, although the cancers originate as scattered isolated tumors among non-cancerous cells. Even with the presence of two expressed oncogenes, the cells must undergo further randomly generated changes to become cancerous.

In follicular B-cell lymphomas, collaboration between *myc* and the *BCL2* gene occurs. If *myc* alone is overexpressed, cells are driven round the cell cycle inappropriately but this does not result in lymphoma because the progeny of such forced divisions die by apoptosis. If *BCL2* is overexpressed at the same time, the excess progeny survive and proliferate as *BCL2* acts as an oncogene by inhibiting apoptosis.

Applications

The ability to stain for c-Myc in tissue sections has understandably been received with great interest, and several attempts to use the oncoprotein as a prognostic marker have been made. For example, in squamous cell carcinoma of the head and neck significant negative correlation has been shown between c-Myc levels and the number of metastatic nodes and clinical stage of disease but no correlation was found with tumor size or degree of differentiation. Other applications have included c-Myc protein expression in prostatic carcinoma, pituitary adenomas, ovary, lung, and colon, among other tumors.

c-Myc overexpression is noted in post-radiation angiosarcoma, especially in the breast, and this helps in the separation from atypical vascular lesions.

The examination of c-Myc as a marker for persons at risk of various types of cancer, including breast carcinoma, is another potentially useful application, and it has been suggested that c-Myc immunostaining is correlated with proliferation index, differentiation, patient age, and estrogen receptor status.

Comments

Clone 9E10 is immunoreactive in formalin-fixed paraffin-embedded tissue sections.

Selected reference

Vastrik I, Makela TP, Koskinen PJ, *et al.* Myc protein: partners and antagonists. *Critical Reviews in Oncology* 1994; 5: 59–68.

Collagen type IV

Sources/clones

Accurate (COL-4), Biodesign (1042, MC4-HA), Biogenesis (2D8/29), Biogenex (CIV22), Biotec (XCD02), Dako (CIV22), ICN (polyclonal, 1042), Immunotech (CIV22), Milab, Sanbio (SB11), Sera Lab (1042), Serotec (CIV22, PHM-12).

Fixation/preparation

Most commercial clones of antibodies are immunoreactive in fixed paraffin-embedded sections, but only following HIER and enzymatic predigestion with trypsin before the application of the primary antibody.

Background

Basal lamina is mostly formed by a dense 40–60 nm-thick layer called the lamina densa and an electron lucent layer adjacent to the cell membrane known as the lamina lucida. A loose layer of connective tissue known as the lamina reticularis may be present under the lamina densa. Type IV collagen localizes exclusively to the lamina densa and by immunoelectron microscopy is found in both lamina densa and lamina lucida. Laminin has the same distribution but appears to be more intensely localized to the lamina lucida. Other components of basal lamina include heparin sulfate proteoglycan, entactin, fibronectin, and type V collagen, the last of these probably a stromal rather than basal lamina component.

Applications

Diagnostic applications of collagen type IV immunostaining have mostly centered around the demonstration of basal lamina in invasive tumors, particularly epithelial tumors, and their changes with tumor invasion and metastasis. In particular, the demonstration of an intact basal lamina has been used to distinguish benign glandular proliferations such as microglandular adenosis and sclerosing adenosis from well-differentiated carcinoma such as tubular carcinoma of the breast. Immunostaining for collagen type IV has also been applied to discriminate between C-cell hyperplasia and microscopic medullary carcinoma of the thyroid. The former showed complete investment of the C cells by a continuous rim of basal lamina, whereas the latter was typified by deficiencies of the basal lamina so that the constituent C cells were extrafollicular in location. There was also focal reduplication of basal lamina, apparently tumor-derived. Studies of collagen type IV in the matrix proteins and basal lamina of glomeruli and tubules have been reported. Immunostaining for basal lamina has been shown to be a rapid and useful way to distinguish major variants of congenital epidermolysis bullosa, especially when electron microscopy is not available. Fragmentation of the basal lamina has been demonstrated with collagen type IV immunostaining in the mucosa of patients with celiac disease, and decreased or discontinuous staining for basal lamina has been employed to distinguish invasive foci of adenocarcinoma from misplaced submucosal epithelial deposits in adenomatous polyps.

Distinctive patterns of basal distribution have been demonstrated in various types of soft tissue tumors, adding to the diagnostic armamentarium for this group of neoplasms, which are often difficult to separate (Appendix 1.25). While the presence of basal lamina cannot be used as an absolute discriminant for blood vessels and lymphatic spaces, the latter lack the reduplication of the basal lamina characteristic of blood vessels and generally show thin and discontinuous staining for collagen type IV and laminin. The distinctive staining observed around blood vessels has been employed as a marker when performing capillary density measurements.

Glomus tumors of the stomach have been shown to be invested by net-like pericellular staining for both collagen IV and laminin, and cytological preparations of the same type of tumor were described to be strongly positive for collagen IV, smooth muscle actin, and muscle-specific actin.

Interestingly, besides being typically a major component of basal lamina, collagen type IV is also expressed in the interstitial stroma of extrahepatic bile duct carcinoma and schirrous gastric carcinoma, where it may play a role in desmoplastic stroma formation.

Comments

Earlier work on basal lamina immunostaining was restricted to the use of immunofluoresence techniques in frozen sections, because of the lack of sensitivity of the available antibodies and techniques. The application of HIER combined with proteolytic digestion makes it possible to produce consistent immunostaining of paraffin-embedded, routinely prepared tissue sections.

Selected reference

Birembaut P, Caron Y, Adnet JJ. Usefulness of basement membrane markers in tumoral pathology. *Journal of Pathology* 1985; 145: 283–96.

CXCL13

Sources/clones

Abcam (rabbit polyclonal), R&D Systems Inc. (goat polyclonal), R&D Systems Inc. (53610, mouse monoclonal), US Biological (mouse monoclonal).

Fixation/preparation

The antigen is preserved in formalin-fixed paraffin-embedded tissues.

Background

C-X-C motif chemokine 13 (CXCL13), also known as B-lymphocyte chemoattractant (BLC), is a cytokine capable of inducing chemotaxis (i.e., a chemokine) in nearby responsive cells. As its alternative name implies, CXCL13 is thought to be selectively chemotactic for B cells. Together with its ligand CXCR5, CXCL13 plays a role in determining the organization of B cells within lymphoid follicles, including during normal lymph node development, and is important for subsequent immune system responses.

Applications

CXCL13 is a relatively specific marker for follicular helper T (TFH) cells, the CD4+ T-cell subset that typically resides in the germinal center and helps coordinate immunologic reactions in this location. In addition to CXCL13, TFH cells characteristically express CD10, Bcl-6, and PD-1. Similar to PD-1, immunohistochemical staining for CXCL13 in reactive lymphoid proliferations will highlight a small subset of the T cells within the germinal centers, as would be expected for TFH cells, as well as occasional TFH cells in the interfollicular areas. By immunohistochemistry, CXCL13 is typically expressed in the cytoplasm, in a granular or perinuclear dot-like pattern. In our experience, immunoreactivity with CXCL13 is highly fixation-dependent and is best interpreted in well-preserved, formalin-fixed paraffin-embedded tissues.

CXCL13 immunohistochemical staining primarily has clinical applications in the diagnostic workup of T-cell non-Hodgkin lymphomas. Angioimmunoblastic T-cell lymphoma (AITL) is a peripheral T-cell lymphoma characterized by numerous high endothelial venules, expanded follicular dendritic cell meshworks, and a proliferation of neoplastic small-/intermediate-sized T lymphocytes with clear/pale cytoplasm and distinct cell membranes (so-called "clear cells"). These neoplastic T cells are derived from TFH cells and consequently variably express CD10, Bcl-6, PD-1, and CXCL13. In AITL, cytoplasmic CXCL13 expression is typically only seen in a subset of the neoplastic cells. While more specific for TFH cells than CD10, Bcl-6, or PD-1, CXCL13 is a less sensitive marker of TFH cells, in part because antigenic preservation appears more tissue fixation-dependent. Cases with cutaneous involvement by angioimmunoblastic T-cell lymphoma also express CXCL13, although only a subset of the cells are usually positive.

Strong expression of CXCL13 is unusual in other T-cell lymphoproliferative disorders, but has been reported in some cases of peripheral T-cell lymphoma not otherwise specified (PTCL-NOS) that are of TFH origin, but lack the characteristic clinical and histologic features of AITL. Similarly, some authors have suggested a provisional category of "primary cutaneous follicular helper T-cell lymphoma" for cases with cutaneous involvement by a T-cell population with a TFH phenotype (including variable expression of CXCL13), in which the patients lack significant adenopathy at the onset of disease or the clinical signs/symptoms suggestive of AITL. CXCL13 is not well described in other cutaneous T-cell lymphomas, although there is at least one report of TFH marker expression in rare cases of mycosis fungoides/Sézary syndrome.

CXCL13 is less often used in the diagnostic workup of B-cell neoplasms, although TFH cells are often seen in the background in tissues involved by nodular lymphocyte-predominant Hodgkin lymphoma (NLPHL), follicular lymphoma, or chronic lymphocytic leukemia/small lymphocytic lymphoma (CLL/SLL). In NLPHL, the neoplastic B cells (so-called "popcorn" or LP cells) are surrounded by rosettes of TFH cells; however, CXCL13 has been shown to have a very low sensitivity for detecting these TFH cells, and PD-1 is considered to be a superior antibody for this application.

TFH cells have been shown to play a role in the proliferation of the neoplastic cells in CLL/SLL, and TFH cells are often present in the lymph nodes of CLL/SLL patients. Of note, PD-1 immunoreactivity among the neoplastic cells has been described in cases of CLL/SLL; however, significant CXCL13 expression has not been reported to our knowledge. CXCL13 staining has also been described in macrophages found in lymph nodes from patients with CLL/SLL. In our experience, CXCL13 immunoreactivity can occasionally be observed on B cells (likely representing CXCL13 bound to its receptor CXCR5 on B cells), and expansions of benign TFH cells can also be seen in a variety of benign immunologic reactions.

There is increasing evidence that TFH cells aberrantly support auto-reactive B cells in autoimmune disease. Several human autoimmune diseases, including systemic lupus erythematosis, autoimmune thyroid disease, myasthenia gravis, ankylosing spondylitis, and rheumatoid arthritis, are associated with increased numbers of TFH cells, and CXCL13 could potentially serve as a biomarker for some autoimmune disorders; however, these applications are outside the scope of this chapter.

Selected references

Burkle A, Neidermeier M, Schmitt-Graff A, *et al.* Overexpression of the CXCR5 chemokine receptor, and its ligand, CXCL13 in B cell chronic lymphocytic leukemia. *Blood* 2007; 110: 3316–25.

Dupuis J, Boye K, Martin N, *et al.* Expression of CXCL13 by neoplastic cells in angioimmunoblastic T cell lymphoma (AITL): A new diagnostic marker providing evidence that AITL derives from follicular helper T cells. *American Journal of Surgical Pathology* 2006; 30: 490–4.

Nam-Cha SH, Roncador G, Sanchez-Verde L, *et al.* PD-1, a follicular T-cell marker useful for recognizing nodular lymphocyte-predominant Hodgkin lymphoma. *American Journal of Surgical Pathology* 2008; 32: 1252–7.

Ortonne N, Dupuis J, Plonquet A, *et al.* Characterization of CXCL13+ neoplastic T cells in cutaneous lesions of angioimmunoblastic T cell lymphoma (AITL). *American Journal of Surgical Pathology* 2007; 31: 1068–76.

Cyclin D1 (Bcl-1)

Sources/clones

Dako (DCS-6), Immunotech (5D4), Novocastra (P2D11F11, DCS-6).

Fixation/preparation

Clone DCS-6 is effective on paraffin wax embedded tissue. We have found that microwave antigen unmasking in Tris buffer produces an optimum immunoreaction. Alkaline pH of 8–10 produces the best results, although tissue sections do not tolerate the higher pH. The combination of superheating to 120 °C and Tris buffer at pH 8 produces optimal immunostaining.

Background

The G1 cyclin gene, cyclin D1 (*PRAD1*, *CCND1*), located on chromosome 11q13, exhibits characteristics of known cellular oncogenes. It plays an integral role in normal cell growth control and a complementary role in the in-vitro transformation of cultured cells. Mechanisms of abnormal 11q13 regulation leading to cyclin D1 overexpression include genomic amplification in a variety of carcinomas, characteristic t(11;14) (q13;q32) reciprocal chromosomal translocations in mantle cell lymphoma, and chromosome 11 pericentric inversions in parathyroid adenomas. Together, cyclin D1 and cyclin-dependent kinase (Cdk) activities are required for completion of the G1/S transition in the normal mammalian cell cycle. Further, cyclin D1 inhibits the growth-suppressive function of retinoblastoma tumor-suppressor protein. Cyclin D1 is a 36 kDa protein, with maximum expression of cyclin D1 occurring at a critical point in mid to late G1 phase of the cell cycle. Recombinant prokaryotic fusion protein is used as the antigen to raise antibody to cyclin D1 (Class IgG2a). In normal tissues, cyclin D1 expression is restricted to the proliferative zone of epithelial tissues, and is absent from several other tissues such as lymph node, spleen, and tonsil.

Applications

Many neoplasms, including mantle cell lymphoma, parathyroid adenomas, and a spectrum of carcinomas including breast, supradiaphragmatic squamous cell, ovarian, and bladder transitional cell carcinomas demonstrate overexpression of cyclin D1 antibody on paraffin sections. Immunohistochemical demonstration of nuclear cyclin D1 protein was observed in 75% of mantle cell lymphoma, and was not found in normal B cells and other B-cell lymphomas (including follicle center cell lymphoma, diffuse large B-cell lymphoma, lymphocytic lymphoma, and MALT lymphoma). More recent interest in this marker involves its potential as a prognostic indicator in a variety of epithelial tumors. Cyclin D1 overexpression has been demonstrated in metastasizing papillary microadenocarcinomas of the thyroid. Overexpression of the protein predicted poor prognosis in estrogen receptor-negative breast cancer patients, recurrence in nasopharyngeal carcinoma, and reduced disease-free survival in papillary bladder carcinoma.

There is diffuse immunoreactivity in high-grade endometrial stromal sarcomas, allowing distinction from low-grade endometrial and undifferentiated uterine sarcoma.

Comments

Cyclin D1 is the main marker currently available to distinguish mantle cell lymphoma from the other small B-cell lymphomas (Appendix 2.8). Breast cancer tissue may be used as positive controls.

Selected reference

Bartkova J, Lukas J, Strauss M, Bartek J. Cell cycle-related variation and tissue-restricted expression of human cyclin D1 protein. *Journal of Pathology* 1994; 172: 237–45.

NOTES

Cytokeratins

Cytokeratins (CKs) belong to a group of proteins known as intermediate filaments (IFs) that constitute the cytoskeletal structure of virtually all epithelial cells. Being intermediate between microfilaments (6 nm) and microtubules (25 nm), the intermediate filaments comprise five characteristic groups based on cellular origin: CKs (epithelium), glial (astrocytes), neurofilaments (nerve cells), desmin (muscle), and vimentin (mesenchymal cells). More recently, these families of cytoskeletal proteins – the intermediate filaments – have been reclassified into six types (Table 1).

Intermediate filament proteins are composed of a 310 amino acid residue central region known as the rod domain, which is flanked by end domains of varying length and sequence, known as the head and tail. It is these flanking sequences that are the most immunogenic, responsible for the different properties and functions of the intermediate filament proteins. Being exposed, these molecules are also sensitive to fixation artifact due to the formation of cross-linkages. It is also important to note that because of the 30–50% sequence homology between the amino acid sequences of intermediate filaments of different types, monoclonal antibodies may cross-react with different intermediate filament types.

CKs are present in both benign and malignant epithelial cells, independent of cellular differentiation. However, CK immunohistochemistry utilizing subset-selective antibodies has extended beyond the typing of epithelial tumors, with recent descriptions of non-epithelial cells and tumors expressing CK.

The CKs are a family of proteins coded by different genes, and the expression in epithelial cells is dependent on the embryonic development and degree of cellular differentiation. In practice, the most important CKs have

Table 1 Classification of intermediate filaments

Type	Intermediate filament protein
I	Acidic cytokeratin (CK9-20)
II	Basic cytokeratin (CK1-8)
III	Vimentin (mesenchymal cells), desmin (muscle), glial fibrillary acid protein (glial cells and astrocytes), peripherin (neuronal cells)
IV	Neurofilaments protein triplet (neurons)
V	Nuclear laminin proteins (nuclear lamina)
VI	Nestin (CNS stem cells)

Table 2 Cytokeratins according to Moll's classification[a]

Moll's cytokeratin groups	Chromosome localization	Molecular weight ($\times 10^{-3}$)	Isoelectric point
K1	12	67	7.8
K2	12	65	6.1
K3	12	64	7.5
K4	12	59	7.3
K5	12	58	7.4
K6	12	56	7.8
K7	12	54	6.0
K8	12	52	6.1
K9	17	64	5.4
K10	17	56.5	5.3
K11	17	56	5.3
K12	17	55	4.9
K13	17	51	5.1
K14	17	50	5.3
K15	17	50	4.9
K16	17	48	5.1
K17	17	46	5.1
K18	17	45	5.7
K19	17	40	5.2
K20	17	46	5.7

[a] Moll R, Franke WW, Schiller DL, Geiger B, Krepler R. The catalog of human cytokeratins: patterns of expression in normal epithelia, tumors and cultured cells. *Cell* 1982; **31**: 11–24.

Table 3 Keratins 1–20, with their molecular weights and most important distributions

Type II	Molecular weight (kDa)	Distribution	Type I	Molecular weight (kDa)
		Epidermis – palms and soles	9	64
1	67	Epidermis, keratinizing squamous epithelia	10	56.5
2	65		11	56
3	63	Cornea	12	55
4	59	Non-keratinizing squamous epithelia (internal organs)	13	51
5	58	Basal cells – squamous and glandular epithelia, myoepithelium, mesothelium	14	50
		Squamous epithelia	15	50
6	56	Squamous epithelia (hyperproliferative)	16	48
7	54	Simple epithelia, basal cells – glandular epithelia, myoepithelium	17	46
8	52	Simple epithelia	18	45
		Simple epithelia, most glandular, some squamous epithelia (basal)	19	40
		Simple epithelia – intestines and stomach, Merkel cells	20	46

Modified from Miettinen M. Keratin immunohistochemistry: update of applications and pitfalls. *Pathology Annual* 1993; **28** (2): 113–43.
Keratin pairs appear on the same line.

Table 4 Summary of the most important keratin subtypes of some epithelial tumors

Carcinoma type	Keratin composition (Moll's catalog)									
	4	5	7	8	13	14	17	18	19	20
Squamous cell carcinoma, skin		+				+			+[a]	
Squamous cell carcinoma of esophagus	+				+	+			+	
Ductal carcinoma of breast			+	+		+[a]	+[a]	+	+	
Malignant mesothelioma		+	+	+		+		+	+	
Adenocarcinoma, lung			+	+				+	+	
Adenocarcinoma, colon				+				+	+	+
Adenocarcinoma, pancreas			+	+				+	+	+[a]
Hepatocellular carcinoma				+				+	+[a]	
Carcinoid tumor/small-cell carcinoma				+				+	+[b]	
Merkel cell carcinoma				+				+	+	+
Renal (cell) adenocarcinoma				+				+	+[b]	
Transitional cell carcinoma, low grade	+		+	+	+			+	+	+[a]
Transitional cell carcinoma, high grade			+	+	+[a]			+	+	
Thyroid carcinoma, papillary				+				+	+	
Thyroid carcinoma, follicular				+				+	+[a]	
Adenocarcinoma of prostate			+[a]	+				+	+	
Adenocarcinoma of ovary			+	+				+	+	+[a]

Modified from Miettinen M. Keratin immunohistochemistry: update of applications and pitfalls. *Pathology Annual* 1993; **28** (2): 113–43.
[a] Occasionally present/minor component.
[b] Often but inconsistently present.

been classified and numbered (Table 2). These CKs were identified by the biochemical properties in two-dimensional gel electrophoresis of tissue extracts, with their identification based on their isoelectric points and molecular weight. Hence, two groups of CKs emerge: type I/A (CK9–20) with an acidic isoelectric point, and type II/B (CK1–8) with a basic-neutral isoelectric point. Apart from a few exceptions, CKs are numbered from the highest to the lowest molecular weight in each group (Table 3).

Table 5 Specificities of selected cytokeratin antibodies

Molecular Weight (kDa)	35βH11	34βE12	AE1	AE3	Anti-Bovine keratin[a]	Anti-Callus keratin[a]	Cam 5.2	KL1	MNF116
39							+		+
40			+					+	
45							+	+	+
48			+	+					
50		+	+						
51				+					
52			+	+					
52.5									
54	+								+
56					+	+	+	+	
56.5		+	+	+					
57		+						+	+
58		+		+	+				
60					+		+		
64						+			
65				+					
65.5									
66					+			+	
67				+					
68		+							

Specificities as supplied by manufacturers.
Antibody sources: 35βH11 and 34βE12 (Dakopatts, California, USA); Anti-Bovine keratin, Anti-Callus keratin (Dakopatts, California, USA); AE1, AE3 (available as AE1/3 cocktail) (Boehringer, Sydney, Australia; Dakopatts, California, USA); Cam 5.2 (Becton Dickinson, California, USA); KL1 (Immunotech, Marseille, France); MNF116 (Dakopatts, California, USA).
[a] Polyclonal antisera.
Other cytokeratin cocktails not included above: Pankeratin cocktail (Bio Tek Solution, Inc., Santa Barbara, CA, USA – cocktail of AE1, AE3, Cam 5.2, and 35βH11); LP34 (Dako Corp, Capinteria, CA, USA – K5, K6, K17, and K19); Pancytokeratin antibodies (Novocastra, Burlingame, CA, USA – K5, K6, K8, and K18); Anti-cytokeratin 5/6 (Chemicon International, Inc., Temecula, CA, USA – K5 and K6).

An interesting phenomenon is the existence of the keratin intermediate filaments as pairs. With some exceptions, all other CKs form polymers with their corresponding member from each type (Table 3). Hence it follows that all epithelial cells contain at least two CKs. For example, while hepatocytes harbor a single pair of CK8 and CK18, keratinocytes may contain as many as 10 CKs.

Thus, these laws governing the expression of various CKs are observed in part by neoplastic cells, forming the basis for the application of antibodies to CKs within neoplastic cells (indicating epithelial differentiation) using immunohistochemical methods. The emergence of selective monoclonal antibodies identifying individual CKs now offers the advantage of immunohistochemical detection with morphological correlation. Monoclonal antibodies to CKs may be divided into two categories: (1) a broad group that recognizes many members of the keratin family and (2) a selective group that reacts with isolated CKs; in this regard, only CKs 7 and 20 will be considered in detail. Nevertheless, Table 4 provides a list of the most important CK subtypes in some epithelial neoplasms. In addition, popular commercially available antibodies to broad groups of CKs are also detailed individually (Table 5). False negativity due to masking of keratin epitopes and loss of antigenicity warrants antigen retrieval in most instances. Hence, the need for extensive and carefully controlled optimization of every new antibody before diagnostic application cannot be overemphasized.

Selected references

Battifora H. Diagnostic uses of antibodies to keratins: a review and immunohistochemical comparison of seven monoclonal and three polyclonal antibodies. In Fenoglio-Preiser CM, Wolff M, Rilke F, eds. *Progress in*

Surgical Pathology, Vol. VIII. Berlin: Springer-Verlag, 1988, pp. 10–15.

Heatley, MK. Cytokeratins and cytokeratin staining in diagnostic histopathology (commentary). *Histopathology* 1996; 28: 479–83.

Miettinen M. Keratin immunohistochemistry: update of applications and pitfalls. *Pathology Annual* 1993; 28 (2): 113–43.

Cytokeratin 5/6 (CK5/6)

Sources/clones

Boehringer Mannheim, Chemicon International, Dako (Clone D5/16B4), Zymed Laboratories.

Fixation/preparation

The antibody is immunoreactive in formalin-fixed tissues, and reactivity is enhanced by heat-stimulated antigen retrieval combined with enzyme digestion.

Background

Cytokeratins 5 and 6 correspond to keratins of 58 and 56 kDa respectively. Clone D5/16B4 is a monoclonal antibody raised against cytokeratin 5 (CK5). CK5 (58 kDa) is a high-molecular-weight basic type of cytokeratin expressed in the basal, intermediate, and superficial layers of stratified epithelia, transitional epithelium and mesothelium. CK6 (56 kDa) is also a high-molecular-weight basic cytokeratin expressed by proliferating squamous epithelium, palmoplantar cell, mucosa, and epidermal appendages. Although this combination of cytokeratins is expressed by a number of different epithelia, its popularity stems from its use in the diagnosis of mesothelioma. Morphologically, the mesothelium is similar to simple epithelium, and, like adenocarcinomas, mesotheliomas express simple epithelial keratins such as CK7, CK8, and CK19. Similar to squamous cell carcinoma, mesotheliomas also express the stratified epithelial keratins such as CK14, CK5/6, and CK17.

Using the AE14 monoclonal antibody that recognizes keratin 5, immunopositivity is seen in 92% (12/13) of epithelial and biphasic mesotheliomas with negative results in pulmonary adenocarcinomas. While recommended as a useful marker to distinguish epithelial mesotheliomas from pulmonary adenocarcinomas, these results were not repeated, probably due to the restricted use of keratin 5 on frozen tissue. More recently, a study using CK5/6 on formalin-fixed paraffin-embedded tissue demonstrated positive immunostaining in 100% of pleural epithelial mesotheliomas, with 81% of pulmonary adenocarcinomas being negative. The remaining adenocarcinomas were weak, equivocal, or focally positive. However, the majority of sarcomatoid or desmoplastic mesotheliomas in this study were negative for CK5/6. Another study produced a 100% cytokeratin 5/6 immunopositivity in epithelial mesotheliomas with reciprocal negativity in pulmonary adenocarcinomas. The frequency of CK5/6 positivity in mesotheliomas varies because of case selection, sarcomatoid mesothelioma being less likely to be positive than biphasic and epithelioid mesothelioma.

Applications

CK5/6 is useful in discriminating between epithelial mesotheliomas and pulmonary adenocarcinomas but does not exclude metastatic carcinomas from some sites, as the latter may be positive for CK5/6. Furthermore, as it is often negative in sarcomatoid mesothelioma, CK5/6 is best utilized in a panel of antibodies for this differential diagnosis. CK5/6 also stains both reactive and neoplastic mesothelium. It has also been suggested for use in the differential diagnosis of squamous cell carcinoma and adenocarcinoma, being positive in basal cells and stratum spinosum cells of squamous epithelium so that the immunoexpression of CK5/6 in a poorly differentiated metastatic carcinoma is highly predictive of a primary tumor of squamous differentiation. It has been reported that intense CK5/6 positivity in ductal hyperplasia and negative staining of most cases of atypical ductal hyperplasia and ductal carcinoma in situ (DCIS) may assist in the differential diagnosis of atypical proliferations of the breast, but this requires confirmation. It should be noted that this marker is of low specificity, as adenocarcinoma of the salivary gland and lung, squamous cell carcinoma of the lung, anus, esophagus, cervix, upper aerodigestive tract, and skin, and carcinomas of the urinary bladder, breast, and pancreas, as well as synovial sarcoma, have been reported to immunoexpress CK5/6.

CK5/6 immunostaining has been employed successfully as a substitute for 34βE12 for the identification of basal cells in benign prostatic glands, allowing their distinction from neoplastic glands.

Comments

CK5/6 demonstrates a diffuse cytoplasm immunopositive reaction. Skin or prostate gland may be a useful source of positive control tissue.

Selected references

Chu PG, Weiss LM. Expression of cytokeratin 5/6 in epithelial neoplasms: an immunohistochemical study of 509 cases. *Modern Pathology* 2002; 15: 6–10.

Chu PG, Weiss LM. Keratin expression in human tissues and neoplasms. *Histopathology* 2002; 40: 403–39.

Cytokeratin 7 (CK7)

Sources/clones

Accurate (LP5K), American Research Products (RCK105), Biodesign, Biogenesis (C-35, C18), Biogenex (OV-TL 12/30), Bioprobe (C-35, C68), Boehringer Mannheim (KS7–18), Chemicon, Cymbus Bioscience (C46, LP5K), Dako (OV-TL 12/30), Intracell Corp (RCK105), Japan Tanner (C-35, C68), Milab (RCK 105), Novocastra (LP5K), Sanbio (OV-TL 12/30, RCK105), Saxon (RCB105), Sera Lab (CK7), Sigma (LD5 68).

Fixation/preparation

CK7 can be used on formalin-fixed paraffin-embedded tissue sections. Enzymatic digestion with proteolytic enzymes such as trypsin should be performed before staining. Pronase digestion has been found to be harsh on CK7. This antibody may also be used on acetone- and/or methanol-fixed cryostat sections or fixed cell smears. It enjoys the additional advantage of being used on cytological preparations already stained by the Papanicolaou stain. For cell smears, the APAAP technique is recommended.

Background

CK7 antibody reacts with the 54 kDa cytokeratin intermediate filament protein isolated from human OTN II ovarian carcinoma cells and other cell lines. Identified as CK7 according to Moll's catalog, it is a basic cytokeratin found in most glandular and transitional epithelia.

In normal tissue CK7 reacts with many ductal and glandular epithelia, but not stratified squamous epithelia. It is also reactive with transitional epithelium of urinary tract. Hepatocytes are negative while bile ducts are positive. In addition, lung and breast epithelia are positive with this antibody, while colon and prostate epithelial cells are negative.

Applications

CK7 is expressed in specific subtypes of ovarian, breast, and lung adenocarcinoma, while carcinomas of the colon are negative. Recent studies have indicated that a CK7+/CK20– immunophenotype is helpful in distinguishing metastatic colonic adenocarcinoma from primary ovarian carcinomas, particularly the endometrioid type (with the exception of the mucinous type) (Appendix 1.14, 1.15). Occasional ovarian mucinous carcinomas may show the same immunophenotype as metastatic colonic carcinomas (CK7–/CK20+). Using the same immunophenotypic profile (together with CK18), CK7 has been shown to assist in determining that most ovarian mucinous tumors in pseudomyxoma peritonei in woman are secondary to appendiceal adenoma.

CK7 is also useful in distinguishing transitional cell carcinomas (CK7+) from prostate cancer (CK7–). The failure of CK7 to interact with squamous cell carcinomas presents the potential for specificity for adenocarcinoma and transitional cell carcinoma.

Comments

We have found the combined use of CK7 and CK20 to be extremely useful in distinguishing ovarian carcinomas (except mucinous) from colonic adenocarcinomas. Serous ovarian carcinoma tissue is recommended for positive control tissue.

Selected reference

Moll R, Franke WW, Schiller DL, Geiger B, Krepler R. The catalog of human cytokeratins: patterns of expression in normal epithelia, tumors and cultured cells. *Cell* 1982; 31: 11–24.

NOTES

Cytokeratin 19 (CK19)

Sources/clones

Abcam (ab15463), Dako (RCK108), Leica Biosystems (NCL-L-CK19), Santa Cruz Biotech (RCK108), Thermo Scientific (RCK108), Ventana (A53-B/A2.26).

Fixation/preparation

The antibody can be used in formalin-fixed paraffin-embedded tissue. Pretreatment of deparaffinized tissue sections with HIER is required.

Background

CK19, like other cytokeratins, is an intermediate filament protein, and a component of the cell cytoskeleton. Cytokeratins have an important mechanical function in maintaining the structural integrity of epithelial cells. They also play a critical role in cell differentiation and are useful markers of tissue specialization. It is this property of cytokeratins that is maintained in malignant transformation and utilized in the characterization of different tumor types.

One of the more abundant cytokeratins, CK19 has a low molecular weight and is normally expressed in the cytoplasm of epithelial cells of the gastrointestinal tract including the appendix, gallbladder, pancreas, tonsil, ureter and bronchus, cervical glands in the ectocervix and endocervix, epithelial cells and Hassall's corpuscles in thymus, basal keratinocytes in tongue, endometrial glandular epithelium, ducts in parotid gland and testis, pneumocytes in lung, bile ducts in liver, glandular epithelium in breast, trophoblasts in placenta, tubules in kidney, and ductal epithelium in skin.

It is also expressed in several malignant neoplasms, including squamous cell carcinomas of the head and neck, cervix, and lung, urothelial carcinoma, papillary thyroid carcinomas, a minority of follicular thyroid carcinomas, infiltrating ductal carcinomas of the breast, adenocarcinomas of the gastrointestinal tract including appendix and colorectum, neuroendocrine tumors and neuroendocrine carcinomas of the gastrointestinal tract, pancreatic adenocarcinoma, cholangiocarcinoma, prostatic adenocarcinoma, mucinous and serous cystadenocarcinoma, clear cell carcinomas of the ovary, endometrial adenocarcinoma, and extramammary Paget's disease (EMPD).

Applications

On a cellular level, CK19 is typically expressed in a cytoplasmic pattern with coexisting complete or partial membranous expression. The other staining pattern noted is paranuclear dot-like accentuation with and without cytoplasmic/membrane staining.

The use of CK19 immunohistochemistry in diagnostic pathology has been mainly to confirm epithelial immunophenotype in undifferentiated-appearing tumors, or to establish pancreaticobiliary ductular origin, usually as part of a larger panel of markers.

In one study, in conjunction with morphological findings, the sensitivity of a panel of anti-human mesothelial cell antibody (HBME-1), CK19, and CD56 was found to be 95.6% in the diagnosis of papillary thyroid carcinoma (classic and follicular variants). CK19 immunostain has also been utilized in thyroid fine needle aspiration specimens, and along with HBME-1 expression has been shown to increase diagnostic accuracy with increased sensitivity and specificity.

In benign liver diseases associated with ductopenia, immunostains for biliary markers such as CK19 and CK7 may be used as a complementary tool to evaluate loss of native interlobular bile ducts.

CK19 positivity is an independent marker of aggressive behavior in pancreatic neuroendocrine tumors, but has been shown to be a favorable marker of tumor cells of EMPD.

Selected references

Ali A, Serra S, Asa SL, *et al.* The predictive value of CK19 and CD99 in pancreatic endocrine tumors. *American Journal of Surgical Pathology* 2006; 30: 1588–94.

Chetty R. An overview of practical issues in the diagnosis of gastroenteropancreatic neuroendocrine pathology. *Archives of Pathology and Laboratory Medicine* 2008; 132: 1285–9.

Deshpande V, Fernandez-del Castillo C, Muzikansky A, *et al.* Cytokeratin 19 is a powerful predictor of survival in pancreatic endocrine tumors. *American Journal of Surgical Pathology* 2004; 28: 1145–53.

Jain R, Fischer S, Serra S, *et al.* The use of cytokeratin 19 (CK19) immunohistochemistry in lesions of the pancreas, gastrointestinal tract, and liver. *Applied Immunohistochemistry and Molecular Morphology* 2010; 18: 9–15.

Nechifor-Boila A, Borda A, Sassolas G, *et al.* Immunohistochemical markers in the diagnosis of papillary thyroid carcinomas: the promising role of combined immunostaining using HBME-1 and CD56. *Pathology, Research and Practice* 2013; 209: 585–92.

Rosai J. Immunohistochemical markers of thyroid tumors: significance and diagnostic applications. *Tumori* 2003; 89: 517–19.

Ryu HS, Lee K, Shin E, *et al.* Comparative analysis of immunohistochemical markers for differential diagnosis of hepatocelluar carcinoma and cholangiocarcinoma. *Tumori* 2012; 98: 478–84.

Cytokeratin 20 (CK20)

Sources/clones

American Research Products (IT-Ks 20.10, IT-Ks 20.3, IT-Ks 20.5), Biodesign, Cymbus Biosciences (Ks 20.8, Ks 20.3, Ks 20.5), Dako (K20.8), Progen (IT-Ks 20.3, IT-Ks 20.5, IT-Ks 20.8).

Fixation/preparation

Formalin-fixed paraffin-embedded tissue is ideally suited for this antibody. Immunoreactivity requires pretreatment with a sodium citrate buffer with heated antigen retrieval. Enzyme pretreatment (trypsin or pronase) should not be used as it abolishes signal. The antibody is not recommended for cryostat sections or cell smears due to cross-reactivity with CK20-negative epithelia.

Background

CK20 is a low-molecular-weight cytokeratin that was originally identified as protein IT in two-dimensional gel electrophoresis of cytoskeletal extracts of intestinal epithelia. The antibody reacts with the 46 kDa cytokeratin intermediate filament isolated from villi of duodenal mucosa.

CK20 is less acidic than other type 1 cytokeratins, and it is particularly interesting because of its restricted range of expression. In normal tissues it is expressed only in gastrointestinal epithelium, urothelium, and Merkel cells. Other epithelial cells, including breast epithelia, do not react with CD20, nor does it recognize other intermediate filament proteins.

Applications

Following extensive testing on both primary and metastatic carcinomas, it was concluded that tumors expressing CK20 were derived from normal epithelia expressing CK20. Hence, colorectal carcinomas consistently express CK20 while gastric adenocarcinomas and other carcinomas of the gastrointestinal tract express this cytokeratin isotype less frequently. In addition, adenocarcinomas of the biliary tree and pancreatic duct, mucinous ovarian tumors, and transitional-cell carcinomas also demonstrate positive immunoreaction. Hence, the application of CK20 antibody for determining the site of origin of carcinomas has been mooted, largely due to absence of CK20 expression in adenocarcinomas of the breast, lung, and endometrium, and in non-mucinous tumors of the ovary (Appendix 1.14, 1.15, 1.20, 1.32). In fact, CK20 has contributed to immunohistochemical evidence supporting the appendiceal origin of pseudomyxoma peritonei in women.

Immunostaining for CK7 and CK20 has been shown to be useful in the differentiation of ovarian metastases from colonic carcinoma and primary ovarian carcinoma. A CK7–/CK20+ immunophenotype was seen in 94% of metastatic colonic carcinomas to the ovary, 5% of primary ovarian mucinous carcinomas, and none of the primary ovarian endometrioid or serous carcinomas.

The almost consistent staining of Merkel cell carcinoma for CK20 and the very low frequency of CK20 reactivity in other small-cell carcinomas (except those of salivary gland origin) can help to resolve the diagnostic dilemma between Merkel cell carcinoma and metastatic small-cell carcinoma presenting in the skin (Appendix 1.20). In fact, it has been shown that CK20 positivity in a small-cell carcinoma of uncertain origin is strongly predictive of Merkel cell carcinoma, especially when the majority of tumor cells are positive. In contrast, a negative CK20 reaction practically rules out Merkel cell carcinoma, provided an effective antigen retrieval technique is used and appropriate immunoreaction obtained with other cytokeratin antibodies.

Finally, CK20 positivity is often encountered in transitional cell carcinomas of the bladder but is rare in squamous carcinomas of that organ or adenocarcinoma of prostate.

Table 1 CK7 and CK20 immunoexpression in epithelial tumors

	CK20+	CK20−
CK20	Bladder Breast Colon Bile duct Ovary mucinous Pancreas Stomach	Cervical Endometrium Esophagus Breast Gastrointestinal tract carcinoid Bile duct Pancreas Kidney Liver Lung carcinoid Neuroendocrine Lung squamous Lung small-cell Mesothelioma Ovary Salivary gland Thyroid
CK7	Merkel cell Stomach Colon	Adrenal cortex Esophagus Gastrointestinal tract carcinoid Germ cell Kidney Liver Lung carcinoid Neuroendocrine carcinoma Lung squamous Lung small-cell Mesothelioma Prostatic Soft tissue epithelioid sarcoma Thymus

Comments

The combined application of CK20 and CK7 allows the separation of a number of epithelial tumors, as shown in Table 1.

CK20 works extremely well in paraffin sections with microwave antigen retrieval in citrate buffer. It is extremely useful for distinguishing between colonic and non-mucinous ovarian adenocarcinomas. Identifying Merkel cell carcinoma from metastatic small-cell carcinoma to the skin is also easily accomplished with CK20. Colonic carcinoma tissue sections should be used as positive control tissue.

Selected reference

Chan JKC, Suster S, Wenig BM, *et al*. Cytokeratin 20 immunoreactivity distinguishes Merkel cell (primary cutaneous neuroendocrine) carcinomas and salivary gland small cell carcinomas from small cell carcinomas of various sites. *American Journal of Surgical Pathology* 1997; 21: 226–34.

Cytokeratins: AE1/AE3

Sources/clones

Dako (AE1/AE3), Zymed (AE1, AE3).

Fixation/preparation

This antibody is suitable for immunohistochemical staining of formalin-fixed paraffin-embedded or frozen tissue sections. Trypsin or pepsin digestion/antigen retrieval is necessary before staining of formalin-fixed paraffin-embedded tissue sections, although pepsin has been found to be superior to trypsin. The Zymed antibody is prediluted and ready to use. However, if 3,3'-diaminobenzidine (DAB) is used as a chromogen for immunodetection, then a further dilution of the primary antibody may be required.

Background

The antibody AE1/AE3 is a mixture of two monoclonal antibodies, raised against human epidermal keratins. AE1 recognizes most of the acidic (type I) keratins with molecular weights 56.5, 50, 48, and 40 kDa. AE3 recognizes all known basic (type II) cytokeratins. This combination shows broad reactivity and is claimed to stain almost all epithelia and their neoplasms. It is also reputed not to cross-react with other members of the intermediate filaments.

Applications

The wide reactivity of AE1/AE3 expressed in simple epithelia and their tumors, including cytokeratins expressed in complex stratified squamous epithelia, permits identification of a wide range of epithelial-derived tumors. Hence, strong staining of AE1/AE3 has been demonstrated in adenocarcinomas (e.g., colorectal, gastric, breast, prostate), renal cell carcinoma, hepatocellular carcinoma, transitional cell carcinoma, small-cell carcinoma, carcinoid tumors, epithelial component of pleomorphic adenoma, and squamous cell carcinoma of the skin (including the spindle cell variant), cervix, and bronchus. Thymomas, mesotheliomas (including the sarcomatoid component), and chordomas consistently stain with AE1/AE3. Non-epithelial tumors that demonstrate AE1/AE3 positivity include germ cell tumors (except seminomas), synovial sarcoma, and epithelioid sarcoma. Cross-reactivity in some leiomyosarcomas has been documented.

In a study of 290 cases of hepatocellular carcinoma, immunohistochemical evidence of biliary differentiation (reactivity with AE1/AE3 or cytokeratin 19) was found in 29.3% of cases. These hepatocellular carcinomas with biliary differentiation showed clinical features of greater aggressiveness with poorer cellular differentiation and higher expression of proliferation markers.

Comments

The pan-keratin marking potential of antibody AE1/AE3 places it in an ideal position to screen for neoplasms of epithelial origin, especially poorly differentiated carcinomas of diverse origin, and to distinguish these from melanoma and lymphoma. Another useful role is the identification of micrometastases, e.g., breast secondaries in lymph nodes and bone marrow.

Selected reference

Battifora H. Diagnostic uses of antibodies to keratins: a review and immunohistochemical comparison of seven monoclonal and three polyclonal antibodies. In Fenoglio-Preiser CM, Wolff M, Rilke F. eds. *Progress in Surgical Pathology*, Vol. VIII. Berlin: Springer-Verlag, 1988, pp. 10–15.

NOTES

Cytokeratins: 34βE12

Sources/clones

Dako, Enzo diagnostics.

Fixation/preparation

34βE12 may be used on formalin-fixed paraffin-embedded tissue sections. Although reactivity on formalin-fixed tissue is obtainable, better consistency is observed on Carnoy's or methacarn-fixed material. Proteolytic treatment with pronase (for prostatic basal cells) and microwave antigen retrieval (for papillary carcinoma of thyroid) is essential for formaldehyde-fixed material. This antibody may also be used on acetone-fixed cryostat sections and fixed cell smears. Incubation of the primary antibody for 1 hour at room temperature is sufficient for prostatic basal cells. However, incubation of primary antibody at 4 °C overnight is necessary for papillary carcinoma of the thyroid gland.

Background

34βE12 identifies keratins of approximately 66 kDa and 57 kDa in extracts of stratum corneum. The antibody reacts with keratins 1, 5, 10, and 14 in Moll's catalog (molecular weights 68 kDa, 58 kDa, 56.5 kDa, 50 kDa respectively). In normal tissue the antibody labels squamous, ductal, and other complex epithelia.

Applications

Perhaps the most useful application for 34βE12 is in the detection of basal cells of the prostatic acini. Demonstration of this high-molecular-weight cytokeratin in the basal cells of prostatic acini is indicative of benignity. Further, 34βE12 is negative in adenocarcinoma of the prostate. In this context 34βE12 is also useful to demonstrate the basal cells in basal cell hyperplasia (partial or atypical) and atypical adenomatous hyperplasia of the prostate, the latter being difficult to distinguish morphologically from prostatic adenocarcinoma.

More recently the role of 34βE12 in diagnostic thyroid pathology has been highlighted (Appendix 1.30). It was shown that 34βE12 positivity was confined to papillary carcinoma of the thyroid, whereas follicular neoplasms and hyperplastic nodules were either negative or showed focal staining.

34βE12 is also consistently positive in squamous cell carcinomas, ductal carcinoma of breast, and in pancreas, bile duct, and salivary gland carcinomas. It has also been demonstrated in transitional cell carcinomas of the bladder, and in nasopharyngeal carcinoma, thymomas, and epithelioid mesotheliomas.

While this antibody has a variable positivity with adenocarcinomas, it is negative in hepatocellular carcinoma, renal cell carcinoma, and endometrial carcinoma. Mesenchymal tumors, lymphomas, melanomas, neural tumors, and neuroendocrine tumors are negative.

Comments

We have found 34βE12 to be extremely useful in both prostatic and thyroid pathology. It should be noted that different incubation protocols need to be followed for these two applications of 34βE12.

Selected reference

Moll R, Franke WW, Schiller DL, Geiger B, Krepler R. The catalog of human cytokeratins: patterns of expression in normal epithelia, tumors and cultured cells. *Cell* 1982; 31: 11–24.

NOTES

Cytokeratins: CAM 5.2

Sources/clones

Becton Dickinson (CAM 5.2).

Fixation/preparation

CAM 5.2 can be applied to both frozen and formalin-fixed paraffin-embedded tissue. Trypsin enzyme pretreatment for antigen retrieval is essential for paraffin sections.

Background

CAM 5.2 was derived from hybridization of mouse cells with spleen cells from BALB/c mice immunized with a human colorectal carcinoma line, HT29. It comprises mouse IgG$_{2a}$ heavy chain and κ light chains from spleen parent and myeloma cell lines. The antibody CAM 5.2 detects human cytokeratin epitopes with molecular weights 52 kDa and 45 kDa, corresponding to Moll's catalog numbers 8 and 18 respectively. In normal tissue CAM 5.2 reacts with secretory epithelia but not stratified squamous epithelium.

Applications

Anti-cytokeratin antibody CAM 5.2 is useful for the detection of adenocarcinomas, mesotheliomas, and certain carcinomas derived from squamous epithelia, the latter including spindle cell carcinomas. It should, however, be noted that some squamous cell carcinomas do not stain with CAM 5.2, e.g., those in the cervix, vagina, and esophagus. The ability of CAM 5.2 to detect epithelial neoplasms but not normal stratified squamous epithelium (e.g., skin) can be exploited to distinguish Paget's disease (both mammary and extramammary) from superficial spreading melanoma. CAM 5.2 is especially useful in the demonstration of subtle metastatic deposits of breast carcinoma cells in lymph nodes and bone marrow. It also successfully reacts with renal cell carcinomas, hepatocellular carcinomas, and cholangiocarcinomas. CAM 5.2 also detects neuroendocrine carcinomas (including small-cell carcinoma and Merkel cell carcinomas), germ cell tumors (with the exception of seminoma showing dot-like cytoplasmic accentuation), and synovial and epithelioid sarcomas. This antibody is also useful for the detection of epithelial cells in thymomas, particularly when masked by lymphocytes. It is reputed not to detect melanomas (except in cryostat sections).

Non-epithelial tissues which react with anti-cytokeratin CAM 5.2 include smooth muscle, rare sarcomas of breast, meningiomas (hyaline bodies or malignant variants), and rosettes of neuroblastomas. B-cell anaplastic large-cell lymphoma, confirmed by immunohistochemistry and immunoglobulin gene rearrangements, has been shown to be immunoreactive with CAM 5.2.

It should also be noted that large-cell lymphoma of B-cell lineage (verified with PCR) has been shown to be rarely reactive for cytokeratin 8.

Comments

Although CAM 5.2 has a narrow range of cytokeratin immunodetection in surgical pathology, it has been proven to be useful as a second-line marker in specific circumstances: for example, in the identification of spindle cell carcinoma of the skin and subtle metastatic deposits of carcinoma in lymph nodes, and to distinguish Paget's disease from superficial spreading melanoma. It also shows strong staining reaction with neuroendocrine carcinomas.

Selected reference

Battifora H. Diagnostic uses of antibodies to keratins: a review and immunohistochemical comparison of seven monoclonal and three polyclonal antibodies. In Fenoglio-Preiser CM, Wolff M, Rilke F. eds. *Progress in Surgical Pathology*, Vol. VIII. Berlin: Springer-Verlag, 1988, pp. 10–15.

NOTES

Cytokeratins: MAK-6

Sources/clones

Triton Diagnostics, Zymed (KA4, UCD/PR 10.11).

Fixation/preparation

MAK-6 works well in routinely fixed paraffin-embedded tissue sections. Trypsin pretreatment is necessary for antigen unmasking. Incubation of the primary antibody for 1 hour at 37 °C or overnight incubation at room temperature yields superior immunostaining. Preincubation with blocking reagents to reduce non-specific background staining has been recommended, but we have found this to be unnecessary.

Background

MAK-6 antibody cocktail contains an optimized mixture of two murine monoclonal antibodies of IgG1 isotype. Antibody UCD/PR 10.11 was produced using shed extracellular antigen purified from MCF-7 tissue culture media and was selected for its specificity to cytokeratin types 8 and 18. Antibody KA4 was produced against human sole epidermis and was selected for its specificity to cytokeratin types 14, 15, 16, and 19.

Applications

MAK-6 is reputed to stain all cases of squamous cell carcinomas and the majority of adenocarcinomas, carcinoid tumors, and undifferentiated carcinomas. Lymphomas, melanomas, gliomas/astrocytomas, and the majority of sarcomas do not demonstrate MAK-6 positivity. The latter is related to the expected cytokeratin expression in synovial sarcomas and epithelioid sarcomas. It should be noted that the majority of ependymomas and basal cell carcinomas of the skin also do not express MAK-6. Caution should be observed in assessing metastatic carcinomas to the brain, since MAK-6 may rarely show cross-reactivity with neural tissue. In these instances application of antibody to glial fibrillary acidic protein (GRAP) would be helpful.

Comments

We have found MAK-6 to be a useful pan-keratin marker. Strong immunoreaction is demonstrated in tissue of epithelial origin. When MAK-6 is used in conjunction with other pan-keratin markers, the majority of neoplasms showing cytokeratin expression may be identified.

Selected reference

Cooper D, Schermer A, Sun TT. Classification of human epithelia and their neoplasms using monoclonal antibodies to keratins: strategies, applications and limitations. *Laboratory Investigation* 1985; 52: 243–56.

NOTES

Cytokeratins: MNF116

Sources/clones

Dako (MNF116), Immunotech (MNF116).

Fixation/preparation

MNF116 performs well on formalin-fixed paraffin-embedded tissue sections. Enzymatic predigestion with proteolytic enzymes such as trypsin and pronase is essential prior to immunodetection, trypsin being superior for MNF116. This antibody may also be applied to acetone-fixed cryostat sections or fixed cell smears. Incubation of the primary antibody for 1 hour at 37 °C yields better immunoreaction.

Background

MNF116 antibody detects an epitope that is present in a wide range of keratins. These comprise a number of discrete polypeptides, whose molecular weights range from 45 to 56.5 kDa. These correspond to Moll's keratin numbers 5, 6, 8, 17, and probably 19. The MNF116 immunogen was derived from a crude extract of splenic cells in a nude mouse engrafted with MCF-7 cells.

In normal tissue, the MNF116 antibody shows a broad pattern of reactivity with epithelial cells from simple glandular to stratified squamous epithelium. Epithelial cells are labeled irrespective of ectodermal, mesodermal, or endodermal origin. However, due to cross-reactivity with the other members of the family of intermediate filaments, this antibody (not unlike other monoclonal anti-keratin antibodies) cross-reacts with non-epithelial cells including smooth muscle, dendritic cells in lymph nodes, syncytiotrophoblasts, some cortical neurons, and a minority of plasma cells.

Applications

MNF116 demonstrates excellent immunopositivity with a wide range of benign and malignant epithelial neoplasms. A strong pattern of staining is observed in squamous cell carcinoma (including nasopharyngeal carcinoma), small-cell carcinoma, sarcomatoid carcinoma, spindle cell carcinoma, adenocarcinoma, and mesotheliomas. A characteristic juxtanuclear globular pattern of staining has been found to be extremely useful in identifying small-cell carcinomas. Both epithelioid and spindle cell components of mesotheliomas react with this antibody.

MNF116 is also useful in confirming the diagnosis in a wide range of soft tissue neoplasms. Monophasic and biphasic synovial sarcomas demonstrate strong positivity (albeit focal in the spindle cells). Vascular neoplasms that react with this broad-range cytokeratin antibody include epithelioid hemangioendothelioma (focal), epithelioid angiosarcoma, and sinonasal hemangiopericytoma. Epithelioid sarcoma (and the proximal variant) require cytokeratin positivity for diagnosis. Other tumors in which cytokeratin positivity is essential for diagnosis include desmoplastic small round-cell tumors, chordomas, and extrarenal rhabdoid tumors, which are consistently positive. Mixed tumors and myoepitheliomas arising in soft tissue have been shown to express pan-keratin.

Among germ cell tumors, embryonal carcinoma and yolk sac tumors are consistently positive with MNF116.

The following neoplasms may demonstrate aberrant staining with MNF116. The co-expression of cytokeratins in smooth muscle tumors is well described. Cytokeratin-positive cells have been revealed in plasmacytoma. A few primitive neuroectodermal tumors may show focal cytokeratin expression. Rarely, myofibroblasts may demonstrate focal cytokeratin positivity. Quite logically all of these potential diagnostic pitfalls may clearly be avoided if relevant panels of immunohistochemical antibodies are applied.

Comments

MNF116 has developed into a first-line antibody in the application of cytokeratins to surgical pathology. It is however necessary to be aware of the aberrant immunoreactions in order to avoid misdiagnosis. It is therefore unwise to arrive at a diagnosis based on the assessment of a single cytokeratin marker without the application of other relevant antibodies used in a diagnostic panel to exclude other possibilities. Any epithelial tissue – glandular or squamous – is suitable for use as positive control for MNF116.

Selected references

Miettinen M. Keratin immunohistochemistry: update of applications and pitfalls. *Pathology Annual* 1993; 28 (2): 113–43.

Moll R, Franke WW, Schiller DL, Geiger B, Krepler R. The catalog of human cytokeratins: patterns of expression in normal epithelia, tumors and cultured cells. *Cell* 1982; 31: 11–24.

Other pan-cytokeratin cocktails

A number of other pan-cytokeratin cocktails are commercially available.

Pankeratin cocktail (Bio Tek Solution, Inc, Santa Barbara, CA, USA) is a cocktail comprising monoclonal antibodies to AE1, AE3, Can 5.2, and 35βH11. This is a useful cocktail which reacts to virtually all epithelia and their corresponding tumors.

Pan-cytokeratin antibodies (Novocastra, Burlingame, CA, USA) contains monoclonal antibodies to CK5, CK6, CK8, and CK18. This cocktail is said to recognize almost all epithelial tissues and their neoplasms.

Clone L34 Antibody (Dako Corp., Carpinteria, CA, USA). A broad-spectrum monoclonal antibody that detects CK5, CK6, CK17, and CK19. It thus labels both simple glandular and stratified squamous epithelium.

Wide-spectrum Screening Antibody (Dako Corp., Carpinteria, CA, USA). This is a useful polyclonal antibody raised to bovine skin that cross-reacts with human keratins.

NOTES

Cytomegalovirus (CMV)

Sources/clones

Accurate (E13, CCH2), American Research Products (1692-18), Axcel (CCH2), Biodesign (084, BM204, BM219, polyclonal), Biogenesis (BM204, polyclonal), Biogenex (BM204, polyclonal), Chemicon, Dako (AAC10, CCH2), EY Labs, Fitzgerald (M2103126, M210312), Sera Lab (E13), Zymed (DDG9/CCH2).

Fixation/preparation

These antibodies are suitable for immunohistochemical staining of paraffin-embedded tissue sections. Enzymatic predigestion with trypsin or pepsin is required for clone CCH2. These antibodies may also be used to detect CMV early nuclear proteins in infected human embryonic fibroblasts 24 hours following inoculation of clinical specimens on cell culture.

Background

The CCH2 clone recognizes a 43 kDa protein, while the DDG9 clone recognizes a 76 kDa protein, both having been demonstrated in glycine-extracted CMV antigen. These proteins are expressed in the immediate early and early stage of CMV replication in infected cells. Early viral proteins are expressed in the nucleus of infected cells within 6–24 hours of infection and prior to viral DNA replication. Several late viral proteins may be demonstrated in the nucleus and the cytoplasm of infected cells. The different viral proteins can be demonstrated in infected cell cultures as well as in infected tissue. These antibodies do not cross-react with adenoviruses or other herpesviruses.

Applications

These antibodies to CMV demonstrate the virus in infected cells, producing a nuclear immunopositive reaction. However, at a later stage, both a nuclear and a cytoplasmic immunoreaction with the early CMV antigen is produced, especially with the Zymed product. Antibodies to CMV have a wide application to diagnostic surgical pathology, especially when characteristic CMV inclusions are not clearly evident. CMV infection (latent or active) may be seen in salivary glands, lungs, kidneys, gastrointestinal tract, and lymph nodes. Awareness of CMV as an opportunistic infection in the context of immunosuppression invokes the use of CMV immunohistochemistry for definitive diagnosis. CMV esophagitis has been observed as a florid aggregate of macrophages without typical inclusions. Conversely, chemotherapy toxicity may mimic CMV gastritis, necessitating CMV immunohistochemistry to exclude false positives. Antibodies to CMV may also be applied for the identification of atypical CMV inclusions in gastrointestinal mucosal biopsy specimens, where classic inclusions are rarely found. The proper recognition of CMV-infected cells in the context of immunosuppression is critical, so that effective therapy is not delayed, preventing further viral dissemination. Immunolabeling for CMV in transbronchial biopsies of transplanted lung shows alveolar epithelial cells and capillary endothelial cells as the major targets of CMV, with rare involvement of ciliated and bronchiolar smooth muscle cells.

Comments

It has been shown that immunohistochemistry with CCH2 detects a higher number of CMV-infected cells than in-situ hybridization. Hence, for routine diagnostic purposes at least, CMV immunohistochemistry would appear to be the method of choice for rapid, sensitive, and specific CMV detection.

Selected references

Swenson PD, Kaplan MH. Rapid detection of cytomegalovirus in cell culture by indirect immunoperoxidase staining with monoclonal antibody to an early nuclear antigen. *Journal of Clinical Microbiology* 1985; 21: 669–73.

Zweygberg WB, Wirgart B, Grillner L. Early detection of cytomegalovirus in cell culture by a monoclonal antibody. *Journal of Virological Methods* 1986; 14: 65–9.

Cytotoxic molecules (TIA-1, granzyme B, perforin)

Sources/clones

TIA-1

Coulter (2G9).

Granzyme B

Coulter (GB7), Sanbio/Monosan (GrB7), Dr. Kummer, Amsterdam, the Netherlands (GB9).

Perforin

Kaimya (KM583), Sumitomo Denko, Osaka, Japan (1B4), T cell Diagnostics (polyclonal).

Fixation/preparation

All antibodies against cytotoxic molecules can be used in formalin-fixed paraffin-embedded tissues. High-temperature antigen retrieval in citrate buffer is essential for staining.

Background

Natural killer (NK) cells and cytotoxic T lymphocytes are characterized by the presence of cytoplasmic granules that are released in response to target cell recognition. Among the wealth of cytotoxic molecules found in cytotoxic cells, perforin and granzyme B are two well-characterized proteins involved in one major pathway leading to apoptosis in target cells. Perforin allows for the entry of granzyme molecules into the target cells, which then activate the apoptotic protease CPP32. The genes for perforin and granzyme B have been cloned, and antibodies directed against these molecules have been generated.

T-cell-restricted intracellular antigen (TIA-1), another molecule found in cytotoxic cells, is recognized by the antibody 2G9. The exact function of TIA-1 has not been elucidated. Since it induces DNA fragmentation of digitonin-permeabilized thymocytes, it may be implicated in the killing induced by cytotoxic lymphocytes. TIA-1 has been demonstrated in many intestinal intraepithelial lymphocytes of normal proximal small intestine, and a corresponding increase of TIA-1 positive cells in active celiac disease.

Applications

The expression of all three cytotoxic molecules appears to be largely restricted to cytotoxic cells. In addition, in-vitro findings have suggested that, with rare exceptions, expression of perforin and granzyme B is also restricted to cytotoxic cells, including NK cells and cytotoxic T cells. Analysis of these antigens in conjunction with other marker molecules can therefore further specify the cellular origin of lymphocytes and lymphoid malignancies. In this regard, granzyme B, TIA-1, and perforin have been demonstrated in the majority of intestinal T-cell lymphomas but not in intestinal B-cell lymphomas and CD8– peripheral nodal T-cell lymphomas. Antibody 2G9, which recognizes TIA-1, proved to be the most sensitive immunohistological marker, being demonstrated in the highest number of cases and also in high numbers of neoplastic cells in positive cases. Hence, the cytotoxic differentiation in intestinal T-cell lymphoma was clearly shown, supporting derivation from intraepithelial cytotoxic T lymphocytes.

T-cell anaplastic large-cell lymphomas (T-ALCLs) have also been shown to express cytotoxic molecules with antibody GB9 to granzyme B, whereas this is not seen in B-cell anaplastic large-cell lymphomas, proving that T-ALCLs are derived from activated cytotoxic T cells. Granzyme B-positive T-cell lymphomas have also been mainly found in mucosa-associated lymphoid tissue, being more often associated with angioinvasion: nasal, gastrointestinal tract; and lung. It has also been shown that immunohistochemical staining with anti-TIA-1 can be used to identify cytolytic T lymphocytes in epidermal lesions of human graft-versus-host disease. Antibodies to cytotoxic molecules have shown that the predominant mechanism of cellular destruction in Kikuchi's lymphadenitis was apoptosis-mediated by cytolytic lymphocytes.

Cutaneous CD8+ and CD56+ lymphomas appear to show different expressions of cytotoxic molecules, with the former expressing only one or two of the cytotoxic proteins while the latter expresses the entire panel of cytotoxic antigens. Such differences may explain differences in their biological behavior. Primary CD30+ cutaneous lymphomas and lymphomatoid papulosis frequently express at least one of the cytotoxic proteins. Sinonasal lymphomas of CD3+/CD56+ phenotype invariably express all three cytotoxic antigens and Epstein–Barr viral RNA but not CD57. In general the aggressive T-cell lymphomas, including gastrointestinal T-cell lymphoma, gastric T-cell lymphoma, hepatosplenic γ/δ-T-cell lymphoma, and some nodal T-cell lymphomas, express varying quantities of the cytotoxic proteins.

Comments

It was impossible to differentiate most functional T-cell subsets, e.g., suppressor and cytotoxic T cells by membrane characteristics on paraffin-embedded tissue. The production of monoclonal antibodies against cytotoxic molecules has enabled the identification of the major components of the cytotoxic granules found in the cytoplasm of activated cytotoxic and natural killer cells. Intestinal T-cell lymphomas provide an ideal positive control for antibodies to cytotoxic molecules.

Selected reference

Anderson P, Nagler-Anderson C, O'Brien C, et al. A monoclonal antibody reactive with a 15-kDa cytoplasmic granule associated protein defines a subpopulation of CD8+ T lymphocytes. *Journal of Immunology* 1990; 144: 574–82.

D2-40

Sources/clones

Podoplanin, D2-40, M2A (Abcam, Genway, Signet, Dako, Nichirei); Mouse monoclonal anti-human (IgG1 isotype).

Background

Podoplanin or D2-40 clone reacts with a transmembrane O-linked sialoglycoprotein (molecular weight 40 kDa) found on lymphatic endothelium, ovarian and testicular germ cells, placenta (endothelium), lung (alveolar epithelium), brain, reticular cells, follicular dendritic cells, and myoepithelial cells. D2-40 clone does not react with vascular endothelium. It is functionally suggested to be involved in cell migration and actin cytoskeletal organization.

Applications

Expressed in endothelial cells of tumors of lymphatic origin (100%), Kaposi's sarcomas (98%), hemangioendothelioma (97%), vascular tumors with lymphatic differentiation, mesotheliomas (84%), and brain tumors such as cerebellar hemangioblastoma, anaplastic ependymomas (100%), some medulloblastomas, glioblastoma, pineal germinoma (100%), craniopharyngioma (100%), choroid plexus papilloma (100%), choroid plexus carcinoma (100%), and meningioma (87%). This antibody is useful to differentiate between choroid plexus carcinoma and metastatic carcinoma, as well as for differentiating mesothelioma from adenocarcinoma. Squamous cell carcinoma of head and neck region, uterine cervix carcinoma, breast carcinoma, skin adnexal tumors, seminomas, dysgerminomas, adrenal cortical carcinoma, schwannoma, epithelioid MPNST, distal epithelioid sarcoma, skeletal myxoid chondrosarcoma, chondroid and chordoid tumors have all been reported to stain positive.

Selected references

Chu AY, Litzky LA, Pasha TL, Acs G, Zhang PJ. Utility of D2-40, a novel mesothelial marker, in the diagnosis of malignant mesothelioma. *Modern Pathology* 2005; 18: 105–10.

Kahn HJ, Bailey D, Marks A. Monoclonal antibody D2-40, a new marker of lymphatic endothelium, reacts with Kaposi's sarcoma and a subset of angiosarcomas. *Modern Pathology* 2002; 15: 434–40.

Kalof AN, Cooper K. D2-40 immunohistochemistry: so far! *Advances in Anatomic Pathology* 2009; 16: 62–4.

NOTES

DBA.44 (hairy cell leukemia)

Sources/clones

Dako, Immunotech.

Fixation/preparation

The antibody is immunoreactive in formalin-fixed paraffin-embedded tissues, with immunoreactivity enhanced by proteolytic digestion but not by HIER.

Background

DBA.44 recognizes an unknown fixation-resistant B-cell differentiation antigen expressed by mantle zone lymphocytes, reactive immunoblasts, monocytoid B cells, and a small proportion of high- and low-grade lymphomas. The monoclonal antibody was one of four generated against a B-lymphoma cell line (DEAU-cell line) grafted in athymic nude mice. Within the group of low-grade B-cell lymphomas, DBA.44 reacted principally with hairy cell leukemia. Among node-based lymphomas, the strongest membrane staining was observed in centroblastic, immunoblastic and monocytoid B-cell lymphomas.

Applications

In a study of bone-marrow specimens from 166 patients with hairy cell leukemia, strong positive staining of the "hairy" surface membranes was observed in routinely fixed and decalcified bone marrow biopsies of nearly all cases. Subsequent studies have proven the usefulness of DBA.44 in the identification of hairy cell leukemia, particularly in the detection of minimal residual disease following treatment. DBA.44 has been successfully applied to peripheral blood cytospin preparations and for ultrastructural labeling.

The antibody has also been successfully applied to methyl-methacrylate embedded bone marrow biopsies.

DBA.44 appears to be a more sensitive marker of hairy cells than the traditional tartrate-resistant acid phosphatase (TRAP) activity which has long been a cornerstone in the diagnosis of hairy cell leukemia. Mantle zone lymphocytes and their corresponding lymphoma were DBA.44- and CD44-positive, with a weaker reaction for CDw75 than marginal zone lymphocytes and monocytoid B cells, whereas monocytoid B-cell lymphoma showed positivity for CD74 and CDw75 with positivity for DBA.44 observed in only occasional cases. Hairy cell leukemia specimens, in contrast, were all positive for DBA.44, with a weak reaction for CD74 and a stronger positivity for CDw75 than either mantle cell lymphoma or monocytoid B-cell lymphoma specimens.

Comments

While useful as a diagnostic marker, DBA.44 is not specific for hairy cells and should be used in a panel of antibodies to separate other B-cell lymphomas such as large-cell lymphoma, mantle cell lymphoma, and paraimmunoblasts of small-cell lymphoma that may express the antigen. In one study that included a variety of neoplastic and non-neoplastic hematological disorders, the combined positivity for DBA.44 and TRAP was found only in hairy cell leukemia when an antibody to TRAP was used.

Selected references

Cordone I, Annino L, Masi S, *et al.* Diagnostic relevance of peripheral blood immunocytochemistry in hairy cell leukaemia. *Journal of Clinical Pathology* 1995; 48: 955–60.

Hounieu H, Chittal SM, al Saati T, *et al.* Hairy cell leukemia. Diagnosis of bone marrow involvement in paraffin-embedded sections with monoclonal antibody DBA.44. *American Journal of Clinical Pathology* 1992; 98: 26–33.

NOTES

Desmin

Sources/clones

Accurate (DEU10, 4B4B2, 33), American Research Products/Research Diagnostics (DEU10), Biodesign (33), Biogenesis (BIO-41H), Boehringer (DEB5), Dako (DE-R-11, D33), Eurodiagnostica (D9), EY Labs, Immunotech (D33, HHF35), Shandon Lipshaw (D33), Sigma (DEU10), Zymed (ZSD1).

Fixation/preparation

Most of the available antibodies are immunoreactive in fixed tissues and are enhanced by HIER. Enzyme digestion is not required if HIER is employed. Clone D33 can be used without enzyme predigestion.

Background

Desmin belongs to the class of "intermediate" (10 nm) filaments and is a cytoplasmic protein, which is characteristically found in myogenic cells. It has a molecular weight of 53 kDa and is composed of an N-terminal "headpiece" and a C-terminal "tailpiece," both of which are non-helical in conformation. The two pieces bracket an α-helical middle domain of about 300 amino acid residues which is highly conserved from species to species, with striking interspecies homology. This homology is even more than that exhibited between intermediate filament proteins in the same species, with cytokeratin, vimentin, glial fibrillary acidic protein, neurofilaments, and desmin exhibiting sequence homology of about 30%.

In smooth muscle cells, desmin is associated with cytoplasmic dense bodies and subplasmalemmal dense plaques, and in striated muscle it is linked to sarcomeric Z disks. Muscle cells depleted of desmin (skeletin) are still able to contract in response to adenosine triphosphate and calcium, suggesting that desmin plays no role in contractility but rather serves to maintain the relationship and orientation of actin and myosin filaments and to anchor them to the plasmalemma. More recent findings suggest that, like other intermediate filaments of non-epithelial cells, desmin also serves a nucleic acid-binding function, is susceptible to processing by calcium-activated proteases, and is a substrate for cyclic adenosine monophosphate-dependent protein kinases. With its shared structural homology to lamins, the proteins of the nuclear envelope, desmin may also serve as a modulator between extracellular influences governing calcium flux into the cell and may have a role in nuclear transcription and translation. These newer roles of the intermediate filaments, including desmin, relegate the supportive cytoskeletal function of intermediate filaments to a secondary role.

Applications

The development of sensitive and specific antibodies to the intermediate filaments including desmin heralded a new era in diagnostic immunohistochemistry, as they allow the subtyping of many seemingly undifferentiated and pleomorphic tumors through intermediate filament analysis. Through the application of judiciously selected panels of antibodies directed to the differential diagnoses derived from the histologic and clinical findings, it is possible to separate the different entities in the diagnostic categories of pleomorphic spindle cell tumors and round cell tumors in soft tissues and skin (Appendix 1.11, 1.23, 1.24, 1.25, 1.26, 1.27). The former group includes rhabdomyosarcoma, leiomyosarcomas, and tumors with focal myogenic differentiation such as Triton tumors and malignant mixed Müllerian tumors. The latter group includes embryonal rhabdomyosarcoma, epithelioid leiomyoma and leiomyosarcoma, and focal myogenic differentiation in small round cell tumors such as desmoplastic small round cell tumors and primitive/peripheral neuroepithelial tumors. All of these tumors may express desmin. In this context, it is important to remember that although myelogenous cells often express desmin, it is also seen in myofibroblasts. Focal staining for desmin will be observed in tumors of myofibroblastic differentiation such as fibromatosis and dermatofibrosarcoma protuberans, and in reactive conditions with abundant myofibroblasts such as inflammatory pseudotumor and postoperative spindle cell nodule (Appendix 1.31). Equally important is the observation that not all muscle cells contain desmin. For example, among mammalian vascular smooth muscle, three immunophenotypes have been observed. Those that display vimentin only, those co-expressing vimentin and desmin, and a third group which expresses desmin only.

Focal staining for desmin may also be seen in tumors with a background of reactive myofibroblasts or with focal myofibroblastic differentiation. Approximately 50% of angiomatoid fibrous histiocytomas are diffusely or patchily desmin-positive.

Desmin has been employed with h-caldesmon, calponin, CD10, CD34, CD99, inhibin, and keratin to separate leiomyomas, leiomyosarcomas, endometrial stromal tumors, and uterine tumors resembling ovarian sex cord tumors. Desmin was positive in all smooth muscle tumors with the exception of the epithelioid type, which were positive in only about half the cases. It also stained areas of smooth muscle differentiation in endometrial stromal tumors and uterine tumors resembling ovarian sex cord tumors.

Reactive mesothelial cells were shown to be strongly positive for desmin in cell block preparations of serous fluids (22/24 cases) but it was not expressed by malignant mesothelioma and adenocarcinoma, suggesting that desmin may be a useful marker to separate these three entities. Other muscle markers including actin, myoglobin, and myogenin were not expressed by the reactive mesothelial cells or any of the tumors.

Comments

While initial antibodies to desmin lacked sensitivity and specificity, current commercial antibodies are more reliable. Both monoclonal and polyclonal antibodies are useful, but as desmin shares some common epitopes with actin and myosin, it should be ensured that the antibody employed does not show cross-reactivity. We employ clones DE-R-11 and D33, both antibodies being enhanced by HIER.

Selected references

Azumi N, Ben-Ezra J, Battifora H. Immunophenotypic diagnosis of leiomyosarcomas and rhabdomyosarcomas with monoclonal antibodies to muscle-specific actin and desmin in formalin-fixed tissue. *Modern Pathology* 1988; 1: 469–74.

Li Z, Colucci E, Babinet C, Paulin D. The human desmin gene: a specific regulatory program in skeletal muscle both in vitro and in transgenic mice. *Neuromuscular Disorders* 1993; 3: 423–7.

Nagai J, Capetanaki YG, Lazarides E. Expression of the genes coding for the intermediate filament proteins vimentin and desmin. *Annals of the New York Academy of Sciences* 1985; 455: 144–55.

Pollock L, Rampling D, Greenwald SE, Malone M. Desmin expression in rhabdomyosarcoma: influence of the desmin clone and immunohistochemical method. *Journal of Clinical Pathology* 1995; 48: 535–8.

Desmoplakins

Sources/clones

American Research Products, Chemicon, Cymbus Bioscience (DP2.15), Biodesign (DP2.15), Boehringer Mannheim (2.15), ICI (DP2.17), Progen (DP2.15), Research Diagnostic Inc (DP2.15), Serotec (polyclonal).

Fixation/preparation

Available antibodies are immunoreactive only in fresh frozen sections or cell preparations.

Background

Epithelial cells contain complexes of cytokeratin filaments (tonofilaments) associated with specific domains of the plasma membrane that appear as symmetrical junctions known as desmosomes, or as asymmetrical hemidesmosomes. These regions of filament–membrane attachment are characterized by 14–20 nm thick dense plaque; these desmosomal plaques comprise a dense mixture of intracellular attachment proteins including plakoglobin and desmoplakins. Transmembrane linker proteins, which belong to the cadherin family of cell-to-cell adhesion molecules, bind to the plaques and interact through their extracellular domains to hold the adjacent membranes together by a Ca^{2+}-dependent mechanism. Desmoplakins I and II (DPI and DPII) are two polypeptides that make up the desmoplakins; they are of molecular weights 46 and 24 kDa respectively, suggesting that DPI may be a dimer in solution and DPII a monomer.

Applications

The widespread presence of desmosomes in epithelial cells and their corresponding tumors makes the presence of desmoplakins a specific marker of epithelial differentiation. Unfortunately, these proteins are fixative-sensitive, restricting the use of antibodies to desmoplakins to fresh cellular preparations or frozen sections. Applications in diagnostic pathology have therefore been limited to some studies in bullous skin diseases. In autoimmune acantholytic diseases such as pemphigus vulgaris and pemphigus erythematosus, desmoplakins are intact even in acantholytic cells, whereas in Hailey–Hailey disease and Darier's disease the normal plasma membrane localization of desmoplakins is lost and the protein is internalized and present diffusely in the cytoplasm.

Desmoplakins have been demonstrated in follicular dendritic cells and their corresponding tumors. More recent studies employing anti-desmoplakins have included the progression of squamous intraepithelial lesions of the uterine cervix, where the assembly of desmosomes has been shown to be affected during progression of atypia with a dramatically decreased expression of desmoplakins and desmogleins.

Comments

Acetone fixation followed by plastic embedding allows the immunostaining of the desmoplakins in permanent sections. Trypsin digestion needs to be employed.

Selected reference

O'Keefe EJ, Erickson HP, Bennett V. Desmoplakin I and desmoplakin II: purification and characterization. *Journal of Biological Chemistry* 1989; 264: 8310–18.

NOTES

DOG1

Sources/clones

Abnova (DOG1.1, polyclonal), A. Menarini Diagnostics (DOG1.1), Amsbio (M3314, polyclonal), Atlas Antibodies (polyclonal), Biocare (DOG1.1), Biogenex (1.1), LifeSpan BioSciences (SP31, DOG1.1), Merck Millipore (1.1), MyBioSource (polyclonal), Novacastra/Leica (K9), Novus (polyclonal), Proteintech (polyclonal), Sanbio (DOG1.1, SP31), Sigma-Aldrich (polyclonal), Thermo Fisher Scientific (1.1, SP31), Ventana Medical Systems (SP31), Zeta Co (1.1).

Fixation/preparation

Several of the antibody clones/polyclonal antibodies to DOG1 are immunoreactive in fixed paraffin-embedded sections. HIER at 120 °C enhances labeling.

Background

Discovered on GIST-1 (DOG1) was identified initially by gene expression profiling of a few sarcoma types. In other contexts, DOG1 was named as the tumor amplified and overexpressed sequence 1 (TAOS2), ORA cancer OVerexpressed 2 (ORAOV2), FLJ10261, TMEM16A/Anoctamin-1 (ANO1). FLJ10261 was identified by analysis of chromosomal region 11q13 and was demonstrated to be expressed in silico in carcinomas of the esophagus, bladder, head and neck, breast, pancreas, and stomach, and in parathyroid tumors. TMEM16A/ANO1 has been demonstrated to be a Ca^{2+}-activated chloride conductance channel. In a seminal study, DOG1 antibody reactivity was found to correlate with overexpression in gastrointestinal stromal tumors.

Applications

Antibodies to DOG1 are useful for diagnosing gastrointestinal stromal tumors (GISTs). DOG1 exhibits high sensitivity for GIST. In two large studies, DOG1 and KIT (CD117) were detected in 87–95% and 74–95% of GIST cases, respectively. Moderate to strong positive nuclear reactivity specific for DOG1 is present in >30% of cells in most GISTs; however, some cases demonstrate delicate cytoplasmic reactivity. DOG1 is often positive in KIT– cases, which often have *PDGFRA* mutations. Aside from smooth muscle tumors, most tumors in the differential diagnosis of GIST (with only a few exceptional cases) demonstrate no DOG1 reactivity, including desmoid tumor, endometrial stromal sarcoma, inflammatory fibroid polyp, inflammatory myofibroblastic tumor, Kaposi's sarcoma, liposarcoma, malignant peripheral nerve sheath tumor, melanoma, PEComa, schwannoma, solitary fibrous tumor, and undifferentiated sarcoma. Areas of dedifferentiation within GIST can lose DOG1 expression.

Non-GIST tumors express DOG1. A subset of benign and malignant smooth muscle tumors of the uterus and gastrointestinal tract are DOG1-positive. DOG1 is positive in chondroblastoma. Focal DOG1 reactivity was found in synovial sarcoma cases. DOG1 reactivity has been demonstrated in carcinoma of the head and neck and esophagus, and in adenocarcinoma (stomach, lung, colon, endometrium), and is detected in salivary gland carcinomas of varying types. Normal tissue DOG1 reactivity has been reported in the gastric foveolar epithelium, basilar cells of squamous epithelia, breast duct epithelium, endometrium, epithelia of the bile duct, dermal eccrine gland, and salivary acinar and intercalated ducts. In one study, DOG1 reactivity was detected more frequently than KIT in cytology cell blocks. Differences in antibody clones, in part, may explain some of the differential specificity described in the literature.

DOG1 has utility in the diagnosis of GIST and may extend the diagnostic sensitivity of *KIT– PDGFRA*-mutated GIST.

Comments

Immunoreactivity appears not to be enhanced by boiling or proteolytic digestion and is best demonstrated following retrieval at 120 °C EDTA buffer at pH 9.0.

Selected references

Chênevert J, Duvvuri U, Chiosea S, *et al.* DOG1: a novel marker of salivary acinar and intercalated duct differentiation. *Modern Pathology* 2012; 25, 919–29.

Choi JJ, Sinada-Bottros L, Maker AV, Weisenberg E. Dedifferentiated gastrointestinal stromal tumor arising de novo from the small intestine. *Pathology Research and Practice* 2014; 210: 264–6.

Espinosa I, Lee CH, Kim MK, *et al.* A novel monoclonal antibody against DOG1 is a sensitive and specific marker for gastrointestinal stromal tumors. *American Journal of Surgical Pathology* 2008; 32: 210–18.

Hemminger J, Iwenofu OH. Discovered on gastrointestinal stromal tumours 1 (DOG1) expression in non-gastrointestinal stromal tumour (GIST) neoplasms. *Histopathology* 2012; 61: 170–7.

Liegl B, Hornick JL, Corless CL, Fletcher CD. Monoclonal antibody DOG1.1 shows higher sensitivity than KIT in the diagnosis of gastrointestinal stromal tumors, including unusual subtypes. *American Journal of Surgical Pathology* 2009; 33: 437–46.

Miettinen M, Wang ZF, Lasota J. DOG1 antibody in the differential diagnosis of gastrointestinal stromal tumors: a study of 1840 cases. *American Journal of Surgical Pathology* 2009; 33: 1401–8.

Sah SP, McCluggage WG. DOG1 immunoreactivity in uterine leiomyosarcomas. *Journal of Clinical Pathology* 2013; 66: 40–3.

DPC4/SMAD4

Sources/clones

Abcam (EP618Y), Gene Tex (IMD-89), Genway (GWB-BBB081), Leica (JM56), Millipore (ABE21).

Fixation/preparation

The antibody can be used in formalin-fixed paraffin-embedded tissue. Pretreatment of deparaffinized tissue sections with HIER is required.

Background

DPC4, also known as *SMAD4*, is a tumor suppressor gene that encodes a member of the Smad family of signal transduction proteins. DPC4 acts as a cofactor that binds transforming growth factor-β (TGF-β) receptor-activated serine threonine receptor kinases, Smad2 and Smad3, thereby generating transcriptional complexes. These complexes then translocate to the nucleus, bind to a specific sequence of DNA, and regulate the transcription of target genes. Consequently, DPC4 plays a pivotal role in Smad-mediated transcriptional activation.

Defects in *DPC4* are a cause of juvenile polyposis syndrome (JPS), an autosomal dominant gastrointestinal hamartomatous polyposis syndrome in which patients are at risk for developing colonic and other gastrointestinal cancers. Defects in *DPC4* are also a cause of juvenile polyposis/hereditary hemorrhagic telangiectasia syndrome (JP/HHT).

Inactivation or deletion of *DPC4* is a late event in the neoplastic progression of pancreatic cancer, and is found in about half the cases.

Applications

Immunohistochemical expression of DPC4 recapitulates the genetic status of *DPC4* in pancreatic adenocarcinoma. Pancreatic cancer patients with retained DPC4 expression have been shown to have significantly longer survival as compared to those lacking DPC4 expression, and loss of DPC4 expression by immunohistochemistry may be used as a marker of poorer prognosis. Loss of DPC4 expression in colonic adenocarcinomas also correlates with the presence of metastatic disease and is associated with lymph node metastases in gastric cancer.

Comments

Selected references

Lagna G, Hata A, Hemmati-Brivanlou A, *et al.* Partnership between DPC4 and SMAD proteins in TGF-beta signalling pathways. *Nature* 1996; 383: 832–6.

Maitra A, Molberg K, Albores-Saavedra J, *et al.* Loss of Dpc4 expression in colonic adenocarcinomas correlates with the presence of metastatic disease. *American Journal of Pathology* 2000; 157: 1105–11.

Wilentz RE, Iacobuzio-Donahue CA, Argani P, *et al.* Loss of expression of Dpc4 in pancreatic intraepithelial neoplasia: evidence that DPC4 inactivation occurs late in neoplastic progression. *Cancer Research* 2000; 60: 2002–6.

Wilentz RE, Su GH, Dai JL, *et al.* Immunohistochemical labeling for dpc4 mirrors genetic status in pancreatic adenocarcinomas : a new marker of DPC4 inactivation. *American Journal of Pathology* 2000; 156: 37–43.

Xia X, Wu W, Huang C, *et al.* SMAD4 and its role in pancreatic cancer. *Tumour Biology* 2014; 36: 111–19.

NOTES

EMA (epithelial membrane antigen)

Sources/clones

Accurate (E29), Biodesign, Biogenesis (2D5/11), Biogenex (E29, Mc-5), Bioprobe (HMFGP1.4), Chemicon, Dako (E29), Diagnostic Biosystems (E29), Immunon (polyclonal, E29), Immunotech (E29, E348KP), Medac, Novocastra, Oncogene (MC5), Sera Lab (HMFG/5/11IC, polyclonal), Serotec, Zymed (ZCE113).

Fixation/preparation

Most antibodies are immunoreactive in fixed paraffin-embedded sections. Immunostaining is enhanced by proteolytic digestion or HIER, the latter producing less background staining.

Background

Anti-epithelial membrane antigen (EMA) antibodies recognize a group of closely related high-molecular-weight transmembrane glycoproteins with high carbohydrate content. The *MUC1* gene, located on chromosome 1 in the 1q21–24 region, encodes EMA. EMA is very similar to the human milk fat globule (HMFG). A heterogeneous population of HMFG proteins can be recovered from the aqueous phase of skimmed milk following extraction in chloroform and methanol. EMA is related to the high-molecular-weight glycoproteins of HMFG, especially to HMFG-2. Preparations of EMA reacted with polyclonal antibodies raised to delipidized HMFG with avid binding to wheat germ agglutinin and peanut agglutinin. A similar mucin-containing glycoprotein was solubilized from HMFG and labeled PAS-O because of reactivity for PAS. PAS-O and EMA represent closely allied glycoprotein moieties, with common antigenic determinants on both proteins. From a practical standpoint, patterns of immunoreactivity for EMA and HMFG are very similar.

EMA reactivity is found in a wide variety of epithelial cells and their corresponding tumors. When present, immunoreactivity is usually limited to apical cell membranes in benign secretory epithelium and well-differentiated carcinomas such as those of the breast, but in poorly differentiated carcinomas cytoplasmic staining is seen and there is loss of staining polarity in the cell membranes. Secretory epithelia and their fetal anlage that show EMA include eccrine sweat glands, sebaceous glands, and apocrine glands, and EMA may be employed with the appropriate panel to separate cutaneous adnexal tumors (Appendix 1.20). EMA is also expressed in salivary gland, exocrine pancreas, gastric mucosa and endometrium, bronchial glands, alveolar cells, and the epithelium of bile ducts, stomach, bronchi, fallopian tube, and vas deferens. In addition to glandular epithelium, EMA has also been demonstrated in non-secretory epithelia such as urothelium, renal distal and collecting tubules, and syncytiotrophoblast.

Applications

Despite the ready availability of anti-cytokeratin as a marker of epithelial differentiation, there is still widespread use of EMA as a marker of epithelial cells. This is fraught with inconsistencies. While EMA is generally not expressed by germ cells, normal hematolymphoid, mesenchymal, neural, and neuroectodermal, it may be expressed by certain non-epithelial tissues such as fetal notochord, arachnoid granulations, ependyma, choroid plexus, epineurial and perineural fibroblasts, histiocytes, and plasma cells, and their corresponding neoplasms. EMA is normally expressed by plasma cells and is conserved and even increased in plasma cell neoplasms, and by ultrastructural examination has been located diffusely on the cell membranes and focally within rough endoplasmic reticulum. Neoplasms from earlier-stage B-cell differentiation do not usually express EMA, and in lymph node-based B-cell lymphomas EMA is found mainly in diffuse large-cell lymphomas and T-cell-rich B-cell lymphomas. EMA is more frequently seen in T-cell neoplasms, occurring in about 20% of all T-cell lymphomas. EMA expression in Reed–Sternberg cells is unusual, although it is frequently found in the L&H cells of nodular lymphocyte-predominant Hodgkin disease. EMA is also found in almost 50% of cases of anaplastic large-cell lymphoma of CD30 phenotype.

In our practice, staining for EMA is not generally employed as a marker of epithelial cells but more often for the identification of certain mesenchymal tumors including synovial sarcoma, anaplastic large-cell lymphoma (CD30+), and perineurioma. Cytokeratin expression in monophasic (spindle) synovial sarcoma may be focal, but EMA is often more extensively positive in such cases, even in the rare pleuropulmonary synovial sarcoma. The expression of EMA in chordoma serves to distinguish from chondroma and chondrosarcoma; E-cadherin is another marker expressed in most chordomas as opposed to chondrosarcoma. EMA is expressed in solitary fibrous tumors. EMA immunostaining may help distinguish ovarian granulosa cell tumors from tumors that mimic their various histological patterns. While keratin may be expressed in granulosa cell tumors, the absence of EMA and immunoreactivity for smooth muscle actin allows distinction from primary and metastatic carcinomas.

Immunostaining for EMA is a valuable adjunct to the examination of effusions and biopsies for malignant mesothelioma (Appendix 1.17). By ultrastructural examination EMA has been demonstrated exclusively on the long microvillous surfaces of the tumor cells with virtually no cytoplasmic labeling. These findings have been transposed to cytologic preparations and biopsies, and careful staining for EMA employing clone E29 shows membranous labeling of malignant mesothelial cells and demonstrates the long microvilli characteristic of the tumor. In contrast, adenocarcinomas display diffuse cytoplasmic staining, with or without membranous enhancement, but long microvilli are not seen.

EMA and vimentin immunostaining was employed to differentiate chromophobe renal cell carcinoma from renal oncocytoma and conventional renal cell carcinoma, but the same phenotype was found in all three tumors. Chromophobe carcinomas co-expressed both antigens, which was present in 75% of renal oncocytoma in 20% of conventional renal cell carcinoma. The absence of this phenotype, however, would preclude the diagnosis of chromophobe carcinoma.

Comments

For diagnostic applications we prefer to use anti-EMA (clone E29) instead of HMFG, both antigens having very similar tissue distribution.

Selected reference

Heyderman E, Strudley I, Powell G, *et al*. A new monoclonal antibody to epithelial membrane antigen (EMA) – E29. A comparison of its immunocytochemical reactivity with polyclonal anti-EMA antibodies and with another monoclonal antibody HMFG-2. *British Journal of Cancer* 1985; 52: 355–61.

Epidermal growth factors: EGFR

Sources/clones

Accurate (21–1, F4), Biodesign (EGFR1, 2E9, L-4451, F5, E5), Biogenesis (C11, EGFR1), Biogenex (E30), Caltag Laboratories (2E9), Chemicon (polyclonal), Cymbus Bioscience (EGFR1), Dako (EGFR1), Fitzgerald (polyclonal), Immunotech (F4), Novocastra (polyclonal), Oncogene (R.1, 225, 455), Pharmingen, Sigma Chemical (29.1, F4), Zymed (Z025)

Anti-EGFR L858R: Ventana (SP125) and Cell Signaling (43B2)

Anti-EGFR E746˙A750: Ventana (SP111) and Cell Signaling (6B6)

Fixation/preparation

- Formalin-fixed paraffin-embedded tissues are suitable.
- Deparaffinize slides using xylene or xylene alternative and graded alcohols.
- Suitable for automated slide staining system.

Background

The epidermal growth factor receptor (EGFR) is a protein encoded by the *EGFR* gene. EGFR is a 170 kDa protein comprising a cell surface ligand-binding transmembrane domain and a highly conserved cytoplasmic tyrosine kinase domain. This is followed by phosphorylation and an increase in cytosolic calcium ions within target cells. The resultant effect is an increased DNA synthesis with proliferation and differentiation of the cell. It is a transmembrane glycoprotein that is a member of the protein kinase superfamily. The EGFR protein is a receptor for members of the epidermal growth factor family. It is a cell surface protein that binds to epidermal growth factor; this induces receptor dimerization and tyrosine autophosphorylation and leads to cell proliferation. Mutations in this gene are associated with pulmonary adenocarcinomas.

Applications

Exon 21 L858R and exon 19 E746_A750 mutations represent about 90% of all EGFR mutations. Antibodies against these two common *EGFR* mutations are available on the market. Several reports have shown excellent correlation between immunohistochemistry and molecular findings. Patients with mutated *EGFR* lung adenocarcinomas do respond to EGFR inhibitor therapy, like gefitinib and erlotinib, so timely determination of EGFR status in lung adenocarcinoma is essential.

Staining pattern

IHC expression in selected neoplasm	IHC staining pattern
Mutated EGFR lung adenocarcinoma	Membranous cytoplasmic

Selected references

Fan X, Liu B, Xu H, et al. Immunostaining with EGFR mutation-specific antibodies: a reliable screening method for lung adenocarcinomas harboring EGFR mutation in biopsy and resection samples. *Human Pathology* 2013; 44: 1499–507.

Lindeman NI, Cagle PT, Beasley MB, et al. Molecular Testing Guideline for Selection of Lung Cancer Patients for EGFR and ALK Tyrosine Kinase Inhibitors: Guideline from the College of American Pathologists, International Association for the Study of Lung Cancer, and

Association for Molecular Pathology. *Archives of Pathology and Laboratory Medicine* 2013; 137: 828–60.

Wen YH, Brogi E, Hasanovic A, *et al.* Immunohistochemical staining with EGFR mutation-specific antibodies: high specificity as a diagnostic marker for lung adenocarcinoma. *Modern Pathology* 2013; 26: 1197–203.

Yousem SA. Role of molecular studies in the diagnosis of lung adenocarcinoma. *Modern Pathology* 2012; 25 (suppl 1): S11–17.

Epidermal growth factors: TGF-α

Sources/clones

Biodesign, Biogenesis (2D7/44, 2D7/45, 8A5/7, Rt, TB21), Chemicon (polyclonal), Oncogene (134A-2B3, 213.4-4, 189-2130.1).

Fixation/preparation

Applicable to formalin-fixed paraffin-embedded tissue, although an antigen retrieval technique should be used prior to immunostaining, e.g., citrate buffer and microwave oven unmasking. May also be applied to cryostat sections or cell smears.

Background

Transforming growth factors (TGFs) were discovered due to their ability to transform fibroblasts to a malignant phenotype. Two distinct polypeptides were subsequently isolated: TGF-α and TGF-β. TGF-α is a polypeptide of 50 amino acids and is acid- and heat-stable. TGF-α belongs to the epidermal growth factor family, members of which share a common amino acid sequence and biological activities. They also bind to a common receptor, epidermal growth factor receptor (EGFR), on target cells. When TGF-α binds to EGFR, tyrosine kinase of the receptor is activated.

TGF-α is a potent growth stimulator and is distributed in both fetal and adult tissues, playing a role in the physiological regulation of normal growth and differentiation.

Applications

There is sufficient evidence showing that TGF-α is an important growth factor for transformation of various cell types to a malignant phenotype. The co-expression of both the ligand (TGF-α) and its receptor (EGFR) has been documented in a variety of carcinomas – both gastrointestinal and non-gastrointestinal carcinomas. This bond is thought to confer autonomy to tumor cells by autocrine or paracrine mechanisms. While coexistent expression of a growth factor and its receptor would be expected to confer increased growth advantage to tumor cells, the ability of certain tumors to express both growth factor and/or the respective receptor may be lost during the carcinogenic transformation.

The EGFR antibody reacts with the majority of squamous cell carcinomas arising from both squamous epithelium and metaplastic squamous epithelium. Studies on breast cancer have shown that the expression of EGFR may also be of prognostic value, although other studies of the expression of EGFR family ligands including EGF and TGF-α showed no association with cancer-specific survival, tumor size, lymph node status, histologic grade, or c-erbB-2 and hormone status.

Comments

Growth factors and their receptors participate in the process of tumorigenesis by promoting the growth of tumor cells. During this process, tumor cells acquire an increasingly aggressive phenotype with loss of the physiological control for growth and differentiation. At the present time the availability of antibodies to growth factors/receptors can only contribute to our understanding of the complex mechanisms involved in tumorigenesis.

Selected references

Carpenter G. Properties of the receptor for epidermal growth factor. *Cell* 1984; 37: 357–8.

Chen WS, Lazar CS, Lund KA, *et al.* Functional independence of the epidermal growth factor receptor from a domain required for ligand-induced internalization and calcium regulation. *Cell* 1989; 59: 33–43.

NOTES

Epstein–Barr virus, LMP

Sources/clones

Accurate (CS1-4), Biodesign (polyclonal), Dako (CS1-4), EY Labs, Novocastra (polyclonal).

Fixation/preparation

Applicable to formalin-fixed paraffin-embedded tissue sections. Enzymatic digestion (e.g., trypsin) is essential to enhance immunopositivity. Microwave irradiation for antigen retrieval has also been used to good effect. This antibody may also be used for labeling acetone-fixed cryostat sections or fixed cell smears.

Background

The antibody (isotype: IgG1κ) has been raised against recombinant fusion protein containing sequences of bacterial β-galactosidase and the EBV-encoded latent membrane protein (LMP-1). LMP is one of the few viral proteins that are expressed in a latent infection. The antibody reacts with a 60 kDa latent membrane protein encoded by the *BNLF* gene of the Epstein–Barr virus. Being a cocktail of clones CS1, CS2, CS3, and CS4, all four anti-LMP antibodies recognize distinct epitopes on the hydrophilic carboxyl region of LMP. These four epitopes are present on the internal aspect of the membrane-associated viral LMP. Therefore the antibody does not react with viable cells, but with fixed cells in paraffin sections, cytological preparations, and cryostat sections, and in immunoblotting.

Applications

The antibody is characterized by its strong positivity with EBV+ lymphoblastoid cell lines and EBV-infected B-cell immunoblasts in infectious mononucleosis. Although EBV is consistently present in nasopharyngeal undifferentiated carcinoma among East Asian patients, LMP-1 antibody is only positive in about 60% of cases. LMP protein expression is especially useful in identifying these cancers in cervical lymph node metastases. This antibody may also be useful in the diagnosis of lymphoepithelioma-like carcinoma of the lung, mediastinum, stomach, and paranasal sinuses.

Post-transplantation lymphoproliferative disorders, arising in patients treated with a variety of immunosuppressive regimens after organ transplantation, usually show a type III latency pattern with LMP-1 expression. The EBV+ AIDS-associated B-cell lymphomas usually demonstrate a latency type III in the large-cell lymphomas, permitting the use of antibody to LMP-1.

Nasal T/NK-cell lymphoma is strongly associated with EBV. However, LMP-1 protein expression has been inconsistent on paraffin sections, although one study consistently demonstrated LMP-1 protein in frozen sections, suggesting a low level of protein expression. LMP-1 immunohistochemistry is positive in 17% of adult T-cell leukemia/lymphoma (ATLL). LMP-1 expression has also been associated with an aggressive clinical course and hepatosplenomegaly in nodal T-cell lymphomas. About 20–30% of CD30 (Ki-1)-positive anaplastic large-cell lymphomas show LMP-1 immunoreaction.

Approximately 50% of Hodgkin disease cases are associated with EBV. In almost all of these positive cases, nearly all of the Reed–Sternberg cells are positive for EBV. Using modern epitope retrieval techniques, an almost 1:1 correlation between the results of LMP-1 paraffin-based immunohistochemistry studies and Epstein–Barr encoding RNA (EBER) in-situ hybridization studies has been demonstrated in Reed–Sternberg cells and Hodgkin cells of EBV-associated Hodgkin disease. A note of caution with respect to antibodies against LMP is advised: strong staining of normal early myeloid and erythroid precursors may be seen despite a total absence of evidence of EBV by PCR.

Attempts to correlate LMP and p53 immunoexpression in adult and pediatric nasopharyngeal carcinoma have produced conflicting results.

Comments

As a research tool, EBV immunohistochemical investigation is superior to PCR, in that it excludes background/resident lymphocytes harboring EBV. It has been suggested that the interpretation of LMP immunostaining is more accurate when combined with EBER, as LMP staining, while usually strong among all Reed–Sternberg cells in Hodgkin disease in a given case, may alternatively be focal and weak. LMP is localized to the cytoplasm and cell membrane.

Selected references

Bruin PCD. Detection of Epstein–Barr virus nucleic acid sequences and protein in nodal T-cell lymphomas: relation between latent membrane protein-1 positivity and clinical course. *Histopathology* 1993; 23: 509–18.

Delecluse H-J, Kremmer E, Rouault JP, *et al.* The expression of Epstein-Barr virus latent proteins is related to the pathological feature of post-transplant lymphoproliferative disorders. *American Journal of Pathology* 1995; 146: 1113–20.

Hording U, Nielsen HW, Albeck H, Daugaard S. Nasopharyngeal carcinoma: histopathological types and association with Epstein-Barr virus. *European Journal of Cancer Clinical Oncology* 1993; 29B: 137–9.

Kanavaros P, Lecsc M-C, Briere J, *et al.* Nasal T-cell lymphoma: a clinicopathologic entity associated with peculiar phenotype and with Epstein-Barr virus. *Blood* 1993; 81: 2688–95.

ERG

Sources/clones

Abcam (EPR3864), Abnova (MAB10018), Acris Antibodies (polyclonal), A. Menarini (EPR3864), Aviva Systems Biology (polyclonal), BioCare (9FY), Biogenex (EPR3864), Biorbyt (polyclonal), Dako (EP111), Gene Tex (EPR3864, polyclonal), LifeSpan BioSciences (polyclonal), Novus (polyclonal), Origene (EPR3864), Proteintech Group (polyclonal), Santa Cruz (C-1), Sigma (polyclonal), Thermo Fisher Scientific (polyclonal), Ventana Medical Systems (EPR3864).

Fixation/preparation

Several of the antibody clones/polyclonal antibodies to ERG are immunoreactive in fixed paraffin-embedded sections. HIER at 120 °C enhances labeling.

Background

ERG (avian v-ets erythroblastosis virus E26 oncogene homolog) is a member of the ETS family of transcription factors characterized by the 98 amino acid sequence containing a basic helix-turn-helix structure of DNA binding proteins. ERG is constitutively expressed in endothelial cells regulating angiogenesis and endothelial apoptosis. ERG immunoreactivity is detected in the nuclei of endothelial cells, subsets of hematopoietic stem cells, and myeloid progenitors, and in fetal mesoderm-derived cells including endothelium and cartilage.

Applications

Antibodies to ERG are used in several diagnostic situations. These include the identification of endothelium of normal tissue and vascular lesions, certain sarcoma types, and prostatic adenocarcinoma subsets containing the *TMPRSS2–ERG* translocation. ERG staining that demonstrates diffuse and strong nuclear reactivity is considered positive. ERG is positive in malignant vascular neoplasms including nearly all (>95%) cases of angiosarcoma, epithelioid hemangioendothelioma, and Kaposi's sarcoma. Essentially all benign vascular proliferations and neoplasms including hemangioma, lymphangioma, and papillary endothelial hyperplasia are positive for ERG. Recently, ERG immunoreactivity has been demonstrated in ~40–50% epithelioid sarcoma cases. ERG nuclear immunoreactivity is detected in most Ewing's sarcoma cases with *EWSR1–ERG* translocations and less commonly with *EWSR1–FLI1* or *EWSR1–NFAT2*.

The *TMPRSS2–ERG* gene translocation is the most frequent large chromosomal aberration in prostatic adenocarcinoma and is present in about half of total prostatic adenocarcinoma cases. The *TMPRSS2–ERG* translocation causes increased expression of ERG, which can be detected immunohistochemically with high sensitivity. In prostate tissue with *TMPRSS2–ERG* prostatic adenocarcinoma, however, benign prostatic tissue and low- and high-grade prostatic intraepithelial neoplasia demonstrate ERG reactivity in addition to prostatic adenocarcinoma.

ERG is also detected in blastic extramedullary myeloid proliferations in a small number of cases. ERG immunoreactivity is negative in almost all other tumor types with rare exceptions. Two tumors out of 643 tested demonstrated focally positive for ERG: one pulmonary large undifferentiated carcinoma, and one mesothelioma. Non-nuclear, cytoplasmic, or membrane ERG immunoreactivity has been noted in some non-endothelial tumors, including gastrointestinal stromal tumors, ductal carcinoma of the breast, and papillary carcinoma of the thyroid.

Together, the findings support the utility of ERG as a marker of benign and malignant vascular proliferations, and in identifying *ERG* gene translocation associated with prostatic adenocarcinoma and Ewing's sarcoma. In the differential diagnosis of epithelioid sarcoma vs. angiosarcoma, ERG should be used in a panel.

Comments

Clone 9FY produces the best results in our hands. Immunoreactivity appears not to be enhanced by boiling or proteolytic digestion and is best demonstrated following retrieval at 120 °C in EDTA buffer at pH 9.0.

Selected references

Birdsey GM, Dryden NH, Amsellem V, *et al.* Transcription factor ERG regulates angiogenesis and endothelial apoptosis through VE-cadherin. *Blood* 2008; 111: 3498–506.

Falzarano SM, Zhou M, Carver P, *et al.* ERG gene rearrangement status in prostate cancer detected by immunohistochemistry. *Virchows Archiv* 2011; 459: 441–7.

Kumar-Sinha C, Tomlins SA, Chinnaiyan AM. Recurrent gene fusions in prostate cancer. *Nature Reviews: Cancer* 2008; 8: 497–511.

Miettinen M, Wang ZF, Paetau A, *et al.* ERG transcription factor as an immunohistochemical marker for vascular endothelial tumors and prostatic carcinoma. *American Journal of Surgical Pathology* 2011; 35: 432–41.

Miettinen M, Wang Z, Sarlomo-Rikala M, *et al.* ERG expression in epithelioid sarcoma: a diagnostic pitfall. *American Journal of Surgical Pathology* 2013; 37: 1580–5.

Sun C, Dobi A, Mohamed A, *et al.* TMPRSS2-ERG fusion, a common genomic alteration in prostate cancer activates C-MYC and abrogates prostate epithelial differentiation. *Oncogene* 2008; 27: 5348–53.

Wang WL, Patel NR, Caragea M, *et al.* Expression of ERG, an Ets family transcription factor, identifies ERG-rearranged Ewing sarcoma. *Modern Pathology* 2012; 25: 1378–83.

Erythropoietin

Sources/clones

Genzyme Diagnostics (EPO, monoclonal), Santa Cruz Biotechnology (EpoR (C–20), polyclonal SC-695).

Fixation/preparation

This antibody is applicable to formalin-fixed paraffin sections. Antigen retrieval is achieved by gentle boiling in water at high power for 5 minutes in a microwave oven.

Background

Erythropoietin (EPO) is a glycoprotein hormone that stimulates erythropoiesis in mammals. Its synthesis is increased in the anemic and hypoxic state. Although the liver is the major source of EPO production in the fetus, the kidney is the major organ of EPO production in adults. The EPO antibody is an immunoglobulin G antibody that binds to an epitope within the first 26 amino acids at the NH_2 terminus of human urinary and recombinant EPO.

The production of EPO is responsible for stimulating polycythemia in various malignancies: renal cell carcinoma, nephroblastoma, hepatocellular carcinoma, and cerebellar hemangioblastoma. Studies attempting to precisely localize the cells responsible for production of EPO have used immunohistochemistry and in-situ hybridization on frozen tissue sections to demonstrate that tumor cells of epithelial origin are the sites of EPO production in renal cell carcinomas associated with polycythemia. A study using monoclonal antibody EPO on paraffin sections achieved success with 16/19 renal cell carcinomas (comprising clear cell and tubulopapillary type) showing cytoplasmic immunopositivity, irrespective of the presence or absence of polycythemia. Hemangioblastomas stained positively with EPO antibody within the cells of the vascular walls. EPO immunopositivity is seen in metastatic renal cell carcinomas.

To date EPO has been reported to be synthesized in the normal brain, placenta, and capillary endothelium, glandular and surface epithelial cells of the normal cervix and endometrium, and oocytes, granulosa, theca interna, and lutein cells of the ovary. A case of uterine myoma with erythropoietin synthesis by tumor tissue and erythrocytosis has been reported. High levels of EPO and EPO receptor expression have been reported in malignant cells and tumor vasculature in breast cancer but not in normal breast tissue.

Applications

EPO immunopositivity is useful in the identification of both primary and metastatic renal cell carcinoma. This is useful to distinguish from other carcinomas; but not from hemangioblastoma, which may also be EPO-positive. EMA helps in this distinction, being positive in renal cell carcinoma, but not in hemangioblastoma.

Selected reference

Acs G, Acs P, Beckwith SM, et al. Erythropoietin and erythropoietin receptor expression in human cancer. *Cancer Research* 2001; 61: 3561–5.

NOTES

Factor VIII RA (von Willlebrand factor)

Sources/clones

Accurate (KG7/30), Axcel/Accurate (F8/86, polyclonal), Biodesign (101, 102, 103), Biogenesis (37–56/3, 21–43, WF7, polyclonal), Biogenex (polyclonal), Dako (F8/86, polyclonal), Sanbio (KG7/30), Serotec (F8, F8/86), Zymed (Z002, polyclonal).

Fixation/preparation

The antigen is fixation-resistant. Proteolytic digestion or HIER enhances immunoreactivity.

Background

Factor VIII-related antigen is more appropriately known as von Willebrand factor. Factor VIII is a glycoprotein and is complexed with factor VIII-related antigen in plasma. Factor VIII is also present in endothelial cells, where it shows a granular pattern of reactivity. It is also present in the cytoplasm of megakaryocytes.

Applications

Factor VIII-related antigen or von Willebrand factor was one of the first markers employed for endothelial cell differentiation in angiosarcomas, but it soon became apparent that von Willebrand factor is seldom expressed in poorly differentiated vascular tumors. Other markers of endothelial cells provide a higher diagnostic yield, and they include CD34, CD31 (Appendix 1.23), and *Ulex europaeus* agglutinin 1 (UEA-1). There is also considerable overlap between the expression of von Willebrand factor in vascular and lymphatic endothelium.

Von Willebrand factor remains a sensitive marker of benign blood vessels and has been used for the study of angiogenesis in neoplasms such as breast cancer.

Comments

Von Willlebrand factor must be used in conjunction with other more sensitive markers of endothelial cells when identifying angiosarcomas. It should be noted that seepage of the antigen may occur from surrounding blood, particularly in hemorrhagic or vascular lesions, and interpretation should be made with caution in such situations. Although von Willebrand factor continues to be used to delineate vessels in studies of tumor angiogenesis, other markers of endothelial cells including CD34 and CD31 serve this purpose better, particularly CD31, which is more sensitive and more specific.

Selected references

Juric G, Zarkovic N, Nola M, *et al.* The value of cell proliferation and angiogenesis in the prognostic assessment of ovarian granulosa cell tumors. *Tumori* 2001; 87: 47–53.

Marder VJ, Mannucci PM, Firkin BG, *et al.* Standard nomenclature for factor VIII and von Willebrand factor: a recommendation by the International Committee on Thrombosis and Haemostasis. *Thrombosis and Hemostasis* 1985; 54: 871–2.

Sehested M, Hou-Jensen K. Factor VII-related antigen as an endothelial cell marker in benign and malignant diseases. *Virchows Archiv A. Pathological Anatomy and Histology* 1981; 391: 217–25.

NOTES

Factor XIIIa

Sources/clones

Biocare (polyclonal), Calbiochem (polyclonal), Cell Marque (polyclonal), Novocastra (polyclonal).

Fixation/preparation

The antibodies are immunoreactive in routinely fixed paraffin-embedded sections. Staining is enhanced by HIER.

Background

Factor XIIIa is a blood proenzyme found in plasma and platelets. The reaction of factor XIIIa with fibrin is the last enzyme-catalyzed step on the coagulation cascade, leading to the formation of a normal blood clot stabilized as a result of fibrin cross-linkage. This transglutaminase exists in two forms, as an extracellular or plasma factor XIIIa subunit attached to a dimer of the carrier protein or factor XIIIb, and as an intracellular factor XIII, which is exclusively the dimer of subunit a only. Intracellular factor XIIIa has been identified in a variety of cells including human dendritic reticulum cells in reactive lymphoid follicles, fibroblast-like mesenchymal cells in connective tissue, and neoplastic fibroblastic and fibrohistiocytic lesions. The dermal dendrocytes have been characterized as factor XIIIa+ dendritic cells of bone marrow origin that are typically found in the adventitia of dermal blood vessels and in the interstitial dermal connective tissues. In one study of dermal dendritic cells using CD34 and factor XIIIa, it was found that antigenic profiles differed among the dendritic cell types. At ultrastructural level, subepidermal dendritic cells (probably identical with lining macrophages) expressed factor XIIIa only, perivascular dermal dendritic cells reacted with both factor XIIIa and CD34, and reticular dermal dendritic cells were negative for factor XIIIa but positive for CD34. However, at light microscopic level, perivascular dermal dendritic cells also expressed CD34.

Applications

The current diagnostic applications of factor XIIIa pertain largely to the identification of dermal dendritic cells and their presence and role in various cutaneous and soft tissue tumors. Factor XIIIa has been described in various so-called fibrohistiocytic tumors including aneurysmal fibrous histiocytoma, malignant fibrous histiocytoma, dermatofibroma, and dermatofibrosarcoma protuberans. In the latter two conditions, factor XIIIa expression appears to be associated with early lesions, with loss of expression in late or "mature" lesions. The marker also shows promise as a diagnostic discriminator for hepatocellular carcinoma from its morphologic mimics cholangiocarcinoma and metastatic carcinoma in the liver.

With increased use of this marker, a large number of tumors have been shown to be positive for factor XIIIa. Among these are calcifying fibrous pseudotumor, dermatofibroma, solitary fibrous tumor, and a number of so-called histiocytic lesions including xanthoma, xanthogranuloma, pigmented villonodular synovitis, fibroblastic reticular cell tumor, malignant fibrous histiocytoma, atypical fibroxanthoma, and epithelioid histiocytic proliferations. Glomus tumor, meningioma, neurothekoma, inflammatory pseudotumor, and cerebellar hemangioblastoma also express this antigen, albeit less frequently.

Comments

Reactivity in frozen sections is generally weak. We employ the polyclonal antibody from Calbiochem for paraffin-section immunostaining.

Selected references

Alawi F, Stratton D, Freedman PD. Solitary fibrous tumor of the oral soft tissues: a clinicopathologic and immunohistochemical study of 16 cases. *American Journal of Surgical Pathology* 2001; 25: 900–10.

Busam KJ, Granter SR, Iversen K, Jungbluth AA. Immunohistochemical distinction of epithelioid histiocytic proliferations from epithelioid melanocytic nevi. *American Journal of Dermatopathology* 2000; 22: 237–41.

Cerio R, Spaull J, Oliver GF, Wilson-Jones E. A study of factor XIIIa and MAC387 immunolabeling in normal and pathological skin. *American Journal of Dermatopathology* 1990; 12: 221–33.

Fucich LF, Cheles MK, Thung SN, *et al*. Primary versus metastatic hepatic carcinoma. An immunohistochemical study of 34 cases. *Archives of Pathology and Laboratory Medicine* 1994; 118: 927–30.

Hill KA, Gonzalez-Crussi F, Chou PM. Calcifying fibrous pseudotumor versus inflammatory myofibroblastic tumor: a histological and immunohistochemical comparison. *Modern Pathology* 2001; 14: 784–90.

Kraus MD, Haley JC, Ruiz R, *et al*. "Juvenile" xanthogranuloma: an immunophenotypic study with a reappraisal of histiogenesis. *American Journal of Dermatopathology* 2001; 23: 104–11.

Leong AS-Y, Lim MHT. Immunohistochemical characteristics of dermatofibrosarcoma protuberans. *Applied Immunohistochemistry* 1994; 2: 42–7.

Mentzel T, Kutzner H, Rutten A, Hugel H. Benign fibrous histiocytoma (dermatofibroma) of the face: clinicopathologic and immunohistochemical study of 34 cases associated with an aggressive clinical behaviour. *American Journal of Dermatopathology* 2001; 23: 419–26.

Nemes Z, Thomaszy V. Factor XIIIa and the classic histiocytic markers in malignant fibrous histiocytoma. *Human Pathology* 1988; 9: 822–9.

Nestle FO, Nickoloff BJ. A fresh morphological and functional look at dermal dendritic cells. *Journal of Cutaneous Pathology* 1995; 22: 385–93.

Nestle FO, Nickoloff BJ, Burg G. Dermatofibroma: an abortive immunoreactive process mediated by dermal dendritic cells? *Dermatology* 1995; 190: 265–8.

Takata M, Imai T, Hirone T. Factor XIIIa-positive cells in normal peripheral nerves and cutaneous neurofibromas of type-1 neurofibromatosis. *American Journal of Dermatopathology* 1994; 16: 37–43.

Zelger BW, Zelger BG, Steiner H, Ofner D. Aneurysmal and hemangiopericytoma-like fibrous histiocytoma. *Journal of Clinical Pathology* 1996; 49: 313–18.

Fas (CD95) and Fas-ligand (CD95L)

Sources/clones

FAS (CD95)

Alexis Corp (SM1/17, SM1/1, SM1/23, APO-1-3), Dako (APO-1, DX2), Pharmingen (DX2, G254-274).

FAS-ligand (CD95L, anti-FAS)

Immunotech (4A5, 4H9), Pharmingen (NOK-1, NOK-2, G247-4).

Fixation/preparation

Several of the antibodies (clones APO-1, DX2) are immunoreactive in fixed paraffin-embedded tissue sections as well as frozen sections and cell preparations.

Background

Fas (CD95) is a cell surface protein that belongs to the tumor necrosis factor family. Cross-linking of Fas and Fas-ligand (FasL) transduces signals, which cumulate in apoptosis in sensitive cells. These proteins therefore have a role in the genesis of neoplasms, and they have been extensively studied in this context. Their expression in certain malignancies has been implicated as a possible key mechanism in the immune privilege of such tumors. FasL is also expressed in immunologically privileged sites in the non-neoplastic state. The induction of apoptosis by FasL in invading lymphocytes acts as a mechanism of immune privilege and is important in preventing graft rejection. The placenta, another immune privileged site, has also been shown to express high levels of FasL. The induction of apoptosis in lymphocytes by invading trophoblasts may account for the immune tolerance of the fetal semi-allograft. Experimentally, FasL can be employed to induce apoptosis in Fas-bearing cells. In celiac disease mucosal flattening is thought to result from an increased enterocyte apoptosis triggered by the Fas/FasL system and perforin cytolytic granules. This is not the case in autoimmune enteropathy, where enterocyte auto-antibody-dependent cellular cytotoxicity is the prevalent mechanism of enterocyte death.

Fas and FasL expression has been studied in a wide variety of tissues and in other diseases besides neoplasms. These include idiopathic pulmonary fibrosis, human cancers following ionizing radiation, Alzheimer's disease, chronic hepatitis, alveolar type II pneumocytes, colonic epithelial cells, inflammatory myopathies, diabetes, and germ cells of the testis.

Applications

Interest in immunostaining for Fas and FasL centers around their role in tumor destruction. Macrophages and lymphocytes express high levels of Fas, and it has been thought that expression of FasL by tumor cells allows destruction of Fas+ lymphocytes, allowing the survival of the tumor cells in vivo. With the discovery that tumors may express both FasL and Fas, it is realized that tumors like melanoma may induce their own apoptosis in an autocrine and/or paracrine fashion, and that the decline of tumor apoptosis rather than the apoptosis of infiltrating lymphocytes may affect prognosis.

Macrophages heavily infected by tuberculosis or leprosy bacteria have been shown to be induced to express high levels of FasL, which may protect them from destruction by Fas-expressing lymphocytes.

Selected references

Bamberger AM, Schulte HM, Thuneke I, et al. Expression of the apoptosis-inducing Fas ligand (FasL) in human first and third trimester placenta and choriocarcinoma cells. *Journal of Clinical Endocrinology and Metabolism* 1997; 82: 3173-5.

De la Monte SM, Sohn YK, Wands JR. Correlates of p53- and Fas (CD95)-mediated apoptosis in Alzheimer's disease. *Journal of Neurological Sciences* 1997; 152: 73–83.

Hellquist HB, Olejnicka B, Jadner M, et al. Fas receptor is expressed in human lung squamous cell carcinomas, whereas bcl-2 and apoptosis are not pronounced: a preliminary report. *British Journal of Cancer* 1997; 76: 175–9.

Kazufumi M, Sonoko N, Masanori K, et al. Expression of bcl-2 protein and APO-1 (Fas antigen) in the lung tissue from patients with idiopathic pulmonary fibrosis. *Microscopy Research Technology* 1997; 38: 480–7.

Lee J, Richburg JH, Younkin SC, Bockelheide K. The Fas system is a key regulator of germ cell apoptosis in the testis. *Endocrinology* 1997; 138: 2081–8.

Nichans GA, Brunner T, Frizelle SP, et al. Human lung carcinomas express Fas ligand. *Cancer Research* 1997; 57: 1007–12.

Nonomura N, Mild T, Yokoyama M, et al. Fas/APO-1-mediated apoptosis of human renal cell carcinoma. *Biochemistry Biophysiology Research Communications* 1996; 229: 945–51.

Sheard MA, Vojtesek B, Janakova L, et al. Up-regulation of Fas (CD95) in human p53 wild-type cancer cells treated with ionizing radiation. *International Journal of Cancer* 1997; 73: 757–62.

Shukuwa T, Katayama I, Koji T. Fas-mediated apoptosis of melanoma cells and infiltrating lymphocytes in human malignant melanomas. *Modern Pathology* 2002; 15: 387–96.

Strater J, Wellisch I, Riedl S, et al. CD95 (APO-l/Fas)-mediated apoptosis in colon epithelial cells: a possible role in ulcerative colitis. *Gastroenterology* 1997; 113: 160–7.

Tachibana O, Lampe J, Kleihues P, Obgaki H. Preferential expression of Fas/APOl (CD95) and apoptotic cell death in perinecrotic cells of glioblastoma multiforme. *Acta Neuropathologica (Berlin)* 1996; 92: 431–4.

Uckan D, Steele A, Wang BY, et al. Trophoblasts express Fas ligand: a proposed mechanism for immune privilege in placenta and maternal invasion. *Molecular Human Reproduction* 1997; 3: 655–62.

Fascin

Sources/clones

Dako (clone 55K-2).

Fixation/preparation

Anti-fascin is applicable to formalin-fixed paraffin-embedded tissue sections. HIER is essential prior to the immunohistochemical staining procedure.

Background

Human fascin is a highly conserved 55 kDa actin-bundling protein. Fascin is encoded by the human homolog for the *hsn* gene and is thought to be involved in the formation of microfilament bundles. The clone 55K-2 was raised against fascin purified and characterized from HeLa cells.

Fascin immunoexpression has been demonstrated in interdigitating reticulum cells, follicular dendritic cells, and interstitial dendritic cells in lymph nodes. In addition, strong immunoreactivity has also been observed in dendritic cells of the thymus and spleen.

Histiocytes, smooth muscle cells, endothelial cells, and squamous mucosal cells may also express fascin. Fascin-expressing dendritic cells are decreased or absent in the neoplastic follicles of germinal centers compared with hyperplastic follicular centers. In contrast, cases of Castleman's disease reveal tight syncytial networks of fascin-positive follicular dendritic cells.

Fascin has been demonstrated in the cytoplasm of most Reed-Sternberg cells and their variants in Hodgkin disease, while only a minority of non-Hodgkin lymphoma was immunoreactive. Fascin immunopositivity has also been shown to highlight Reed-Sternberg cells in follicular Hodgkin lymphoma. Follicular dendritic cell tumors and juvenile xanthogranulomas have demonstrated uniform immunopositivity with fascin. However, only 75% of interdigitating dendritic cell sarcomas were fascin positive.

Applications

Fascin immunoreactivity in Hodgkin disease may serve to complement CD15 and CD30 to identify Reed-Sternberg cells (Appendix 2.3). Similarly, addition of fascin to CD21 and CD35 would be useful to identify follicular dendritic cell tumors (Appendix 2.7).

Selected references

Biddle DA, Ro JY, Yoon GS, *et al.* Extranodal follicular dendritic cell sarcoma of the head and neck region: three new cases, with a review of the literature. *Modern Pathology* 2002; 15: 50–8.

Dako Corporation. Anti-human fascin, 55K-2 (data sheet).

Duh FM, Latif F, Weng Y, *et al.* cDNA cloning and expression of the human homolog of the sea urchin fascin and Drosophila singed genes which encodes an actin-bundling protein. *DNA and Cell Biology* 1994; 13: 821–7.

Gaertner EM, Tsokos M, Derringer GA, *et al.* Interdigitating dendritic cell sarcoma. A report of four cases and review of the literature. *American Journal of Clinical Pathology* 2001: 115: 589–97.

Kansal R, Singleton TP, Ross CW, *et al.* Follicular Hodgkin lymphoma: a histopathologic study. *American Journal of Clinical Pathology* 2002; 117: 29–35.

Kraus MD, Haley JC, Ruiz R, *et al.* "Juvenile" xanthogranuloma: an immunophenotypic study with a reappraisal of histogenesis. *American Journal of Dermatopathology* 2001; 23: 104–11.

Mosialos G, Birkenbach M, Ayehunie S, *et al.* Circulating human dendritic cells differentially express high levels of 55-kd actin-bundling protein. *American Journal of Pathology* 1996; 148: 593–600.

Pinkus GS, Pinkus JL, Langhoff E, *et al.* Fascin, a sensitive new marker for Reed-Sternberg cells of Hodgkin's disease: evidence for a dendritic or B-cell derivation? *American Journal of Pathology* 1997; 150: 543–62.

Said JW, Pinkus JL, Shintaku IP, *et al.* Alterations in fascin-expressing germinal center dendritic cells in neoplastic follicles of B-cell lymphomas. *Modern Pathology* 1998; 11: 1–5.

Yamashiro-Matsumura S, Matsumura F. Purification and characterization of an F-actin-bundling 55-kilodalton protein from HeLa cells. *Journal of Biological Chemistry* 1985; 260: 5087–97.

Ferritin

Sources/clones

American Research Products (047A1703), Axcel/Accurate (polyclonal), Biodesign (ME.110, S1, S2, 501, 502, 503, 504, polyclonal), Biogenesis (05, 7D3/7, polyclonal), Biogenex (M-3.170, polyclonal), Chemicon (polyclonal), Dako (polyclonal), Fitzgerald (M94156, M94157, M94159, M94160, M94212, M94258, polyclonal), Serotec (polyclonal), Zymed (ZMFE1).

Fixation/preparation

Ferritin is resistant to formalin fixation, and immunoreactivity is enhanced following HIER.

Background

Ferritin, the iron storage protein, plays a key role in iron metabolism, and its ability to sequester iron gives ferritin the dual functions of iron detoxification and iron reserve. The distribution of ferritin is ubiquitous among living species, and its three-dimensional structure is highly conserved. All ferritins have 24 protein subunits arranged in 432 symmetry to give a hollow shell with an 80 A diameter cavity capable of storing up to 45,000 Fe (III) atoms as an inorganic complex. Subunits are folded as four-helix bundles each having a fifth short helix at roughly 60 degrees to the bundle axis.

Applications

Ferritin was one of the first markers employed for the identification of hepatocytes and their neoplastic counterparts, but it proved to be of low sensitivity and low specificity, being found in a wide range of benign and neoplastic tissues. Ferritin is expressed in hepatoid tumors such as those in the ovary and hepatoblastomas. Ferritin is employed as a marker of hemorrhage in the brain and is employed as a marker of microglia. In bone marrow biopsies, ferritin has been found to correlate with marrow hemosiderin as detected by the Perls' stain and is advocated as a more sensitive tool for the evaluation of body iron stores. In the skin, ferritin is localized to the outer layer of the eccrine duct, and in sweat gland neoplasms two distinct patterns have been noted. In syringoma the antibody decorated the outermost layer of cells in the epithelial cords of the tumor so that a characteristic ring was produced in cross sections, whereas only sparse staining was observed with other eccrine duct tumors such as dermal duct tumor and eccrine poroma. Syringoma showed diffuse staining, as did acrospiroma and a number of other adnexal carcinomas.

The presence of ferritin in epithelial cells often indicates increased cell permeability, and this property has been exploited in the demonstration that hyaline globules associated with a variety of tumors are the product of apoptotic cell death; the name "thanatosomes" has been proposed for such hyaline globules.

Comments

The diagnostic applications of this marker are limited, and except perhaps for the assessment of bone marrow iron stores, ferritin immunostaining is never employed alone.

Selected references

Abenoza P, Manivel JC, Wick MR, Hagen K, Dehner LP. Hepatoblastoma: an immunohistochemical and ultrastructural study. *Human Pathology* 1987; 18: 1025–35.

Carter RL, Hall JM, Corbett RP. Immunohistochemical staining for ferritin in neuroblastomas. *Histopathology* 1991; 18: 465–8.

Fleming S. Immunocytochemical localization of ferritin in the kidney and renal tumors. *European Urology* 1987; 13: 407–11.

Harrison PM, Arosio P. The ferritins: molecular properties, iron storage function and cellular regulation. *Biochemia Biophysiologica Acta* 1996; 1275: 161–203.

Imoto M, Nishimura D, Fukuda Y, *et al.* Immunohistochemical detection of alpha-fetoprotein, carcinoembryonic antigen, and ferritin in formalin-fixed sections from hepatocellular carcinoma. *American Journal of Gastroenterology* 1985; 80: 902–6.

Johnson DE, Powers CN, Rupp G, *et al.* Immunocytochemical staining of fine needle aspiration biopsies of the liver as a diagnostic tool for hepatocellular carcinoma. *Modern Pathology* 1992; 5: 117–23.

Kaneko Y, Kitamoto T, Tateishi J, Yamaguchi K. Ferritin immunohistochemistry as a marker for microglia. *Acta Neuropathologica (Berlin)* 1989; 79: 129–36.

Momotani E, Wuscger N, Ravisse P, Rastogi N. Immunohistochemical identification of ferritin, lactoferrin and transferrin in leprosy lesions of human skin biopsies. *Journal of Comparative Pathology* 1992; 106: 213–20.

Navone R, Azzoni L, Valente G. Immunohistochemical assessment of ferritin in bone marrow trephine biopsies: correlation with marrow hemosiderin. *Acta Hematologica* 1988; 80: 194–8.

Nogales FF, Concha A, Plata C, Ruiz-Avila I. Granulosa cell tumor of the ovary with diffuse true hepatic differentiation simulating stromal luteinization. *American Journal of Surgical Pathology* 1993; 17: 85–90.

Ozawa H, Nishida A, Mito T, Takashima S. Immunohistochemical study of ferritin-positive cells in the cerebellar cortex with subarachnoid hemorrhage in neonates. *Brain Research* 1994; 65: 345–8.

Papadimitriou JC, Drachenberg CB, Brenner DS, *et al.* "Thanatosomes": a unifying morphogenetic concept for tumor hyaline globules related to apoptosis. *Human Pathology* 2000; 31: 1455–65.

Penneys NS, Zlatkiss I. Immunohistochemical demonstration of ferritin in sweat gland and sweat gland neoplasms. *Journal of Cutaneous Pathology* 1990; 17: 32–6.

Tuccari G, Rizzo A, Crisafulli C, Barresi G. Iron-binding proteins in human colorectal adenomas and carcinomas: an immunohistochemical investigation. *Histology and Histopathology* 1992; 7: 543–7.

Fibrin

Sources/clones
Accurate (T2G1), Biodesign (polyclonal), Biogenesis (2F7), Serotec (E8).

Fixation/preparation
The antigen is resistant to formalin fixation, and proteolytic digestion or HIER enhances immunoreactivity.

Background
Proteolytic conversion of fibrinogen to fibrin results in self-assembly to form a clot matrix that subsequently becomes cross-linked by factor XIIIa to form the main structural element of the thrombus in vivo. The roles of fibrin and its precursor have been extensively studied both in vitro and in vivo.

Applications
Diagnostic applications of fibrin are mainly limited to the study of glomerulopathy, with sporadic use of anti-fibrin to identify fibrin deposits and thrombi in extrarenal sites.

Comments
The diagnostic applications of anti-fibrin are limited to specific situations. Applications in nephropathology, particularly with immunofluoresence techniques, are still extensive.

Selected references
Bini A, Kudryk BJ. Fibrinogen and fibrin in the arterial wall. *Thrombosis Research* 1994; 75: 337–41.

Blomback B. Fibrinogen structure, activation and polymerization and fibrin gel structure. *Thrombosis Research* 1994; 75: 327–8.

Blomback B. Fibrinogen and fibrin: proteins with complex roles in hemostasis and thrombosis. *Thrombosis Research* 1996; 83: 1–75.

Bonsib SM. Differential diagnosis in nephropathology: an immunofluorescence-driven approach. *Advances in Anatomic Pathology* 2002; 9: 101–14.

Dowling JP. Immunohistochemistry of renal diseases and tumours. In Leong AS-Y, ed. *Applied Immunohistochemistry for Surgical Pathologists*. London: Edward Arnold, 1993, pp. 210–59.

Gaffhey PJ. Structure of fibrinogen and degradation products of fibrinogen and fibrin. *British Medical Bulletin* 1997; 33: 245–51.

Imokawa S, Sato A, Hayakawa H, *et al*. Tissue factor expression and fibrin deposition in the lungs of patients with idiopathic pulmonary fibrosis and systemic sclerosis. *American Journal of Respiratory and Critical Care Medicine* 1997; 156: 631–6.

Kahng HC, Chin NW, Opitz LM, Pahuja M, Goldberg SL. Cellular angiolipoma of the breast: immunohistochemical study and review of the literature. *Breast Journal* 2002; 8: 47–9.

Lorand L. Physiological roles of fibrinogen and fibrin. *Federation Proceedings* 1965; 24: 784–93.

Mosessan MW. The roles of fibrinogen and fibrin in hemostasis and thrombosis. *Seminars in Hematology* 1992; 29: 177–88.

Mosessan MW. Fibrinogen and fibrin polymerization: appraisal of the binding events that accompany fibrin generation and fibrin clot assembly. *Blood Coagulation and Fibrinolysis* 1997; 8: 257–67.

Takahashi H, Shibata Y, Fujita S, Okabe H. Immunohistochemical findings of arterial fibrinoid necrosis in major and lingual minor salivary glands of primary Sjogren's syndrome. *Anatomical and Cellular Pathology* 1996; 12: 145–57.

NOTES

Fibrinogen

Sources/clones

Accurate (2C2G7, 85D4), Axcel/Accurate (polyclonal), American Qualex (polyclonal), Biodesign (PA), Biogenesis (2D 1–2, polyclonal), Biogenex (2D 1–2, polyclonal), Calbiochem (polyclonal), Caltag Laboratories, Chemicon, Coulter (D1G10VL2, E3F8E5), Dako (polyclonal), EY Labs, Immunotech (D1G10VL2, E3F8E5), Sera Lab (polyclonal), Sigma (85D4, FG21).

Fixation/preparation

Fibrinogen is fixative-resistant.

Background

Fibrinogen is a 340 kDa multi-subunit glycoprotein present in plasma and tissue of all classes of vertebrates. Fibrinogen has a variety of physiologically important functions, most of which, if not all, are assigned to certain structures of fibrin including double-stranded fibrin protofibrils and highly cross-linked fibrin networks. Its role in hemostasis and thrombosis has been extensively studied.

Applications

Diagnostic applications of fibrinogen are largely limited to the identification of fibrinogen deposition and breakdown products in glomerular diseases.

Comments

Immunostaining for fibrin/fibrinogen deposits is employed for the detection of microthrombi.

Selected references

Blomback B. Fibrinogen and fibrin -proteins with complex roles in hemostasis and thrombosis. *Thrombosis Research* 1996; 83: 1–75.

Dowling JP. Immunohistochemistry of renal diseases and tumours. In Leong AS-Y, ed. *Applied Immunohistochemistry for Surgical Pathologists*. London: Edward Arnold, 1993, pp. 210–59.

Gaffney PJ. Structure of fibrinogen and degradation products of fibrinogen and fibrin. *British Medical Bulletin* 1997; 33: 245–51.

Henschen A. On the structure of functional sites in fibrinogen. *Thrombosis Research* 1983; 5 (Suppl): 27–39.

Mosesson MW. The roles of fibrinogen and fibrin in hemostasis and thrombosis. *Seminars in Hematology* 1992; 29: 177–88.

Mosesson MW. Fibrinogen and fibrin polymerization: appraisal of the binding events that accompany fibrin generation and fibrin clot assembly. *Blood Coagulation and Fibrinolysis* 1997; 8: 257–67.

Shafer JA, Higgins DL. Human fibrinogen. *Critical Reviews in Clinical Laboratory Science* 1988; 26: 1–41.

Stewart FA, Te Poele JA, Van der Wal AF, *et al*. Radiation nephropathy: the link between functional damage and vascular mediated inflammatory and thrombotic change. *Acta Oncologica* 2001; 40: 952–7.

NOTES

Fibronectin

Sources/clones

Accurate (2B6F9, 568), Axcel/Accurate (polyclonal), Biodesign (1601, 1602, 120-5), Biogenesis (BIO-FIBTN-001, Bo, Rt, polyclonal), Biogenex (2755-8), Calbiochem (3E1, polyclonal), Caltag Laboratories, Cymbus Bioscience (FN4), Dako (polyclonal), EY Labs, Fitzgerald (polyclonal), Harlan Sera Lab/Accurate (2.3F9), Novocastra (polyclonal), Serotec (polyclonal), Sigma Chemical (FN-15, FN3-E2), Zymed (Z068, FN12-8).

Fixation/preparation

The antibody is well suited for both formalin-fixed paraffin-embedded sections and cryostat sections. Proteolytic predigestion with protease or pepsin of formalin-fixed tissue is recommended.

Background

Fibronectin is a non-collagenous connective tissue glycoprotein found in association with both basement membranes and interstitial connective tissue. The exact ultrastructural localization of fibronectin within the basement membrane is controversial. Fibronectin is a β-glycoprotein with a molecular weight of 44 kDa, comprising two nearly identical sub-chains. It is widely distributed throughout many normal tissues including connective tissues, blood vessel walls, and basement membranes. Some of the properties of fibronectin include forming cross-links with fibrin in blood clots through factor XIII and binding to heparin and collagen. It is also thought to play a role in cellular adhesion, wound healing, and tissue repair. Antiserum to human fibronectin was produced from purified human material isolated from a pool of normal human plasma.

Applications

Fibronectin (and laminin) has been demonstrated to line cystic lumina and around tumor islands in adenoid cystic breast and salivary gland carcinomas. This pattern of distribution has been recommended as an aid to the diagnosis of these tumors, while its absence may have important prognostic implications, pointing to an aggressive outcome. Fibronectin immunoreactivity in breast adenoid cystic carcinomas is also useful in distinguishing them from cribriform carcinomas, the latter being negative.

In a comparative study of epithelial neoplasms of gastrointestinal and salivary gland origin, the difficulty in distinguishing between fibronectin of epithelial and fibroblastic origin was emphasized. In addition, carcinoma fibronectin was sometimes, but not invariably, lost from epithelial cell surfaces, suggesting that loss of cell surface fibronectin was unlikely to serve as a useful diagnostic marker for malignancy. In soft tissue tumors, fibronectin was found to be most abundant in the stroma, both benign and malignant. Fibronectin failed to be useful in the identification of vitality of human skin injuries because of low sensitivity of immunohistochemical staining, although it was shown to be useful with immunofluoresence techniques, as for the demonstration of decreased basement membrane in the intestinal mucosa of patients with celiac disease.

Comments

The major role of fibronectin is in the diagnosis of adenoid cystic carcinoma of the salivary gland and breast, with the latter being distinguished from cribriform carcinoma. Either adenoid cystic carcinoma or connective tissue stroma may be used as a positive control.

Selected references

D' Arderme AJ, Burns J, Skyes BC, Bennett MK. Fibronectin and type III collagen in epithelial neoplasms of gastrointestinal tract and salivary gland. *Journal of Clinical Pathology* 1983; 36: 756–63.

D'Ardenne AJ, Kirkpatrick P, Sykes BC. The distribution of laminin, fibronectin and interstitial collagen type III in soft tissue tumors. *Journal of Clinical Pathology* 1984; 37: 895–904.

D'Ardenne AJ, Kirkpatrick P, Wells CA, Davies JD. Laminin and fibronectin in adenoid cystic carcinoma. *Journal of Clinical Pathology* 1986; 39: 138–44.

Kirkpatrick P, d'Ardenne AJ. Effects of fixation and enzymatic digestion on the immunohistochemical demonstration of laminin and fibronectin in paraffin embedded tissue. *Journal of Clinical Pathology* 1984; 37: 639–44.

Laurie GW, Leblond CP, Martin GR. Localization of type IV collagen, laminin, heparan sulfate proteoglycan and fibronectin to the basal lamina of basement membranes. *Journal of Cell Biology* 1982; 95: 340–4.

Mosher DF, Fiocht L. Fibronectin: review of its structure and possible functions. *Journal of Investigative Dermatology* 1981; 77: 175–80.

Ortiz-Rey JA, Suarez-Penaranda JM, da Silva EA, *et al.* Immunohistochemical detection of fibronectin and tenascin in incised human skin injuries. *Forensic Science International* 2002; 126: 118–22.

Stenman S, Vaheri A. Distribution of a major connective tissue protein, fibronectin in normal human tissues. *Journal of Experimental Medicine* 1978; 147: 1054–64.

Verbeke S, Gotteland M, Fernandez M, *et al.* Basement membrane and connective tissue proteins in intestinal mucosa of patients with celiac disease. *Journal of Clinical Pathology* 2002; 55: 440–5.

Fli-1

Sources/clones

Abbexa (polyclonal), Abcam (polyclonal), Abnova (polyclonal), Acris (BV4), Amsbio (polyclonal), Aviva Systems Bio (polyclonal), Biorbyt (polyclonal), Bio S B (G146-222), Bioss (polyclonal), Boster Immunoleader (polyclonal), Cell Marque/Leica (MRQ-1), Creative Biomart (polyclonal), Enzo Life Sciences (NF6), Gene Tex (polyclonal), Lifespan Biosciences (EPR4646, polyclonal), Novus (polyclonal), Santa Cruz (SC-356, polyclonal), Thermo Scientific Pierce Products (polyclonal), United States Monoclonal (F4550–05B, 6D397).

Fixation/preparation

Several of the antibody clones and polyclonal antibodies to Fli-1 are immunoreactive in fixed paraffin-embedded sections. HIER at 120 °C enhances labeling.

Background

Human Friend leukemia virus integration 1 (Fli-1) is a member of a family of transcription factor proteins that share a conserved DNA-binding region, the E26 transformation-specific (ETS) domain. That peptide sequence is 98 amino acid residues long, and it bears a molecular resemblance to the helix-turn-helix motif of DNA-binding proteins. Fli-1 is a sequence-specific transcriptional activator involved in cell proliferation. It recognizes the DNA sequence 5′-C(CA)GGAAGT-3′ and is encoded by a gene on the long arm of chromosome 11 (11q24). In rodents, the *FLI1* gene locus is a common site of viral nucleic acid integration in virus-driven leukemogenesis. In all vertebrates, the *FLI1* gene regulates the development of hematopoietic precursors and endothelial cells. In endothelial cells, Fli-1 interacts with the proximal promoter of the *LMO2* gene.

Ewing's sarcoma/primitive neuroectodermal tumor (ES/PNET) is characterized in approximately 90% of cases by a reciprocal translocation t(11;22)(q24;q12) which results in the fusion of the *EWS* gene on chromosome 22 to the *FLI1* gene on chromosome 11. The *FLI1* gene encodes for a truncated transcription factor belonging to the avian ETS family of DNA-binding transcription factors, which is involved in cellular proliferation and tumorigenesis. The resultant fusion protein may play a role in the evasion of cellular senescence.

Applications

Fli-1 is expressed in diverse tumor types. Fli-1 is expressed in most cases of Ewing's sarcoma (71–100%). The initial study of Fli-1 immunoreactivity showed high sensitivity (94%) among vascular tumors including hemangiomas, hemangioendotheliomas, angiosarcoma, and Kaposi's sarcoma, and absent immunoreactivity in non-vascular tumors. Follow-up studies have expanded the spectrum of Fli-1 immunoreactivity to also include certain types of carcinoma, lymphoma, juvenile granulosa cell tumor, melanoma, anaplastic large-cell neuroblastoma, and sarcomas. In the differential diagnosis of cutaneous angiosarcoma of the head and neck, strong, diffuse nuclear Fli-1 reactivity was highly sensitive for angiosarcoma (100%), but specificity was low at only 29% given the high frequency of Fli-1 expression detected in squamous cell carcinoma (90%), atypical fibroxanthoma (90%), melanoma (60%), and atypical intradermal smooth muscle neoplasms (20%). These observations limit the utility of Fli-1 in the diagnosis of vascular neoplasms. Given the wide availability of *EWSR1* FISH adjunctive testing for Ewing's sarcoma/primitive neuroectodermal tumor (ES/PNET), the role of Fli-1 diagnostic testing is confined to the small subset of Ewing's sarcoma cases lacking *EWSR1*. It should also be pointed out that in previously decalcified specimens that are considered unsuitable for FISH, Fli-1 can be detected in some cases.

Since normal lymphocytes and endothelial cells demonstrate nuclear localization of Fli-1, interpretation can be challenging in some cases and caution is recommended to avoid overinterpretation of positive Fli-1 reactivity in neoplastic cells.

Using a polyclonal antibody raised against the carboxyl terminal of Fli-1 protein, workers have demonstrated Fli-1 immunopositivity in cytologic preparations of ES/PNET cell lines known to contain an *EWS/FLI1* fusion gene, and 5/7 formalin-fixed paraffin-embedded ES/PNET. Evaluating small, blue, round cell tumors, the following immunopositivity using formalin-fixed paraffin-embedded tissue was seen: positive for ES/PNET, lymphoblastic lymphomas, desmoplastic round cell tumor; negative for poorly differentiated synovial sarcomas (PDSS), rhabdomyosarcomas (RMS), neuroblastomas, esthesioneuroblastomas, Wilms tumor, mesenchymal chondrosarcoma. Fli-1 protein expression is seen in 95% of benign and malignant vascular tumors, including angiosarcomas, hemangioendotheliomas, hemangiomas, and Kaposi's sarcomas.

Comments

Fli-1 nuclear transcription factor appears to be a relatively sensitive and specific marker for ES/PNET. However, a note of caution in the differential diagnosis of small round blue cell tumors is that the great majority of lymphoblastic lymphomas are also positive with Fli-1 protein. Nevertheless, Fli-1 protein is useful to distinguish ES/PNET from other CD99+ tumors such as PDSS and RMS (Appendix 1.3). The Fli-1 immunopositivity in vascular tumors appears to equal or exceed those of established vascular markers such as CD31, CD34, and FVIII.

Being a transcription factor, Fli-1 immunopositivity is nuclear in location. Clone MRQ-1 produces the best results. Immunoreactivity appears not to be enhanced by boiling or proteolytic digestion and is best demonstrated following retrieval at 120 °C in EDTA buffer at pH 9.0.

Selected references

Cuda J, Mirzamani N, Kantipudi R, *et al.* Diagnostic utility of Fli-1 and D2-40 in distinguishing atypical fibroxanthoma from angiosarcoma. *American Journal of Dermatopathology* 2013; 35: 316–18.

Folpe AL, Chand EM, Goldblum JR, Weiss SW. Expression of Fli-1, a nuclear transcription factor, distinguishes vascular neoplasms from potential mimics. *American Journal of Surgical Pathology* 2001; 25: 1061–6.

Folpe AL, Hill CE, Parham DM, *et al.* Immunohistochemical detection of FLI-1 protein expression: A study of 132 round cell tumors with emphasis on CD99-positive mimics of Ewing's sarcoma/primitive neuroectodermal tumor. *American Journal of Surgical Pathology* 2000; 24: 1657–62.

Nilsson G, Wang M, Wejde J, *et al.* Detection of EWS/FLI-1 by immunostaining. An adjunctive tool in diagnosis of Ewing's sarcoma and primitive neuroectodermal tumor on cytological samples and paraffin-embedded archival material. *Sarcoma* 1999; 3: 25–32.

Turc-Carel C, Aurias A, Mugneret F, *et al.* Chromosomes in Ewing's sarcoma. I: an evaluation of 85 cases of remarkable consistency of t(11; 22)(q24; q12). *Cancer Genetics and Cytogenetics* 1988; 32: 229–38.

Zucman J, Delattre O, Desmaze C, *et al.* Cloning and characterization of the Ewing's sarcoma and peripheral neuroepithelioma t(11; 22) translocation breakpoints. *Genes Chromosomes and Cancer* 1992; 5: 271–7.

FMC-7

Sources/clones

Monoclonal antibody FMC-7 (Immunotech, Beckman Coulter Company).

Fixation/preparation

This antibody has been largely utilized by flow cytometry with FMC-7-FITC. Its role in immunophenotyping of mature B-cell lymphomas has been utilized in the recent World Health Organization classification of lymphomas.

Background

The monoclonal antibody FMC-7, developed at the Flinders Medical Centre (Australia) by somatic hybridization against the human B-cell line HRIK, appears to define a subset of normal human B lymphocytes. It is also useful to distinguish mature B-cell leukemias from immature variants. The antibody FMC-7 detects an antigen on certain subgroups of neoplastic and normal B cells that have arisen from cells in later stages of B-cell maturation. However, some studies indicate that the use of FMC-7 antibody in immunophenotypic studies of lymphomas does not contribute any additional information or diagnostic reliability.

FMC-7 and CD23 expression pattern was evaluated in B-cell lymphoma, and the CD23−/FMC-7+ pattern was most common in large-cell, mantle, and marginal zone lymphomas. The CD23/FMC-7/CD5 co-expression pattern permitted accurate classification of all cases of small lymphocytic, mantle cell, and marginal zone lymphomas. The widest variation of patterns was with follicular cell lymphomas. The CD23 and FMC-7 antigen expression pattern was predictive of subtypes in more than 95% of lymphoma cases and could narrow the differential diagnosis in the remaining cases.

Applications

It would appear that FMC-7 expression in combination with CD23 facilitates accurate and reproducible classification of B-cell lymphomas in flow cytometric analysis.

Selected references

Catovsky D, Brooks D. Bradley J, et al. Heterogeneity of B-cell leukemias demonstrated by the monoclonal antibody FMC-7. *Blood* 1981; 58: 406–8.

Drexler HG, Menon M, Gaedicke G, Minowada J. Expression of FMC7 antigen and tartrate-resistant acid phosphatase isoenzyme in cases of B-lymphoproliferative diseases. *European Journal of Cancer and Clinical Oncology* 1987; 23: 61–8.

Garcia DP, Rooney MT, Ahmad E, Davis BH. Diagnostic usefulness of CD23 and FMC-7 antigen expression patterns in B-cell lymphoma classification. *American Journal of Clinical Pathology* 2001; 115: 258–65.

Hubl W, Iturraspe J, Braylan RC. FMC7 antigen expression on normal and malignant B-cells can be predicted by expression of CD20. *Cytometry* 1998; 34: 71–4.

Huh YO, Pugh WC, Kantarjian HM, et al. Detection of subgroups of chronic B-cell leukemias as FMC7 monoclonal antibody. *American Journal of Clinical Pathology* 1994; 101: 283–9.

Menon M. Drexler HG, Minowada J. Heterogeneity of marker expression in B-cell leukemias and its diagnostic significance. *Leukemia Research* 1986; 10: 25–8.

Zola H, McNamara PJ, Moore HA, et al. Maturation of human B lymphocytes: studies with a panel of monoclonal antibodies against membrane antigens. *Clinical and Experimental Immunology* 1983; 52: 655–64.

Zola H, Moore HA, Hohmann A, Hunter IK. The antigen of mature human B cells detected by the monoclonal antibody FMC7: studies on the nature of the antigen and modulation of its expression. *Journal of Immunology* 1984; 133: 321–6.

NOTES

Forkhead box L2 (FOXL2)

Sources/clones

Santa Cruz (H-43, 262C1a), Imgenex (polyclonal).

Fixation/preparation

Antibodies are immunoreactive in fixed paraffin-embedded tissues.

Background

FOXL2 is a forkhead transcription factor that is active in multiple tissues including eyelid, ovary, and pituitary gland. It is expressed as a nuclear protein mainly in the adult ovary and is important for the development of granulosa cells in the ovary. Ovarian sex cord–stromal tumors (SCSTs) are uncommon neoplasms. Adult granulosa cell tumors (aGCTs) are the most common type of malignant SCST, and it has been reported that 97% of aGCTs harbor a mutation in the *FOXL2* gene (*402G*). The mutation was found to be absent in 49 SCSTs of other types and in 329 unrelated or breast tumors. Also, the mutation is occasionally present in a very small proportion of thecomas and juvenile granulosa cell tumors (jGCTs). Testing for FOXL2 mutation (*402G-C*) is not widely available at present, and therefore FOXL2 immunostaining, which gives a nuclear pattern of staining, is useful.

Applications

Ovarian SCSTs are a heterogeneous group of tumors that have varied appearances which can lead to difficulties in diagnosis. FOXL2 staining is present in almost all SCSTs with a *FOXL2* mutation, and also in a majority of SCSTs without a mutation. Testing for FOXL2 immunoexpression can serve to distinguish between SCST and non-SCST. Studies have shown that FOXL2 expression is highly specific for SCST (99%). Within the SCST category, FOXL2 expression is present strongly in all subtypes except in Sertoli–Leydig cell tumor in which FOXL2 expression is seen in only 50% of those tumors. Regardless of growth pattern (solid, cystic, trabecular, gyriform, cystic, pleomorphic), FOXL2 expression is similar among all aGCTs. FOXL2 staining can help distinguish spindle cell tumors of sex cord origin from other mesenchymal tumors. In the fibrothecoma group, FOXL2 immunoexpression is seen in 91% of cases, in contrast to no reactivity in non-ovarian mesenchymal lesions.

Of note, female adnexal tumors of probable Wolffian origin (FATWO), which usually occur in the broad ligament and may be confused with SCSTs, are also immunoreactive for FOXL2.

Selected references

Al-Agha OM, Huwait HF, Chow C, *et al.* FOXL2 is a sensitive and specific marker for sex cord–stromal tumors of the ovary. *American Journal of Surgical Pathology* 2011; 35: 484–94.

Shah SP, Kobel M, Senz J, *et al.* Mutation of FOXL2 in granulosa-cell tumors of the ovary. *New England Journal of Medicine* 2009; 360: 2719–29.

Stewart CJ, Alexiadis M, Crook ML, Fuller PJ. An immunohistochemical and molecular analysis of problematic and unclassified ovarian sex cord–stromal tumors. *Human Pathology* 2013; 44: 2774–81.

NOTES

GATA binding protein 3 (GATA3)

Sources/clones

Clone HG3-31 Mouse monoclonal anti-GATA3 antibodies, Santa Cruz Biotechnology, CA.
Clone L50-823 Mouse monoclonal anti-GATA3 antibody, Biopcare Medical, Concord, CA.

Fixation/preparation

Standardized for formalin-fixed paraffin-embedded tissue. Nuclear staining.

Background

The name GATA is given to a family of transcription factors whose members bind the DSA sequence (A/T) GATA (A/G) via 2 zinc-finger domains with consensus sequence CX2C17–18CX2 C. The family comprises six members that are divided into two subgroups on the basis of their tissue distribution, structure, and function. Members of the first group are GATA1, GATA2, and GATA3, which have an overwhelming association with hematopoietic lineage and the development of nervous system. The second group is composed of GATA4, GATA5, and GATA6 and associated with a large variety of mesoderm and endodermal-derived tissues including parts of the genitourinary system, lungs, parts of gastrointestinal tract organs including stomach and intestine, and vasculature. The GATA family (with the exception of GATA5) plays an obligatory developmental role. They influence cell-fate specification, differentiation, proliferation, and movement.

GATA3, also known as endothelial transcription factor 3, is a ~48 kDa protein comprising 443 amino acids encoded by a gene located on chromosome 10p15. It is expressed in early-stage erythrocytes and T cells. It is extensively expressed in embryonic tissue such as brain, parathyroid, skin, inner ear, adrenal glands, liver, and placenta. Normal adult tissues including lung, parotid gland, stomach, small intestine, colon, pancreas, liver, thyroid, prostate, seminal vesicle, ovary, and endometrium are negative. In normal adult cells GATA3 is expressed in T lymphocytes, luminal glandular epithelial cells of breast, parathyroid glands, and urothelium. In the kidney GATA3 has been reported to be expressed in distal tubules but absent in proximal tubules. GATA3 is expressed strongly in a large majority of urothelial (67% to ~80%) and breast (~70%) carcinomas. Differences may be partially due to the difference in antibody clones used in these studies. GATA3 expression in urothelial carcinoma is diffuse with strong intensity usually.

GATA3 is more sensitive than uroplakin III, but less sensitive than S100P, thrombomodulin, or p63. GATA3 is a more specific urothelial marker than S100P, thrombomodulin, or p63, but less specific than uroplakin. In addition to urothelial epithelium, GATA3 is positive in various putative urothelial cell proliferations such as Walthard nests and benign Brenner tumors.

Applications

Tumors involving male and female genitourinary tract

1. High-grade prostatic adenocarcinoma vs. high-grade urothelial carcinoma

    While the majority of prostate cancers can be clinically and morphologically distinguished from urothelial carcinoma (UC), this distinction may be difficult if not impossible in poorly differentiated tumors that involve the bladder neck. In the setting of a transurethral resection of bladder neck tumor this differentiation may be particularly challenging. While most prostate cancers are composed of atypical yet uniform populations of cells with a sheet-like growth pattern, UC tends to show a more nested growth pattern with atypical pleomorphic cells. Subtle cribriforming can be seen in both prostatic adenocarcinoma and UC. Additionally, rarely, prostate cancers may appear to grow in a nested pattern with pleomorphic cells: the so-called "pleomorphic giant cell adenocarcinoma." A precise and concise panel in working up such a differential diagnosis consists of GATA3, prostate-specific antigen (PSA), prostate-specific membrane antigen (PSMA), p501S (Prostein), and NKX3.1.

In cases where both PSA and PSMA are lost in high-grade prostatic adenocarcinoma, additional prostatic adenocarcinoma markers and GATA3 are helpful in teasing out the differences.

2. High-grade urothelial carcinoma vs. spread from uterine cervical or anal squamous cell carcinoma

Primary squamous cell carcinoma (SCC) of the urinary bladder is rare, and associated with specific etiologic events. The differential diagnosis of SCC in bladder includes primary urothelial SCC or a secondary involvement of bladder via extension from SCC of the uterine cervix or anus. In such cases GATA3 should not be used, as its expression is only seen in about 5% of primary SCC of bladder; on the other hand SCC arising from uterine cervix or anus can be positive in approximately 6% and 7% of cases, respectively. The use of GATA3 may therefore spuriously suggest urothelial origin. Additional stains including p16 or in-situ hybridization for high-risk HPV may be considered to accurately differentiate the two.

3. Urothelial carcinoma vs. primary renal cell carcinoma

High-grade, poorly differentiated urothelial carcinoma of the renal pelvis that extensively invades the renal parenchyma may be difficult to distinguish from a poorly differentiated primary renal cell carcinoma. An immunohistochemical panel with GATA3 (67–88%), S100P (another marker commonly expressed in UC) and PAX-8 (expressed in all subtypes of renal cell carcinomas, but absent in UC) will help differentiate the two.

Metastatic urothelial carcinoma

1. Urothelial carcinoma and its variants. 67–80% of conventional UCs show GATA3 expression, with 90% concordance between matched primary and metastatic UC. Among the variants of UC, micropapillary and plasmacytoid UC are positive in 57% and 44% of cases respectively. Sarcomatoid and small-cell variants express GATA3 weakly and only in 16% and 5% of cases respectively. Thus, while GATA3 expression is helpful in identifying the urothelial origin of micropapillary and plasmacytoid UC in the workup of metastatic carcinomas, it has limited if any usefulness in the workup of sarcomatoid UC and small-cell carcinoma.

2. GATA3 is highly expressed in breast carcinomas across all histological subtypes. When compared to other available markers including GCDFP-15 and mammaglobin, GATA3 has been found to be a more sensitive immunohistochemical marker for breast cancer. GATA3 therefore is a useful marker when the differential diagnosis of metastatic breast cancer does not include UC. Additionally, low expression of GATA3 has been associated with a poorer prognosis for invasive carcinoma.

3. Secondary involvement of bladder by adenocarcinoma from prostate, colon, endometrium, breast, or lung is uncommon, but more common than primary adenocarcinoma of bladder. The distinction is very important, as treatment of primary adenocarcinoma of bladder is surgical whereas metastases are treated systemically. GATA3 is positive in 40% of primary urothelial signet ring carcinomas, 10% of signet ring cancers with extracellular mucin, and 5% of conventional urothelial adenocarcinomas. GATA3 therefore has some utility when the differential diagnosis includes signet ring cell carcinoma originating from the gastrointestinal tract vs. those arising as primary bladder adenocarcinoma.

4. GATA3 positivity has also been noted in trophoblastic tumors and mesonephric adenocarcinoma of the uterine cervix.

Selected references

Chang A, Amin A, Gabrielson E, *et al.* Utility of GATA3 immunohistochemistry in differentiating urothelial carcinoma from prostate adenocarcinoma and squamous cell carcinomas of the uterine cervix, anus, and lung. *American Journal of Surgical Pathology* 2012; 36: 1472–6.

Ellis CL, Chang AG, Cimino-Mathews A, *et al.* GATA-3 immunohistochemistry in the differential diagnosis of adenocarcinoma of the urinary bladder. *American Journal of Surgical Pathology* 2013; 37: 1756–60.

Liu H, Shi J, Prichard JW, Gong Y, Lin F. Immunohistochemical evaluation of GATA-3 expression in ER-negative breast carcinomas. *American Journal of Clinical Pathology* 2014; 141: 648–55.

Liu H, Shi J, Wilkerson ML, Lin F. Immunohistochemical evaluation of GATA3 expression in tumors and normal tissues: a useful immunomarker for breast and urothelial carcinomas. *American Journal of Clinical Pathology* 2012; 138: 57–64.

Ordonez NG. Value of GATA3 immunostaining in tumor diagnosis: a review. *Advances in Anatomic Pathology* 2013; 20: 352–60.

Simon MC. Gotta have GATA. *Nature Genetics* 1995; 11: 9–11.

Yoon NK, Maresh EL, Shen D, *et al*. Higher levels of GATA3 predict better survival in women with breast cancer. *Human Pathology* 2010; 41: 1794–801.

NOTES

Glial fibrillary acidic protein (GFAP)

Sources/clones

Accurate (GA-5, 6F2, polyclonal), Amersham, Biodesign (DP46.10, GF-01), Biogenesis (GF-01, polyclonal), Biogenex (GA-5, polyclonal), Chemicon (monoclonal, polyclonal), Cymbus Bioscience (polyclonal), Dako (6F2, polyclonal), Enzo, EY Labs, ICN (polyclonal), Immunotech (DP46.10), Milab (polyclonal), Novocastra, Sanbio (6F2, polyclonal), Saxo (polyclonal), Sera Lab (GA-5), Serotec (GA-5, MIG-G2), Sigma (GA-5, polyclonal), Signet, Zymed (ZSGFAP2, ZCG29).

Fixation/preparation

Glial fibrillary acidic protein (GFAP) is relatively resilient to fixation, and most antibodies are immunoreactive in routinely fixed and processed tissue sections. GFAP staining seems more consistent after fixation in Bouin's fixative. Monoclonal antibodies are more fixative-sensitive, and polyclonal antibodies show more intense and more extensive staining. GFAP immunoreactivity is mildly enhanced by HIER.

Background

GFAP is an intermediate filament (IF) protein of astroglia and belongs to the type III subclass of IF proteins. Like other IF proteins, GFAP is composed of an amino-terminal head domain, a central rod domain, and a carboxyl terminus tail domain. GFAP, with a molecular weight of 50 kDa, has the smallest head domain among the class III IF proteins. Despite its insolubility, GFAP is in dynamic equilibrium between assembled filaments and unassembled subunits. As with other IF proteins, assembly of GFAP is regulated by phosphorylation–dephosphorylation of the head domain by alteration of its charge. The frequent co-polymerization of GFAP with vimentin IF in immature, reactive, or radial glial indicates that vimentin has an important role in the build-up of the glial architecture. The human GFAP gene is localized to chromosome 17.

Applications

In the central nervous system, astrocytes, rare ependymal cells, and cerebellar radial glia express GFAP (Appendix 1.2). Mature oligodendrocytes do not express GFAP. GFAP or a GFAP-like protein is also found in Schwann cells, enteric glia, cells in all portions of the pituitary, cartilage, the iris and lens epithelium, and the fat-storing cells of the liver. While monoclonal antibodies are said to recognize the GFAP epitope exclusively, there may be cross-reactivity with common epitopes shared by other IFs like neurofilaments and vimentin.

Immunohistochemical staining of GFAP has proven use in the identification of benign astrocytes and neoplastic cells of glial lineage. Its application to the developing nervous system has contributed to our understanding of the histogenesis of neural tissue, and its identification in various forms of injury and neoplasia has helped in the understanding of the role of astrocytes in these processes.

While it was initially thought that the GFAP expression in salivary gland tissues and pleomorphic adenomas was in myoepithelial cells, more recent evidence from developmental and cell culture studies indicates that GFAP is expressed in the epithelial cells, the myoepithelial cells being uniformly negative for the antigen. GFAP has been demonstrated in cartilage cells in culture but does not appear to occur in chondrosarcomas and mesenchymal chondrosarcomas, and in-vivo and immunohistochemical detection of GFAP is used to identify chordomas. Choroid plexus tumors and ependymomas express GFAP in addition to S100 protein, and occasionally cytokeratin and epithelial membrane antigen. In the setting of vacuolated clear cell tumors occurring in the retroperitoneal space, GFAP positivity would serve to distinguish chordoma and ependymoma from other mimics, including renal cell carcinoma and colorectal carcinoma.

Comments

Polyclonal antibodies to GFAP produce more intense and more extensive staining than monoclonal antibodies. GFAP and S100 are sensitive markers of glial differentiation. GFAP is useful in the identification of intracranial and intraventricular tumors (Appendix 1.7, 1.35), and in the differential diagnosis of small-cell tumors in the brain (Appendix 1.36).

Selected reference

Inagaki M, Nakamura Y, Takeda M, *et al.* Glial fibrillary acidic protein: dynamic property and regulation by phosphorylation. *Brain Pathology* 1994; 4: 239–43.

Glut-1

Sources/clones

Glut-1 clone SPM 498: Thermo Fisher Scientific, Kalamazoo, MI

Polyclonal goat anti-Glut-1 antibodies, 1:500 dilution: Santa Cruz Biotechnology, CA

Polyclonal rabbit anti-glucose transporter antibodies reactive with Glut-1 (brain/erythrocyte) (diluted 1:500): East Acres Biological, Southbridge, MA

Polyclonal rabbit GLUT 1 antibody: Dako, Carpenteria, CA

Background

A 38–55 kDa erythroid/brain-type carboxyl terminal of hexose transporter GLUT-1 protein (member of sodium independent glucose transporter gene superfamily) was originally reported by immunofluorescence studies in rat brain and liver tissues; and later in normal rat kidney cells, with increased expression in glucose-deprived cells.

Applications

This was followed by the detection of increased expression in breast cancer cells, biopsied glioblastoma, pancreatic neoplasms, small cell and non-small-cell lung cancer, head and neck squamous cell carcinoma, gastric carcinomas, rhabdomyosarcoma, choriocarcinoma, invasive urothelial carcinoma, embryonal neoplasms of CNS, borderline and malignant ovarian neoplasms, fallopian tube carcinoma, uterine carcinoma, cervical carcinoma colorectal adenomas and carcinomas, malignant thyroid nodules, cholangiocarcinoma, juvenile hemangioma, renal cell carcinoma, perineurioma, epithelioid and sarcomatoid mesotheliomas, and thymic carcinoma.

Comments

Glut-1 is positive in many neoplasms, and relative utility has been noted if the differential is between reactive benign or malignant neoplasms.

Selected references

Brown RS, Wahl RL. Overexpression of Glut-1 glucose transporter in human breast cancer: an immunohistochemical study. *Cancer* 1993; 72: 2979–85.

Haber RS, Weiser KR, Pritsker A, Reder I, Burstein DE. GLUT1 glucose transporter expression in benign and malignant thyroid nodules. *Thyroid* 1997; 7: 363–7.

Kato Y, Tsuta K, Seki K, et al. Immunohistochemical detection of GLUT-1 can discriminate between reactive mesothelium and malignant mesothelioma. *Modern Pathology* 2007; 20: 215–20.

Lyons LL, North PE, Mac-Moune Lai F, et al. Kaposiform hemangioendothelioma: a study of 33 cases emphasizing its pathologic, immunophenotypic, and biologic uniqueness from juvenile hemangioma. *American Journal of Surgical Pathology* 2004; 28: 559–68.

Mentzel T, Kutzner H. Reticular and plexiform perineurioma: clinicopathological and immunohistochemical analysis of two cases and review of perineurial neoplasms of skin and soft tissues. *Virchows Archiv* 2005; 447: 677–82.

Sakashita M, Aoyama N, Minami R, et al. Glut1 expression in T1 and T2 stage colorectal carcinomas: its relationship to clinicopathological features. *European Journal of Cancer* 2001; 37: 204–9.

NOTES

Glypican-3

Sources/clones

Abcam (ab66596), Proteintech (25175-1-AP), Santa Cruz Biotech (IG12), Spring Bioscience (E1887), Thermo Scientific/Pierce Antibody Products (SP86), Ventana (GC33).

Fixation/preparation

The antibody can be used in formalin-fixed paraffin-embedded tissue. Pretreatment of deparaffinized tissue sections with HIER is required.

Background

Glypican-3 is a glycosylphosphatidylinositol-anchored heparan sulfate cell surface proteoglycan. One of the six glypicans, glypican-3 regulates several developmental signaling pathways by acting as a co-receptor for many heparin-binding growth factors, such as fibroblast growth factors, Hedgehogs and Wnts. GPC3 is mutated in Simpson–Golabi–Behmel syndrome, which is characterized by tissue overgrowth and an increased risk of embryonal malignancies. It is widely expressed in a variety of tissues during development, including fetal liver and placenta, but is suppressed in most adult tissues. It is also involved in the modulation of growth in predominantly mesodermal tissues and organs.

Glypican-3 is overexpressed in hepatocellular carcinoma (HCC) cells and tissues and stimulates the growth of HCC cells by increasing autocrine/paracrine canonical Wnt signaling. Benign liver lesions including cirrhotic nodules are negative for Glypican-3. Glypican-3 is also a sensitive but not specific marker for testicular and ovarian yolk sac tumors. It is expressed in placental site nodules and placental site trophoblastic tumors. Glypican-3 is expressed in rhabdomyosarcomas but not adult spindle cell and pleomorphic sarcomas.

Applications

Immunohistochemical expression of Glypican-3 when used in a panel with other markers such as heat shock protein 70, glutamine synthetase, and reticulin has shown high specificity for HCC, especially poorly differentiated HCC.

In fine needle aspiration specimens, Glypican-3 immunohistochemistry has been demonstrated to be a useful marker for HCC.

Glypican-3 may be used to distinguish placental site trophoblastic tumors from non-trophoblastic tumors. Its expression by immunohistochemistry has also been noted in ovarian clear cell carcinoma, gastric adenocarcinoma, pancreatic acinar cell carcinoma, Merkel cell carcinoma, small-cell neuroendocrine carcinoma, squamous cell carcinomas from various primary sites, and urotheial carcinoma, and therefore must be interpreted with caution when determining site of origin of an unknown primary malignancy.

Selected references

Akutsu N, Yamamoto H, Sasaki S, et al. Association of glypican-3 expression with growth signaling molecules in hepatocellular carcinoma. *World Journal of Gastroenterology* 2010; 16: 3521–8.

Capurro M, Wanless IR, Sherman M, et al. Glypican-3: a novel serum and histochemical marker for hepatocellular carcinoma. *Gastroenterology* 2003; 125: 89–97.

Capurro MI, Xiang YY, Lobe C, et al. Glypican-3 promotes the growth of hepatocellular carcinoma by stimulating canonical Wnt signaling. *Cancer Research* 2005; 65: 6245–54.

He H, Fang W, Liu X, et al. Frequent expression of glypican-3 in Merkel cell carcinoma: an immunohistochemical study of 55 cases. *Applied Immunohistochemistry and Molecular Morphology* 2009; 17: 40–6.

Maeda D, Ota S, Takazawa Y, *et al.* Glypican-3 expression in clear cell adenocarcinoma of the ovary. *Modern Pathology* 2009; 22: 824–32.

Ou-Yang RJ, Hui P, Yang XJ, *et al.* Expression of glypican 3 in placental site trophoblastic tumor. *Diagnostic Pathology* 2010; 5: 64.

Shafizadeh N, Kakar S. Diagnosis of well-differentiated hepatocellular lesions: role of immunohistochemistry and other ancillary techniques. *Advances in Anatomic Pathology* 2011; 18: 438–45.

Ushiku T, Uozaki H, Shinozaki A, *et al.* Glypican 3-expressing gastric carcinoma: distinct subgroup unifying hepatoid, clear-cell, and alpha-fetoprotein-producing gastric carcinomas. *Cancer Science* 2009; 100: 626–32.

Zynger DL, McCallum JC, Luan C, *et al.* Glypican 3 has a higher sensitivity than alpha-fetoprotein for testicular and ovarian yolk sac tumour: immunohistochemical investigation with analysis of histological growth patterns. *Histopathology* 2010; 56: 750–7.

Gross cystic disease fluid protein 15 (GCDFP-15, BRST-2)

Sources/clones

Biogenex (GCDFP-15), Signet (GCDFP-15).

Fixation/preparation

The antigen is fixation-stable and can be detected in paraffin-embedded sections as well as fresh frozen sections and cell preparations. HIER enhances immunostaining and proteolytic digestion is unnecessary. Cytologic preparations should be fixed in 10% formalin or Bouin's solution. Alcohol-fixed preparations are not immunoreactive.

Background

Gross cystic disease fluid protein 15 (GCDFP-15) is one of four major component proteins found in the cystic fluid obtained from patients with fibrocystic changes of the breast. GCDFP-15 is a marker of apocrine glandular differentiation in both benign and malignant mammary epithelium. This protein has widespread distribution in apocrine glands elsewhere in the axillary and perianal tissues, as well as in the sublingual and submaxillary salivary glands. The GCDFP-15 protein is a 15 kDa glycoprotein shown to be prolactin-inducible, the GCDFP-15 gene having been recently cloned. Ultrastructurally, the GCDFP-15 protein has been localized in Golgi vesicles and cytoplasmic granules. The protein is released by exocytosis at the apices of the mammary epithelial cells.

Applications

Carcinoma of the breast is a treatable disease with a variable prognostic outcome. Its recognition is therefore of great therapeutic importance, but in metastatic sites identification of breast carcinoma can often be difficult. A marker of mammary epithelial differentiation would be of diagnostic importance. GCDFP-15 goes some way towards fulfilling this role and is currently the best marker to identify breast cancer metastases. GCDFP-15 was identified by immunostaining in 55–75% of cases of breast carcinoma and has a higher rate of sensitivity and specificity than α-lactalbumin as a marker of both primary and metastatic breast cancer. Besides mammary carcinomas, the major tumor types that express GCDFP-15 are salivary glands, sweat glands, bronchial glands, prostate, and seminal vesicle. It is also a marker of apocrine differentiation in the skin (particularly in combination with lysozyme) and can be suitably applied for the separation of cutaneous adnexal tumors (Appendix 1.20). A case of signet ring carcinoma of the eyelid was shown to immunoexpress GCDFP-15 in addition to estrogen and progesterone receptors and was negative for CK20 and Her-2, supporting an apocrine differentiation. It is worth noting that the expression of GCDFP-15 varies among the histologic subtypes of breast carcinoma, with the highest incidence in infiltrating lobular carcinoma with signet ring cell differentiation (90%), compared to 70% in ordinary infiltrating ductal carcinoma and 75% in those subtypes showing apocrine differentiation. Expression of the GCDFP-15 gene was significantly associated with relapse-free survival and was suggested to represent a marker of prognostic relevance. GCDFP-15 expression appears to be androgen receptor-mediated and can be inhibited by anti-androgens; androgen receptor, in turn, appears to be involved with apocrine differentiation in neuroendocrine carcinomas of the breast.

Antibodies to GCDFP-15 have been used successfully to identify metastases from breast carcinoma in the brain, ovary, lung, and other sites. Immunodistinction of metastasis from breast cancer and eccrine and apocrine tumors in the skin can be difficult, as the latter two tumors also express this antigen. However, as with other metastatic sites, the highest diagnostic yield was obtained when anti-GCDFP-15 was employed together with other antibodies in a diagnostic panel. Similarly, when used in conjunction with estrogen and progesterone receptors, CA125, CK7, CD20, and CEA, it provided discriminant analysis between primary adenocarcinomas of the ovary and ovarian metastases of colonic and breast origin.

GCDFP-15 is also a suitable marker in cytological specimens, and the best results are obtained following fixation in 10% formalin or Bouin's solution, alcohol-fixed samples showing no immunoreactivity for this antigen.

Comments

The immunoreactivity of monoclonal antibodies and polyclonal antisera to GCDFP-15 appears to be the same, HIER enhancing immunoreactivity of both antibodies.

Selected references

Fiel MI, Cernainu G, Burstein DE, Batheja N. Value of GCDFP-15 (BRST-2) as a specific immunocytochemical marker for breast carcinoma in cytologic specimens. *Acta Cytologica* 1996; 40: 637–41.

Haagensen DE, Dilley WG, Mazoujian G, Wells SA. Review of GCDFP-15. An apocrine marker protein. *Annals of the New York Academy of Sciences* 1990; 586: 161–73.

HBME-1 (mesothelial cell)

Sources/clones

Dako (HBME-1).

Fixation/preparation

The antibody is immunoreactive in formalin-fixed paraffin-embedded tissue sections and in frozen sections and cell preparations.

Background

The antibody reacts with an antigen present in the membrane of mesothelial cells and their neoplastic counterparts, particularly epithelioid mesotheliomas. In initial testing the antibody failed to decorate epithelial cells of the kidney, lung, liver, ovary, and pancreas. The antibody was derived from human epithelioid mesothelioma cells.

Applications

The antibody was designed primarily for the identification of normal and neoplastic mesothelial cells from metastatic carcinoma and is useful in this context. The antibody HBME-1 has met with limited success. Both HBME-1 and CA125 were not sufficiently specific to be employed on their own as mesothelial markers but made a contribution when used in an appropriate panel. No staining for HBME-1 makes the diagnosis of mesothelioma unlikely. HBME-1 reactivity is seen in the serous membranes of all reactive and malignant mesothelial cells, and in 25% of metastatic carcinomas and 85% of ovarian carcinomas. HBME-1 does not label sarcomatous malignant mesothelioma.

HBME-1 produces a thick pattern of immunoreactivity of the cell surfaces, often including the intracytoplasmic lumina, and is said to show excellent correlation with the presence of abundant long microvilli with electron microscopy. There is usually no cytoplasmic labeling, and although adenocarcinoma cells may show membrane staining, they do not display the characteristic "thick" membranes and may show cytoplasmic staining. A similar pattern of immunoreactivity with anti-epithelial membrane antigen (anti-EMA) has been described, corresponding to the labeling of the cell membranes and long microvilli characteristic of mesothelioma cells. The microvillous processes that are visible with EMA immunostaining are not only abnormally long, but the circumferential distribution around the cell is aberrant in nature and signifies malignancy. A comparison of EMA and HMFG-2 immunostaining in mesothelioma and adenocarcinoma concluded that membranous staining by EMA had a sensitivity of 65% and a specificity of 86% for the identification of malignant mesothelioma, but HMFG-2 membranous staining was not a useful discriminator.

Ultrastructural examination with immunogold reveals labeling of the membranes of the long microvilli. These ultrastructural findings are very similar to those described with EMA. HBME-1 has been recognized to stain adenocarcinoma. When HBME-1 is compared to thrombomodulin, the latter may be of greater discriminatory value in separating mesothelioma from adenocarcinoma. So too MOC-31, which is positive or equivocal in only 5% of mesotheliomas and positive in 90% of adenocarcinomas (reactive meothelium being negative), suggesting that it may be a useful addition to the panel for the diagnosis of mesothelioma vs. carcinoma.

HBME-1 membranous staining along with CK19 positivity is a useful diagnostic pointer to papillary thyroid cancer.

Comments

As with EMA, immunostaining with HBME-1 is aimed at highlighting the cell membranes and the long microvilli characteristic of mesothelioma. We have not identified any difference in the staining patterns or sensitivity of these two antibodies. Optimal dilutions of the antibody have to be determined before use in diagnostic panels, as high concentrations will result in cytoplasmic staining of both mesothelioma and adenocarcinoma cells, reducing the usefulness of HBME-1 as a diagnostic discriminator between the two entities. HBME-1 may be used as a substitute for EMA in the panel to distinguish mesothelioma from carcinoma (Appendix 1.17).

Selected references

Ascoli V, Carnovale-Scalzo C, Taccogna S, Nardi F. Utility of HBME-1 immunostaining in serous effusions. *Cytopathology* 1997; 8: 328–35.

Attanoos RL, Goddard H, Gibbs AR. Mesothelioma-binding antibodies: thrombomodulin, OV 632 and HBME-1 and their use in the diagnosis of malignant mesothelioma. *Histopathology* 1996; 29: 209–15.

Helicobacter pylori

Sources/clones

Biodesign (51-13), Biogenesis (1G6, CP15), Biogenex (UM01), Dako (polyclonal), Sanbio/Monosan (51-13).

Fixation/preparation

Applicable to 10% neutral buffered formalin or Bouin's fixed tissue.

Background

Helicobacter pylori (HP) is a spiral bacillus that can colonize the human gastric mucosa and induce a specific humoral immunologic reaction in the host. Colonization of the gastric mucosa by HP is a very common finding in gastric ulcers and active chronic gastritis. HP is increasingly recognized as one of the most prevalent human pathogens worldwide, and possibly plays a pathogenetic role in gastric carcinogenesis and primary gastric lymphogenesis. The details of the interaction between bacteria, epithelial cells, and inflammatory cells are being explored. As effective specific treatment for HP-associated gastroduodenal disorders emerges, surgical pathologists are requested to identify the organism in endoscopic biopsies. Histologic identification of HP (with special staining methods) has been shown to be as accurate as microbiologic culture techniques.

Applications

Bacteria lying within the mucus and on the epithelial surface can be seen on sections stained with hematoxylin–eosin (H&E). However, organisms closely adherent to cells, insinuated in intercellular spaces, or intimately associated with and perhaps phagocytosed by inflammatory cells are frequently difficult to identify.

There are several published special stains that demonstrate HP efficiently in the histologic sections. However, the use of immunohistochemical methods is highly specific and has an important role in selected situations. For example, small gastric biopsies with a very low density of *H. pylori*, post-treatment biopsy specimens to assess therapeutic success, or specimens in which abundant debris or mucus is present on gastric surface and pits may benefit from identification of *H. pylori* with immunohistochemistry. A concordance of 95% is seen between touch smear cytology and immunohistochemical identification of *H. pylori*, and fixation in Carnoy's fixative has been shown to allow immunohistochemical identification of the organism both in the surface mucus gel layer and in surface mucus cells in patients with peptic ulceration.

Comments

Immunohistochemical methods for the detection of *H. pylori* are highly specific and play an important role in selected situations, but cannot be advocated for the routine diagnosis of *H. pylori* gastritis. HP-infected gastric tissue is recommended as positive control tissue.

Selected references

Cartun RW, Kryzmowski GA, Pedersen CA, *et al.* Immunocytochemical identification of *H. pylori* in formalin-fixed gastric biopsies. *Modern Pathology* 1991; 4: 498–502.

Genta RM, Robason GO, Graham DY. Simultaneous visualization of *Helicobacter pylori* and gastric morphology: a new stain. *Human Pathology* 1994; 25: 221–6.

NOTES

Hep Par 1 (hepatocyte marker)

Sources/clones

Dako (OCH 1E5).

Fixation/preparation

The antibody is immunoreactive in fixed paraffin-embedded sections and immunoreactivity is slightly enhanced following HIER.

Background

Hep Par 1 (hepatocyte paraffin 1) is an IgGκ antibody to both normal and neoplastic hepatocytes. Hep Par 1 detects an antigen that is localized to the hepatocyte cytoplasm and produces no staining of bile ducts or other non-parenchymal cells. The staining is granular, occasionally ring-like, and is seen diffusely throughout the hepatocyte cytoplasm, without canalicular accentuation. There is no apparent zonal preference in normal liver. Hepatoblastomas have demonstrated uniform immunoexpression of the antigen.

Applications

The highest diagnostic yield is obtained with Hep Par 1 when it is employed in a panel of antibodies in the context of the differential diagnosis (Appendix 1.8). Its main diagnostic application would be for the distinction of HCC from CC and metastatic adenocarcinoma in the liver. When employed with CK19 and CK20, it is able to provide useful diagnostic information to allow the separation of these three entities. CK19 is largely limited to bile duct epithelium and corresponding neoplasms including CC, whereas CK20 is a marker of gastrointestinal carcinomas, particularly those from the colon and less consistently the upper gastrointestinal tract and pancreas.

Comments

As the staining of Hep Par 1 is heterogeneous and may be focal within HCCs, caution should be exercised in interpretation, as small biopsies such as needle cores may produce false-negative results. Despite its limitations, Hep Par 1 is still the best antibody for use in the context of the differential diagnosis of liver carcinomas. The OCH 1E5 antibody cross-reacts with canine hepatocytes.

Selected references

Fasano M, Theise ND, Nalesnik M, *et al.* Immunohistochemical evaluation of hepatoblastomas with use of the hepatocyte-specific marker, hepatocyte paraffin 1, and the polyclonal anti-carcinoembryonic antigen. *Modern Pathology* 1998; 11: 934–8.

Leong AS-Y, Sormunen RT, Tsui WM-S, Liew CT. Immunostaining for liver cancers. *Histopathology* 1998; 33: 318–24.

NOTES

Hepatitis B core antigen (HBcAg)

Sources/clones

Accurate/Axcel (polyclonal), American Research Products (1734-17), Biodesign (1841), Biogenesis (polyclonal), Biogenex (ESP512, polyclonal), Boehringer Mannheim (BW35A/312), Dako (polyclonal, B586), Fitzgerald (M29091, M22131), Immunon (polyclonal), Novocastra (polyclonal), Zymed (polyclonal).

Fixation/preparation

These antibodies are applicable to formalin-fixed paraffin-embedded tissue. No antigen unmasking is required. However, caution is advised when using the ABC immunodetection method, as hepatocytes contain biotin that may cross-react with the ABC system.

Background

The complete hepatitis B (HB) virus (Dane particle) is a 42 nm double-stranded DNA virus (Hepadnavirus), composed of a 27 nm core particle and envelope 7 nm in thickness, and it is immunolocalized within endoplasmic reticulum of liver cells. The HB core protein of 183 amino acids is encoded by the gene C. It is self-assembling and has binding sites for HBV-RNA, which is encapsulated together with viral polymerase. Immunolocalization of HBcAg is cytoplasmic, cytoplasmic and membranous, and nuclear. Antibodies are raised against HBcAg obtained from recombinant core DNA of HB virus, purified from lysates of *E. coli* clones. HBcAg is expressed predominantly in the nuclei of liver cells, although variable immunoreaction may also be seen in the perinuclear cytoplasm.

Applications

Antibody to HBcAg detects the replicative form of the virus found in the nucleus of HB-infected cells. Perinuclear cytoplasmic immunolocalization is sometimes observed. In very actively replicating infections, cells with cytoplasmic reactivity may outnumber those with nuclear labeling. The presence of HBcAg on immunohistochemistry is usually correlated with complete viral synthesis, as proved by positivity for viral DNA in both liver and blood, as well as circulating Dane particles in blood. Demonstration of HBcAg in liver cells therefore reflects failure to eliminate cells with active viral replication. This is often associated with signs
of active disease (piecemeal necrosis or chronic lobular hepatitis) with a membranous pattern of HBsAg. HBcAg is seen with the greatest frequency in immunosuppressed patients with chronic hepatitis. Excess accumulation of core particles can be recognized in an H&E stain in rare cases as "sanded" nuclei.

HBcAg expression in liver biopsies of children with chronic hepatitis B showed a significant decrease after treatment with interferon-α, whereas HBsAg expression either increased or remained unchanged. Periportal piecemeal necrosis and intralobular confluent and spotty necrosis decreased, but the extent of fibrosis and scoring of portal inflammation remained unchanged after treatment.

Comments

It is assumed that viral DNA active in HBcAg production is episomal and not integrated into the host genome.

Selected reference

Burns J. Immunoperoxidase localization of hepatitis B antigen (HB) in formalin-paraffin processed liver tissue. *Histochemistry* 1975; 44: 133–5.

NOTES

Hepatitis B surface antigen (HBsAg)

Sources/clones

Accurate (BM51), American Research Products/EY Labs, Axcel/Accurate (polyclonal), Becton Dickinson, Biogenesis (1044-329, polyclonal), Biogenex (SI201), Calbiochem, Dako (polyclonal, 3E7), Fitzgerald (M94172, M94173, M94253, M94254, polyclonal), Harlan Sera Lab/Accurate (V2.5G4, V2.6E4), Novocastra (1044/341), Pharmingen (S1-210), Zymed (ZCH16, ZMHB5).

Fixation/preparation

These antibodies are applicable to formalin-fixed paraffin-embedded tissues. No antigen unmasking is required. However, caution is advised when using the ABC immunodetection method, as liver cells contain biotin and may cross-react with the ABC system.

Background

The complete hepatitis B (HB) virus (Dane particle) is a 42 nm double-stranded DNA virus (Hepadnavirus), composed of a 27 nm core particle and envelope 7 nm in thickness, and it is immunolocalized within endoplasmic reticulum of liver cells. The glycosylated surface protein of the HB virus is composed of three gene products: the small, middle, and large HBs-protein, governed by the S-, pre S2- and pre S1- domains respectively.

Applications

These antibodies react with antigen-positive cells in patients with type B viral hepatitis, cirrhosis, and hepatocellular carcinoma. Immunoreaction may occur in seropositive as well as seronegative patients. HBsAg in human liver biopsies has two expression patterns with apparently different biological implications:

1. Membranous HBsAg is strongly associated with HBcAg expression and is an indirect indication of replicative HBV infection.
2. Intracytoplasmic HBsAg in excess is visible by H&E staining as a homogeneous ground-glass appearance of the cytoplasm, and is an indicator of chronic elimination insufficiency for this antigen but is an unreliable marker of active replication. In contrast, membrane-associated HBsAg should always raise suspicion of active viral replication.

Children with chronic hepatitis B showed a significant decrease in HBcAg immunoexpression after treatment with interferon-α, whereas HBsAg expression either increased or remained unchanged.

In patients with IgA nephropathy and HBV antigenemia, polyclonal antibodies have demonstrated HBcAg and HBsAg in the nuclei of glomerular mesangial cells, suggesting immune complex deposition as a possible mechanism of the nephropathy. In-situ hybridization studies of HBV DNA in such patients showed co-expression of HBV DNA and HBsAg and/or HBcAg, suggesting the expression of HBsAg in situ in infected renal cells.

Comments

Liver tissue from known patients with hepatitis may be used as control tissue for both HBcAg and HBsAg.

Selected reference

Gudat F, Bianchi L. HGsAg: a target antigen on the liver cell? In Popper H, Bianchi L, Reutter W, eds. *Membrane Alterations as Basis of Liver Injury*. Lancaster: MTP Press, 1977, pp. 171–8.

NOTES

Herpes simplex virus I and II (HSV I and II)

Sources/clones

Polyclonal HSV I and HSV II

Biodesign, Biogenesis, Biogenex, Chemicon, Dako (polyclonal), Fitzgerald, Immunon, Pharmingen.

Monoclonal antibody

Accurate (A321, M22253A, HP2M222M53A), American Research Products (1697-151, 1589-136, 1645-18), Biodesign (203, 206, 016, 017), Biogenesis (CHA437, 10527, H62), Biogenex (G16, E10, 023A1909, 045A1930B), EY Labs, Fitzgerald (M22254, M22255, M2110155, M2110156), Sera Lab (CHA437).

Fixation/preparation

Both antibodies 302M and 303M are applicable to frozen cryostat sections as well as fixed paraffin-embedded tissue sections. The latter require microwave pretreatment to eliminate nonspecific background staining.

Background

The antigens used in the production of these antibodies comprise detergent solubilized HSV I- and HSV II-infected whole rabbit cornea cell. The 302M antibody reacts with HSV I-specific antigens, while the 303M antibody reacts with HSV II-specific antigens. Both antibodies react with antigens common for HSV I and II, all major glycoproteins present in the viral envelope, and at least one core protein. There is no demonstrable cross-reactivity with Varicella zoster virus, cytomegalovirus, or Epstein–Barr virus.

Applications

Both antibodies 302M and 303M detect the presence of HSV I and HSV II, respectively, in tissue sections, e.g., skin and brain. A diffuse intranuclear signal is produced, often coinciding with the ground-glass intranuclear inclusions of HSV. Similar intranuclear inclusions, associated with biotin accumulation, have been observed in glandular epithelia of gestational endometrium. Hence, to the unwary, any attempt to demonstrate HSV in these biotin inclusions may produce a false-positive immunoreaction, especially when the avidin–biotin complex (ABC) immunodetection system is utilized. The application of prewashing with 0.05% free avidin and 0.05% free biotin does not eliminate this cross-immunoreactivity. It is therefore recommended that the PAP or APAAP immunodetection system be used for any HSV immunohistochemical investigation of gestational endometrium.

Localized herpes simplex lymphadenitis which resulted in rapid lymph node enlargement clinically indistinguishable from Richter's transformation has been described in a patient with chronic lymphocytic leukemia, emphasizing the need to make the correct diagnosis. Such infected nodes show marked germinal center and paracortical hyperplasia with foci of necrosis. Viral inclusions may be present, and HSV antigen may be demonstrated immunohistologically.

Comments

Biotin-like activity has been observed in thyroid lesions as well. Hence, awareness of this interference is crucial to avoid misinterpretation of immunohistochemical investigations, especially with the ABC immunodetection system. Genital lesions with typical multinucleated giant cells with "ground-glass" intranuclear inclusions should be used as positive control tissue.

Selected reference

Miliauskas J, Leong AS-Y. Localized herpes simplex lymphadenitis: report of three cases and review of the literature. *Histopathology* 1991; 19: 355–60.

NOTES

HHV-8 LANA-1

Sources/clones

Abbiotech (polyclonal), Advanced Biotechnologies (LNA-1), Biorbyt (polyclonal), Calbiochem/Novocastra/Leica (13B10), Fitzgerald (AT4C11), Gennova (13B10), MBL International Corporation (A23-9), Santa Cruz Biotechnologies (LN35).

Fixation/preparation

Several of the antibody clones/polyclonal antibodies to human herpesvirus 8 (HHV-8) latency-associated nuclear antigen 1 (LANA-1) are immunoreactive in fixed paraffin-embedded sections. HIER at 120 °C enhances labeling.

Background

Kaposi's sarcoma herpesvirus (KSHV) or human herpesvirus 8 (HHV-8) was isolated from Kaposi's sarcoma lesions from patients with the acquired immunodeficiency syndrome (AIDS). Differential expression analysis comparing lytic and latent stages of infection demonstrated that the HHV-8 open reading frame 73 encodes LANA-1, which is a useful marker for HHV-8 infection since it is constitutively expressed in all infected cells. The LANA-1 protein is predominantly expressed during viral latency and appears to play a role in viral integration into the host genome. LANA-1 interacts with p53 and interferes with p53-dependent apoptosis.

Applications

Antibodies to HHV-8 LANA-1 are used in several diagnostic situations. LANA-1 is best known for its diagnostic utility in the identification of Kaposi's sarcoma, but it is also used as adjunctive diagnostic evidence to support certain lymphoid proliferative disorders. Patch-stage Kaposi's sarcoma is morphologically recognizable and demonstrates expression of lymphoendothelial-type markers. In the nodular stage, spindle cells can lose lymphatic endothelial marker expression. The demonstration of immunoreactivity to LANA-1 distinguishes the diagnosis of Kaposi's sarcoma from other morphologic stimulants including various types of hemangioma/lymphangioma, cellular angiolipoma, cutaneous angiosarcoma, dermatofibrosarcoma protuberans, vascular transformation of lymph node, pilar leiomyoma, stasis dermatitis, pyogenic granuloma, kaposiform hemangioendothelioma, myopericytoma, and spindle cell melanoma. The nuclear localization of LANA-1 provides additional specificity to the immunohistochemical reactivity of infected cells. Staining of tumor cells can vary from focal ($<25\%$) to diffuse ($>75\%$). Nuclear localization is readily apparent, although cytoplasmic reactivity can also be present. LANA-1 has been demonstrated in rare tonsillar lymphoid cells in patients between the ages of 2 and 20 years. LANA-1 demonstrates high sensitivity for Kaposi's sarcoma ($>95\%$ overall).

Utilization of LANA-1 immunohistochemistry as a standalone test for the diagnosis of Kaposi's sarcoma is not recommended. Instead, integration with morphologic features and/or other markers is recommended. With respect to the latter, markers of lymphatic endothelium such as CD31 and podoplanin/D2-40 are of diagnostic utility.

HHV-8 LANA-1 can be detected in a subset of multicentric Castleman's disease patients and primary effusion lymphoma.

Comments

Clone 13B10 produces the best results in our hands. Immunoreactivity appears not to be enhanced by boiling or proteolytic digestion and is best demonstrated following retrieval at 120 °C in citrate buffer at pH 6.0.

Selected references

Cesarman E, Chang Y, Moore PS, Said JW, Knowles DM. Kaposi's sarcoma-associated herpesvirus-like DNA sequences in AIDS-related body-cavity-based lymphomas. *New England Journal of Medicine* 1995; 332: 1186–91.

Kazakov DV, Schmid M, Adams V, *et al.* HHV-8 DNA sequences in the peripheral blood and skin lesions of an HIV-negative patient with multiple eruptive dermatofibromas: implications for the detection of HHV-8 as a diagnostic marker for Kaposi's sarcoma. *Dermatology* 2003; 206: 217–221.

McDonagh DP, Liu J, Gaffey MJ, *et al.* Detection of Kaposi's sarcoma-associated herpesvirus-like DNA sequence in angiosarcoma. *American Journal of Pathology* 1996; 149: 1363–8.

Soulier J, Grollet L, Oksenhendler E, *et al.* Kaposi's sarcoma-associated herpesvirus-like DNA sequences in multicentric Castleman's disease. *Blood.* 1995; 86: 1276–80.

HLA-DR

Sources/clones

Accurate (917D7, CLBHLADR, DR), Axcel/Accurate (DK22), Biogenesis (HL-12, polyclonal), Biogenex (Q513), Biosource (BF1), Boehringer Mannheim (CR3-43), Coulter (12, 13), Cymbus Bioscience (DDII, IQU9, TAL1B), Dako (DK22, TAL.1B5), Harlan/Sera Lab/Accurate (MID3, YD1-63.4.10), Immunotech (B8.12.2), Novocastra (polyclonal), Pharmingen (TU36), Research Diagnostics (CLB-HLA-DR), Sanbio/Monosan (HL39), Sanbio/Monosan/Accurate (HL39), Sigma chemical (HA14), Zymed (LN3).

Fixation/preparation

These antibodies are applicable to B5 or formalin-fixed paraffin-embedded tissue sections. In addition, cryostat sections and cell smears may also be used with the antibodies.

Background

HLA molecules are highly polymorphic glycoproteins with a single binding site for immunogenic peptides. The complex formed by HLA-DR molecules and peptides is the entity specifically recognized by the antigen receptor of CD4+ helper T lymphocytes. This biological function has been linked to the constitutive cell surface expression of HLA molecules on antigen-presenting cells, which provide immunogenic peptides through denaturation, or fragmentation of antigen.

The HLA-DR is a member of the 11β subclass of HLA (the other member is HLA-DQ). B cells of the germinal centers and mantle zones express the HLA-DR antigen. It is also expressed by macrophages, monocytes, and antigen-presenting cells such as interdigitating reticulum cells and Langerhans cells of the skin. Activated T cells may express the HLA-DR antigen, but not inactive T cells. Some endothelial and epithelial tissues may also express HLA-DR.

Applications

Anti-HLA-DR may be useful in distinguishing B-cell follicle center lymphomas from T-cell lymphomas. The antibody also detects class II antigens which may be expressed de novo or increased in certain pathological states e.g., autoimmune diseases.

Similarly, it will demonstrate aberrant expression of class II antigen in various malignant cell types. Expression of HLA-DR has been demonstrated in bladder carcinoma and may have a role in the treatment of such tumors with intravesicle Bacillus Calmette–Guérin. The expression of HLA-DR molecules on crypt epithelial cells of jejunal biopsies of patients with Hashimoto's thyroiditis together with other signs of mucosal T-cell activation has been interpreted to suggest the potential of developing celiac disease.

Comments

Tonsil or skin may be used as positive control tissue.

Selected references

Crumpton MJ, Bodmer JC, Bodmer WF, et al. Biochemistry of class II antigens: workshop report. In Albert ED, Mayr WR, eds. *Histocompatibility Testing*. Berlin: Springer-Verlag, 1984, pp. 29–37.

Jendro M, Goronzy JJ, Weyand CM. Structural and functional characterization of HLA-DR molecules circulating in the serum. *Autoimmunity* 1991; 8: 289–96.

NOTES

HMB-45 (melanoma marker)

Sources/clones

Axcel/Accurate, Biodesign, Biogenesis, Biogenex, Dako, Enzo, Immunotech.

Fixation/preparation

The antibody is immunoreactive in paraffin-embedded tissue as well as frozen sections. Immunoreactivity is stronger in ethanol-fixed tissues than following formalin fixation, with immunoreactivity diminishing significantly following prolonged fixation in the latter. Sensitivity is enhanced following HIER. Mercury-based fixatives result in a high degree of nonspecific staining.

Background

The HMB-45 monoclonal antibody was generated to a whole-cell extract of a heavily pigmented lymph node deposit of human melanoma and has been shown to be a highly specific and sensitive reagent for the identification of melanoma. The designation HMB is derived from the immunogen employed, i.e., human melanoma, black. The antigen is intracytoplasmic, and ultrastructural studies suggest that the antibody reacts with melanosomes before melanin deposition, with HMB-45 binding to stage 1 and 2 melanosomes and to the non-melanized portion of stage 3, whereas stage 4 melanosomes and melanosome complexes found in macrophages and keratinocytes have been negative. The antibody appears to label premature and immature melanosomes in retinal pigment epithelium from fetuses and neonates but not from adults, leading to the suggestion that this "oncofetal" pattern of expression may indicate a role in melanocytic cell proliferation. This thesis has not been confirmed, and the sequential expression of the HMB-45 antigen in melanocytes may relate to activation by specific growth factors, resulting in alterations in protein glycosylation during various ontogenic and pathologic states of melanocytes. The epitope recognized by HMB-45 appears to be, in part, the oligosaccharide side chain of a sialated glycoconjugate, as the immunoreactivity can be abolished with neuraminidase treatment.

The gene corresponding to the HMB-45-defined proteins was cloned and designated gp 100-cl. This gene encodes the melanocyte lineage-specific antigens recognized by HMB-45 and HMB-50 (one of two other monoclonal antibodies to melanocytes initially obtained with HMB-45) as well as another monoclonal antibody, NKI-beteb. These three antibodies appear to recognize different epitopes of the same antigen; the melanosomal matrix protein or Pmel 17 gene product defined by them is apparently related by differential splicing.

Applications

Immunoreactivity for HMB-45 is seen in normal fetal and neonatal melanocytes but not in adult resting melanocytes. Reactive or proliferating melanocytes in inflamed adult skin, wound healing, increased vascularity, and in skin overlying certain dermal neoplasms may label for HMB-45 as a result of activation and stimulation by growth factors and "re-expression" of the antigen. HMB-45+ melanocytes have been demonstrated in the anal squamous zone and transitional zone but not in the colorectal zone. Increased numbers of such melanocytes can be present adjacent to primary anal melanomas.

The staining for HMB-45 in melanocytic nevi depends on their location within the skin. Junctional nevi and the junctional components of compound nevi are HMB-45-positive. In contrast, intradermal nevi and the dermal components of compound nevi are consistently negative. Thus, HMB-45 does not provide distinction between benign and malignant melanocytic proliferations, and the difference in reactivity supports the concept, based on differences in morphology, enzyme activity, and other immunological reactivity, that junctional and dermal cells are not identical. Junctional nevus cells are in an activated or proliferative state compared to their quiescent dermal counterparts, and their immunoreactivity with HMB-45 is analogous to the proliferating fetal melanocytes that are positive for the antigen while quiescent adult melanocytes are nonreactive.

Dysplastic nevi, in contrast, usually express HMB-45 in both the junctional nevus cells and in the dysplastic cells in the superficial dermis. Nevus cells within the deeper dermis do not usually react with HMB-45. In one study, minimally dysplastic nevi displayed intense immunolabeling of the junctional melanocytes but no staining of dermal nevus cells, whereas, with the moderately and severely dysplastic nevi, the dermal melanocytes showed focal cytoplasmic immunoreactivity. The likelihood of expression of HMB-45 paralleled the degree of dysplasia of the nevi. Common blue nevi and cellular blue nevi are generally HMB-45-positive, as are malignant blue nevi. Other nevi such as spindle and epithelioid cell nevi, congenital nevi, and other nevi occurring in hormonally reactive sites show immunostaining in nevus cells in the deep dermis as well as those near the dermal–epidermal junction. Less common benign melanocytic proliferations such as plexiform spindle cell nevi, Spitz nevi, and atypical melanocytic hyperplasias are also HMB-45-positive.

Malignant melanoma shows strong cytoplasmic positivity for HMB-45 in the majority of cases (65–95%), with the proportion of positive tumor cells ranging from a few to 100%. When the expression of the antigen is weak, staining may appear as a fine granularity similar to that seen in cytologic preparations. The positivity for HMB-45 is seen in almost all types of primary and metastatic melanoma, including amelanotic melanoma, spindle cell melanoma, and acral lentiginous melanoma (Appendix 1.10). One important exception is desmoplastic malignant melanoma, which consistently displays a much lower rate of positivity and may be completely negative. When positive, reactivity is usually seen in the superficial epithelioid cell rather than the dermal spindle cells, which only rarely stain for HMB-45. The newer markers of melanoma including tyrosinase, MiTF, and Melan-A do not appear to stain HMB-45+ desmoplastic melanomas. There is greater sensitivity of tyrosinase, MiTF, and Melan-A over HMB-45.

Attesting to the specificity of the antigen, HMB-45 reactivity has been demonstrated in malignant melanomas of diverse morphology such as signet ring melanoma, myxoid melanoma, small-cell melanoma, and balloon cell melanoma, and in melanomas of different anatomic sites such as the gallbladder, urinary bladder, anorectal region, vulva, sinonasal region, uterine cervix, other mucosal sites, and bone. Melanomas and melanocytic proliferations occurring in complex tumors such as pulmonary blastoma have also been HMB-45-positive.

HMB-45 staining has also application in the separation of melanin-containing macrophages from melanoma cells, allowing the accurate determination of tumor thickness and depth of invasion. Similarly, labeling for the antigen helps the identification of recurrence or residual spindle melanoma cells from desmoplastic fibroblasts at resection sites.

As HMB-45 immunoreactivity is melanocyte-specific, positivity can be encountered in lesions with melanin production such as adrenal pheochromocytoma, melanotic neuroectodermal tumor of infancy (progonoma), melanin-containing hepatoblastoma, malignant epithelioid schwannoma of the skin, pigmented carcinoid tumor, and esthesioneuroblastoma.

HMB-45 positivity has been reported in a variety of lesions: angiomyolipoma, lymphangiomyomatosis, and sugar tumor of the lung. While these tumors consistently manifest HMB-45 immunoreactivity, they do not display obvious pigmentation. However, ultrastructural studies confirm the presence of premelanosomes, and all three lesions also manifest evidence of smooth muscle differentiation. The reactivity for HMB-45 can be a useful diagnostic discriminator especially in the case of clear cell or sugar tumor, which resembles metastatic renal cell carcinoma and clear cell carcinoma of the lung (Appendix 1.9). Similarly, immunoreactivity for HMB-45 can be helpful in the identification of lymphangiomyomatosis in transbronchial biopsies, obviating the need for an open biopsy for definitive diagnosis.

The expression of this antigen in angiomyolipoma and lymphangioleiomyomatosis, both manifestations of the tuberous sclerosis complex, has been linked by the recent demonstration of HMB-45 immunoreactivity in cardiac rhabdomyoma, brain lesions, and other mesenchymal as well as neural lesions found in the tuberous sclerosis complex. These lesions have also shown ultrastructural granules suggestive of melanosome formation, which is in agreement with previous suggestions that a smooth muscle cell with unusual features links the various lesions of tuberous sclerosis. HMB-45 immunoreactivity in these lesions now provides another common denominator. This group of tumors has been expanded to comprise angiomyolipoma, lymphangiomyoma, lymphangioleiomyomaosis, renal capsuloma, clear cell myomelanocytic tumor of the falciform ligament, and clear cell "sugar" tumor, and they are known as PEComas because of their differentiation towards putative perivascular epithelioid cells. The PEComas are characterized by strong immunoreactivity for HMB-45 and variable expression of muscle markers. A monotypic epithelioid angiomyolipoma has been described which showed HMB-45 immunoreactivity.

Comments

Immunoreactivity of formalin-fixed tissue is enhanced following heat-induced antigen retrieval. Enzyme pretreatment does not significantly improve immunostaining for HMB-45. As in other diagnostic situations, heavily pigmented melanocytic lesions may pose a problem in differentiating melanin in other cells, such as macrophages, from tumor cells with true brown immunoreactivity when 3,3′-diaminobenzidine (DAB) is used as the chromogen. This problem can be simply eliminated by employing azure B as a substitute for hematoxylin as the counterstain. Azure B renders melanin granules blue-green, contrasting against the brown granules resulting from positive immunoreactivity.

The HMB-45 antibody has been reported to rarely show false-positive staining in non-melanomatous tumors and some normal tissues. These include breast carcinoma and normal breast epithelium, sweat gland tumors and normal counterparts, pheochromocytomas, hepatocellular carcinoma, chordoma, adenocarcinomas, lymphoma, plasmacytoma, and plasma cells. This spurious staining is usually apical or perinuclear in location and granular in nature. This false positivity has been attributed to contamination of commercial ascites fluid preparations with nonspecific antibodies, and the culture supernatant fluid of the hybridoma cell line, now available from Dako, has been shown to eliminate this false positivity with HMB-45.

Mercury-based fixatives such as B5 should be avoided, as their use results in extensive false-positive staining of mesenchymal cells including vessels, fibroblasts, and inflammatory cells.

Selected reference

Bacchi CE, Bonetti, Pea M, Martignoni G, Gown AM. HMB-45. A review. *Applied Immunohistochemistry* 1996; 4: 73–85.

NOTES

hMLH1 and hMSH2 (mismatch repair proteins)

Sources/clones

Anti-hMLH1: Becton Dickinson/PharMingen (monoclonal G168-15)
Anti-hMSH2: Becton Dickinson/PharMingen (monoclonal G219-1129), Oncogene Research Products (monoclonal FE11)

Fixation/preparation

Both antibodies are applicable to formalin-fixed paraffin-embedded tissues. Microwave antigen retrieval in a citrate buffer is necessary pretreatment.

Background

The deoxyribonucleic acid (DNA) mismatch repair system comprises six genes and is required for the correction of DNA mismatches that occur during replication. Inactivation of DNA mismatch repair (MMR) genes most commonly involve *hMLH1* (human *mutL* homolog 1) and *hMSH2* (human *mutS* homolog 2). The understanding of the role of mismatch repair in human neoplasia resulted from the study of colorectal carcinomas arising in patients with hereditary non-polyposis colorectal cancer (HNPCC). This disorder is responsible for 1–5% of all colorectal carcinomas. These patients have a lifetime risk of 80–90% for developing colorectal carcinoma in the fourth and fifth decade. Patients with HNPCC are also at an increased risk for developing other types of tumors: endometrium, ovary, small intestine, stomach, pancreas, biliary tract, bladder, and ureter.

Germline mutations of *hMLH1* or *hMSH2* result in loss of protein function, accounting for 80–90% of observed mutations in HNPCC and Muir–Torre patients with MMR-deficient cancers. *hMLH1* is localized to chromosome 3p21 and encodes a 756 amino acid protein, while *hMSH2* is localized to chromosome 2p21–22 and encodes a 935 amino acid protein. With development of tumor, the second (wild-type) allele of these genes is also inactivated, resulting in MMR deficiency. This leads to an increased rate of mutations in microsatellite regions, so-called microsatellite instability (MSI). Such mutations also affect crucial genes that regulate growth, differentiation, and apoptosis. The present definition of replication error (RER)-positive tumors is that 30–40% of MSI markers tested need to show rearrangements in order to justify the designation RER+ tumor.

Colon cancers in HNPCC patients typically occur in right colon (in the absence of multiple polyps) and show poor differentiation with a cribiform pattern and a lymphoid inflammatory infiltrate, but carry a better prognosis than "conventional tumors." DNA mismatch repair genes also play a role in approximately 10–15% of sporadic colon cancers. However, these genes are inactivated by somatic hypermethylation rather than germline mutations, with the latter only identified occasionally in tumor DNA. Hence, it is not only the HNPCC cases, but also a significant number of sporadic colorectal carcinomas, that share the molecular mechanisms with the familial counterparts as well as pathologic, clinical, and, more importantly, prognostic features – these being "early-onset" (<50 years) right-sided cancers with an improved survival rate. Further, similar to HNPCC patients, the sporadic colorectal carcinomas with MMR defects have an increased incidence of synchronous and metachronous tumors.

MSI testing requires the services of a molecular diagnostic laboratory, but these tumors may alternatively be recognized with immunohistochemical staining. The absence of *hMLH1* or *hMSH2* nuclear expression may identify tumors with MMR deficiency. Immunohistology can discriminate accurately between MSI and microsatellite-stable tumors. Loss of MLH1 or MSH2 is detected in 90% of MSI-high carcinomas, whereas all MSI-low and MS-stable tumors show normal expression of both proteins. Lack of MLH1 nuclear staining is observed more frequently than absence of MSH2. The finding of carcinomas on the left side of the colon with absence of staining for one MMR protein (some also later develop a second colorectal carcinoma), has resulted in the recommendation that all colorectal carcinomas be screened for loss of immunoexpression for *hMLH1* and *hMSH2*, irrespective of the HNPCC status.

Applications

It is important to identify patients with HNPCC for genetic counseling, screening, and prevention. It is equally important to stratify sporadic MSI tumors for future chemotherapeutic protocols. This would also identify patients who may be at a higher risk of developing a second carcinoma, including those of the endometrium, ovary, and urinary bladder. The immunohistochemical detection of MMR gene proteins (*hMLH1* and *hMSH2*) places the pathologist at the center of this decision-making process.

Comments

The ability to identify HNPCC with immunostaining has allowed the correlation of clinicopathological features of such tumors. MSI-high MLH1/MSH2+ carcinomas are more often located in the distal colon, are more frequently typed as ordinary adenocarcinoma, and are more likely to be well or moderately differentiated, p53+, and <7 cm in diameter than MLH1− and MSH2− carcinomas. Antibodies to other MMR gene proteins that are immunoreactive in fixed paraffin-embedded tissues include anti-PMS2 and anti-MSH6, but abnormalities of these proteins are less common in HNPCC

Selected references

Jiricny J. Eukaryotic mismatch repair: an update. *Mutation Research* 1998; 409: 107–21.

Lanza G, Gafa R, Maestri I, *et al.* Immunohistochemical pattern of MLH1/MSH2 expression is related to clinical and pathological features in colorectal adenocarcinomas with microsatellite instability. *Modern Pathology* 2002; 15: 741–9.

Human immunodeficiency virus (HIV)

Sources/clones

American Research Products (HIV1-1, HIV1-12), Biosource (LOHIV1-1), Dako (Kal-1), Harlan Sera Lab/Accurate (1HIVp24).

Fixation/preparation

Applicable to formalin-fixed paraffin-embedded tissue sections. Pretreatment with proteolytic enzymes such as pronase improves immunoreactivity. May also be used for labeling cryostat sections and fixed cell smears. Although the manufacturers provide working dilutions, optimization in individual laboratories is necessary. We have found that sections require a dual pretreatment with 0.5% trypsin (37 °C, 15 minutes) followed by microwave treatment in citrate buffer.

Background

Kal-1 reacts with the HIV type 1 capsid protein p24 and its precursor p55, as demonstrated by immunohistochemistry, immunoprecipitation, ELISA, and immunoblotting using lysates of purified virus and lysates of HIV type 1 infected cells. The antibody detects an epitope of the p24 protein, which is resistant to fixation and paraffin embedding. It does not cross-react with HIV type 2 or simian immunodeficiency virus (SIV), as shown by immunoblotting. During the phase of persistent generalized lymphadenopathy and subsequent stages of disease leading to development of AIDS, follicular dendritic cells forming the framework of lymphoid follicles degenerate. The expression of HIV-1 proteins by follicular dendritic cells (FDCs) in germinal centers in situ, and the presence of HIV-1 mRNA-positive cells in germinal follicles, suggests that FDCs are infected and able to produce HIV-1. Such infection may contribute significantly to the destruction of the FDC network during the lymphadenopathy phase after HIV-1 infection. Kal-1 reacts with the p24 protein in cells infected with HIV-1, i.e., lymphocytes, monocytes and macrophages, Langerhans cells of the skin, FDCs, and brain cells of monocyte/macrophage or microglia lineage.

In formalin-fixed paraffin-embedded tissue, Kal-1 antibody produces a positive immunoreaction of HIV-infected dendritic reticulum cells in the germinal centers of lymph nodes. The dendritic processes are highlighted, producing the typical network pattern within germinal centers. Occasional positive mononuclear cells and lymphocytes may be observed in the interfollicular areas of the lymph node. However, only immunopositivity confined to the follicular dendritic cells in lymph nodes should be considered as specific.

Comments

Interpretation of a positive lymph node biopsy with this antibody should always be confirmed with a serological assay or Western blot. In some countries an informed consent is required from the patient before testing for HIV status. Hence, histopathologists should be cautious in the reporting of p24+ node biopsies.

Selected references

Daugharty H, Long EG, Swisher BC, et al. Comparative study with in situ hybridization and immunocytochemistry in detection of HIV-1 in formalin-fixed paraffin-embedded cell cultures. *Journal of Clinical Laboratory Analysis* 1990; 4: 283–8.

Kaluza G, Willems WR, Lohmeyer J, et al. A monoclonal antibody that recognizes a formalin-resistant epitope on the p24 core protein of HIV-1. *Pathology Research and Practice* 1992; 188: 91–6.

NOTES

Human papillomavirus (HPV)

Sources/clones

Accurate (polyclonal), American Research Products (1535-18, 1501-17, 1502-17, 1505-17), Biodesign, Biogenesis (HUB, 16L1, C1P5), Biogenex (CH0613), Cymbus Bioscience (BF7), Cymbus Bioscience/Pharmingen (CAM-VIR1), Dako (polyclonal to HPV-1), Novocastra (4C4/F10/H7/83, 5A3/C8), Pharmingen (7H7, TVG401, TVG402, p16INK4 clone G175-405), Santa Cruz (16-E7 clone TVG710Y, 180E6 C-20).

Fixation/preparation

Antibodies to HPV are applicable to formalin-fixed paraffin-embedded tissues and frozen/cryostat sections.

Background

The most extensively studied area of human papillomavirus (HPV) infection has been in epithelia of the anogenital tract, particularly the uterine cervix. Over 25 HPV genotypes have been isolated to date from the female genital tract. HPV genotypes have enabled specific types to be correlated with morphological lesions, e.g., HPV-6/11 being commonly associated with condylomata, while HPV-16/18 is frequently associated with high-grade cervical intraepithelial neoplasia (CIN) and invasive squamous cell carcinoma. It has been demonstrated that over 90% of cervical squamous cell carcinomas harbor a high-risk HPV, the genome of which is usually integrated into the host DNA. Hence, in conjunction with epidemiological data showing that HPV infection and cervical squamous cell carcinoma share several risk factors, the association between high-risk HPV and cervical cancer is now firmly established. Although only a small proportion of high-grade CINs progress to invasive carcinoma, it is thought that HPV detection may assist in predicting the invasive potential of high-grade CIN.

Applications

The detection of HPV in clinical samples depends on the demonstration of viral components within cells and tissues. This entails the detection of either protein or nucleic acid. Viral proteins may be visualized with immunohistochemical techniques using either polyclonal or monoclonal antibodies. Antibodies directed to viral proteins are dependent on the expression/synthesis of the latter by the virus, which is dependent on transcription/translation of the viral genome within the nucleus. Polyclonal antibodies raised to bovine papillomavirus capsid protein are applicable to HPV types in human biopsy specimens, as they cross-react with several human subtypes. The synthesis of bacterial fusion proteins and their use as immunogens in mice has led to the generation of monoclonal antibodies to specific viral proteins to achieve viral specificity. The use of the HPV-16L1 (capsid) protein has led to the production of several antibodies of varying specificity. The immunoreactivity of antibodies to HPV capsid protein is dependent on active viral replication, which is closely correlated with keratin production. This therefore produces an intranuclear signal in the upper third of the squamous epithelia harboring the virus. Apart from the cervix, the use of antibodies to HPV is applicable to the vulva, penis, anus, oral cavity, larynx, and esophagus.

Clone E6H4 (MTM Laboratories, Heidelberg, Germany) has been applied to ThinPreps, and overexpression of $p16^{INK4A}$ has been employed as a specific marker for dysplastic and neoplastic cervical epithelial cells, and a combination of $p16^{INK4A}$ with cyclin E and Ki-67 has been proposed as a surrogate biomarker for HPV-related preinvasive squamous cervical disease.

Comments

With the advent of advanced in-situ hybridization technology for the detection of HPV DNA, the demand for

HPV immunohistochemistry has fallen. Non-isotope in-situ hybridization techniques are easily accessible and readily applicable to the routine diagnostic histopathology laboratory. Squamous epithelium showing the typical morphological features of HPV infection is recommended for use as a positive control. Staining should be mainly intranuclear, with some perinuclear staining of koilocytes.

Selected references

Cooper K, McGee J O'D. Human papillomavirus, integration and cervical carcinogenesis: a clinicopathological perspective. *Molecular Pathology* 1997; 50: 1–3.

Patel D, Shepherd PS, Naylor JA, McCance DJ. Reactivities of polyclonal and monoclonal antibodies raised to the major capsid protein of human papillomavirus type 16. *Journal of Virology* 1989; 70: 69–77.

Human parvovirus B19

Sources/clones
Chemicon, Dako (polyclonal), Novocastra (R92F6), Vector Laboratories (R92F6).

Fixation/preparation
Applicable to archival formalin-fixed paraffin-embedded tissue sections. Before immunostaining, sections should be subjected to HIER at 100 °C for 20 minutes.

Background
Human parvovirus B19 was accidentally discovered in 1975 in human serum being screened for hepatitis B surface antigen. Since its discovery, this virus has been found to be the causative agent in erythema infectiosum, chronic anemia in immunosuppressed patients, fetal death associated with hydrops, and acute arthralgia/arthritis in adults.

Parvovirus B19, which is cytotoxic to erythroid progenitor cells in vivo and in vitro, enters the erythroid precursor cell via the blood group P antigen. Human parvovirus B19 has been reported as a cause of severe and persistent anemia in patients immunocompromised from organ transplantation, autoimmune disease, hematologic malignancies, chemotherapy and congenital or acquired immunodeficiency states including HIV infection.

The R92F6 monoclonal antibody is directed against the VP1 and VP2 capsid proteins of parvovirus B19.

Applications
On bone marrow smears and trephine biopsies the presence of giant erythroblasts and small erythroid precursors with nuclear inclusions (lantern cells) establishes the diagnosis. However, the inexperienced observer may easily overlook these cells, and the use of antibody to parvovirus B19 may be useful in establishing the diagnosis. A high index of suspicion when assessing bone marrow smear/biopsies in immunocompromised patients with chronic severe anemia is required. Some have found anti-parvovirus B19 antibody to be less sensitive than in-situ hybridization (ISH). Good correlation between R92F6 antibody staining and B19 DNA has been found. Immune complex-type glomerulonephritis may also be caused by parvovirus B19 antigen–antibody complexes.

Comments
Parvovirus B19 infection should be considered in any unexplained chronic persistent anemia in an immunocompromised patient.

Selected references
Brown KE, Anderson SM, Young NS. Erythrocyte P antigen: cellular receptor of B19 parvovirus. *Science* 1993; 262: 114–17.

Liu W, Ittmann MD, Liu J, *et al.* Human parvovirus B19 in bone marrows from adults with acquired immunodeficiency syndrome: a comparative study using in situ hybridization and immunohistochemistry. *Human Pathology* 1997; 28: 760–6.

Morey AL, O'Neill HJ, Coyle PV, *et al.* Immunohistological detection of human parvovirus B19 in formalin-fixed, paraffin-embedded tissues. *Journal of Pathology* 1992; 166: 105–8.

NOTES

Human placental lactogen (hPL)

Sources/clones

Accurate (KIHPL3-489D5F3, polyclonal), American Research Products (polyclonal), Biogenesis (LIP603), Chemicon (polyclonal), Dako (polyclonal), Fitzgerald (M310198, M310199, polyclonal), Sera Lab (polyclonal), Zymed (polyclonal).

Fixation/preparation

The antigen is resistant to formalin fixation and immunoreactivity is enhanced by proteolytic digestion.

Background

Human placental lactogen (hPL) is a member of an evolutionarily related gene family that includes human growth hormone (hGH) and human prolactin. hPL together with human chorionic gonadotropin and pregnancy-specific β1-glycoprotein (SP1) are the three major proteins produced by the placenta. Although its expression is limited to the placenta, its physiological actions are far-reaching. hPL has a direct somatotropic effect on fetal tissues. It alters maternal carbohydrate and lipid metabolism to provide for fetal nutrient requirements, and aids in the stimulation of mammary cell proliferation. Two hPL genes (*hPL3* and *hPL4*) encoding identical proteins are responsible for the production of up to 1–3 g hPL hormone per day.

Applications

Several studies have employed hPL and other placental markers for distinguishing intrauterine from extrauterine pregnancies. The presence of cytokeratin and hPL was found to be useful in identifying trophoblastic elements in endometrial curettings, with a sensitivity of 75%. hPL can also be employed in a panel for the distinction of trophoblastic proliferations (Appendix 1.5, 1.33, 1.34, 1.37).

Complete hydatidiform mole showed strong expression of human chorionic gonadotropin (hCG) and weak expression of placental alkaline phosphatase (PLAP), whereas partial mole showed weak hCG and strong PLAP. Choriocarcinoma, on the other hand, showed strong hCG and weak hPL and PLAP. All tissues were positive for cytokeratin but negative for vimentin. Focal expression of hCG and diffuse expressions of hPL and PLAP was a profile not observed in complete moles.

hPL has also been employed as a marker of intermediate trophoblasts (ITs) together with pregnancy-specific glycoprotein, but cytokeratin and vimentin are more reliable markers. Extravillous trophoblasts are diffusely and strongly positive for hPL, in contrast to the focal staining in villous trophoblasts. There appear to be three subpopulations of IT with distinct morphologic and immunohistochemical features, this accounting perhaps for the differences in immunophenotype reports for placental site tumors. Chorionic-type IT was found to comprise two populations – one with eosinophilic and the other with clear (glycogen-rich) cytoplasm. The former tended to be larger with more pleomorphic nuclei, compared to the smaller more uniform nuclei of the clear cell type. Both cell types were diffusely positive for placental alkaline phosphatase but only focally positive for hPL, Mel-CAM (CD146), and oncofetal fibronectin. These cells corresponded to those found in placental site nodule and its neoplastic counterpart, epithelioid trophoblastic tumor, the latter also staining for α-inhibin. In contrast, implantation site IT cells were strongly positive for hPL, Mel-CAM, and oncofetal fibronectin, corresponding to cells in an exaggerated placental site and its neoplastic counterpart, placental site trophoblastic tumor.

Comments

Various tumors that show trophoblastic differentiation may express hPL.

Selected references

Brescia RJ, Kurman RJ, Main CS, *et al.* Immunocytochemical localization of chorionic gonadotropin, placental lactogen, and placental alkaline phosphatase in the diagnosis of complete and partial hydatidiform moles. *International Journal of Gynecological Pathology* 1987; 6: 213–29.

Cheah PL, Looi LM. Expression of placental proteins in complete and partial hydatidiform moles. *Pathology* 1994; 26: 115–18.

Immunoglobulins: Igκ, Igλ, IgA, IgD, IgE, IgG, IgM

Sources/clones

Both monoclonal and polyclonal antibodies to immunoglobulins of the various types are available from a wide variety of sources. Affinity-isolated F (ab')$_2$ fragments to Igκ and Igλ are also available.

Igκ

Accurate (EA2-38), Becton Dickinson (TB28-2), Biodesign/Pharmingen (polyclonal), Biogenesis (HK3, polyclonal), Biosource (LOHK3), Calbiochem (HP6062, polyclonal), Cymbus Bioscience (24K6), Dako (R10-21-F3, A8B5, polyclonal), Immunotech (G6.42), Pharmingen (polyclonal, G20-193), Research Diagnostics (6KA4G7), Sanbio/Monsan/Accurate (2B7), Zymed (HP6053).

Igλ

Accurate (AG7.47), Becton Dickinson (1-155-2), Biogenesis (polyclonal), Biosource (LOHL2), Caltag Laboratories/Sigma Chemical (HP6054), Cymbus Bioscience (24L6), Harlan Sera Lab/Accurate (Lam2.G4), Pharmingen (JDC12, polyclonal), Zymed (HP6054).

IgA

Accurate (GAI, SB14, Al-18), Accurate/Sigma Chemical (GA112), Becton Dickinson (1-155-1), Biodesign (polyclonal), Biogenesis (polyclonal, 15D6, 2E2), Biosource (LOHA8), Cymbus Bioscience (M24A), Dako 6E2C1, polyclonal), EY Labs (polyclonal), Immunotech (NIF2), Pharmingen (polyclonal), Sanbio/Monsan/Accurate (JV1H14-1), Sigma Chemical (Al-18), Zymed (WAN741).

IgD

Becton Dickinson (TA4.1), Biogenesis (polyclonal), Biogenex (NI158, polyclonal), Biosource (LOHD11), Dako (IgD26, polyclonal), EY Labs (polyclonal), Harlan Sera Lab/Accurate (1AD86), Immunotech (JA11), Sera Lab Ltd (12.1), Sigma Chemical (HJ9).

IgE

Accurate (GE1, AMD-E), Accurate/Sigma Chemical (GE1), Biodesign (polyclonal), Biogenesis (0257), Dako C1A-E-7.12, El, polyclonal), EY Labs (polyclonal).

IgG

Accurate (polyclonal, 4.22D10, A57H, SL13), Accurate/Sigma Chemical (GG4), Becton Dickinson (C3-124), Becton Dickinson/Biodesign (polyclonal), Biodesign (polyclonal), Biogenesis (polyclonal, 2D7), Dako (A57H, polyclonal), EY Labs (polyclonal, NL16, GB7B), Harlan Sera Lab/Accurate (ISE503, C3-8-80, C27-15), Pharmingen (G7-18, G18-145, G18-21, G18-3, polyclonal), Sanbio/Monosan/Accurate (MH25-1, BL-G4-1), Sigma Chemical (SH21, SK44).

IgG F(ab)

Accurate/Sigma Chemical (SG16), EY Labs (HP6014).

IgM

Accurate (AMD-u, SB17), Accurate/Sigma Chemical (MB11), Becton Dickinson (145-8), Biogenesis (polyclonal), Dako (Rl/69, polyclonal), EY Labs (polyclonal), Pharmingen (G20-127, polyclonal).

Fixation/preparation

Immunostaining of cytoplasmic immunoglobulin (Cig) can be performed in formalin-fixed paraffin-embedded sections, fresh frozen sections, and cytologic preparations. Other fixatives and processing procedures such as AMEX and freeze-drying have been suggested to produce effective immunoglobulin staining.

Background

Surface membrane immunoglobulin (SIg) expression is the classic and specific marker of B lymphocytes and serves as the antigen recognition molecule for this lymphocyte population. Each of the heavy chain classes of Ig can be expressed on the B-cell membrane, and more than one heavy chain class can be expressed on the same cell, the majority of peripheral B cells expressing IgM with or without IgD, less than 10% expressing IgD or IgA.

IgM is the first heavy chain class to appear in B-cell ontogeny, with the majority of immature B cells expressing IgM in high density. This decreases in density with maturation, and increasing amounts of IgD appear on the cell membrane. The IgM and IgD molecules that coexist in the same membrane cap exist independently but share the same idiotype and have the same light chain. Following B-cell activation and differentiation, there is loss of IgM and IgD as the result of a productive isotype gene rearrangement switch. With the progression to antibody-forming plasma cells, different subpopulations of SIgM- and/or SIgG-bearing memory B cells may appear.

Clonality of a given B-cell population can be inferred from the uniformity of light chain class expression, as individual B cells can express either κ or λ light chains but not both; the ratio of κ- to λ-bearing B cells being 2 to 1. A vast predominance of κ or λ light-chain-bearing B cells indicates monoclonality, generally implying a neoplastic proliferation, whereas a mixture of light-chain-bearing cell types suggests polyclonality and a reactive or non-neoplastic proliferation of B cells.

Direct immunofluorescent staining with heterologous antisera raised against whole or Fab fragments of human Ig molecules is the simplest method of identifying SIg. Class-specific antisera monospecific for individual heavy and light chain determinants (monovalent antisera) may be employed to determine the precise isotype of the SIg, but these procedures require fresh cell preparations. Alternatively, immunoenzyme techniques can be used on cytocentrifuge preparations and imprints as well as frozen sections. The latter procedures have suffered from a high level of background staining, which can make interpretation difficult.

Ideally, the aim would be to be able to perform consistent staining of immunoglobulin in fixed paraffin-embedded tissues, allowing the advantage of retrospectivity as well as optimal cytomorphology. While many attempts have been made with special fixatives such as B5 and other mercury-based fixatives, and the application of various enzymatic digestions, they have not met with much success.

Coupled with the introduction of HIER, the use of 4 M urea as the retrieval solution has produced consistent results, with the claim that the procedure allows the demonstration not only of CIg but also of SIg. We have taken the method further, and have employed HIER in 4 M urea solution in combination with proteolytic digestion prior to antigen retrieval. This has resulted in the consistent demonstration of cellular immunoglobulin in routinely fixed paraffin-embedded sections revealing a number of patterns of immunoglobulin localization. Perinuclear staining of endoplasmic reticulum was the most consistent pattern, often with associated staining of the Golgi. Membrane staining was also possible, as was cytoplasmic staining, the latter as distinct globular heterogeneous deposits of immunoglobulin rather than the homogeneous staining seen in false-positive staining. Stringent washing in between each incubation step results in a clean background in the case of follicular lymphomas.

Applications

About 80% of non-Hodgkin lymphoma in Western countries are of B-cell lineage, and the majority express monotypic SIg. The examination of lymphoid proliferations for the presence and clonal nature of SIg expression is a common practice and forms the basis for traditional immunophenotypic analysis. By convention, it is assumed that monoclonal B-cell proliferations are neoplastic. This analysis has traditionally been carried out by flow cytometry on cell suspensions, in cytospin preparations of disaggregated cells, or in frozen tissue sections. The SIg isotypes expressed by B-cell non-Hodgkin lymphoma and lymphoid leukemias parallel those of normal B cells. The most common heavy chain class is IgM, with or without associated IgD, and IgG and IgA are expressed much less frequently. The ratio of Igκ- to Igλ-bearing lymphomas is about 2 to 1.

Comments

When staining terminally differentiated B cells such as plasma cells, it is important to remember that unlike SIg, which is detectable in viable cells in suspension or in minimally fixed frozen sections, the staining of CIg requires permeabilization of the cell membrane by the fixative to allow penetration of the anti-Ig reagents. Therefore, sections fixed by a gentle fixative such as acetone will not allow the demonstration of CIg and plasma cells may show false-negative staining. Alcohol and formalin are suitable fixatives for the demonstration of CIg in cell preparations and tissue sections respectively. We have found that fixation of freshly prepared or air-dried smears and cell preparations followed by HIER in 4 M urea produces excellent staining of CIg in lymphoid cells through a wide range of differentiation. Formalin-fixed paraffin-embedded sections also show consistent staining for both CIg as well as SIg following a combination of trypsin digestion and HIER in 4 M urea.

Selected references

Leong AS-Y, Forbes IJ. Immunological and histochemical techniques in the study of the malignant lymphomas: A review. *Pathology* 1982; 14: 247–54.

Merz H, Pickers O, Schrimel S, *et al.* Constant detection of surface and cytoplasmic immunoglobulin heavy and light chain expression in formalin-fixed and paraffin-embedded material. *Journal of Pathology* 1993; 170: 257–64.

NOTES

IgG4

Sources/clones

Cell Marque (clone MRQ-44, mouse monoclonal antibody).

Fixation/preparation

The antigen is preserved in formalin-fixed paraffin-embedded tissue.

Background

Immunoglobulin γ (IgG) is the most common of the immunoglobulins. Among the IgGs, there are a variety of isotypes, including IgG1, IgG2a, IgG2b, IgG3, and IgG4. The rarest of the immunoglobulins is IgG4. However, despite its rarity, increased IgG4 production has been associated with a variety of pathologic processes, most notably IgG4-related disease (IRD). A key clinical reason to have a low threshold for evaluating IgG4 in sclerotic lymphoplasmacytic infiltrates is the remarkable responsiveness of IRD to corticosteroid therapy.

Increased IgG4+ plasma cells were first described in type 1 autoimmune pancreatitis, which shows the typical histologic features of IRD. Subsequently, IRD was found to encompass much more than autoimmune pancreatitis, and now has been found to involve a large number of tissues, including secreting glands of other types (lacrimal, salivary), soft tissue (sclerosing mediastinitis, retroperitoneal fibrosis), and lung, kidney, and lymph node. IRD at any of these sites shows three major histologic features: (1) dense lymphoplasmacytic infiltration; (2) fibrosis, typically showing at least a focal storiform pattern; (3) obliterative phlebitis.

Applications

Because the histopathologic diagnosis of IRD requires comparison of the IgG4+ plasma cells to the total IgG+ plasma cells in the same section(s), evaluation for IRD requires staining for IgG4 and total IgG on sister sections. While the anti-IgG4 monoclonal antibody noted above is highly sensitive and specific for this isotype, poly-anti-IgG polyclonal antibodies tend to have lower sensitivity and specificity, leading to occasional difficulties in interpreting the total IgG stain. Therefore, in our laboratory, we routinely perform total IgG staining in two different concentrations of antibody, in the hope that one of those two concentrations proves relatively straightforward to quantify.

In terms of scoring IgG4/total IgG immunohistochemistry, the typical threshold required for the diagnosis of IRD is >40% IgG4+ forms among the total IgG+ cells in the appropriate histologic setting. The absolute number of IgG4+ plasma cells can vary greatly among different anatomic sites involved by IRD.

Selected references

Deshpande V, Zen Y, Chang JK, et al. Consensus statement on the pathology of IgG4-related disease. *Modern Pathology* 2012; 25: 1181–92.

Wallace ZS, Deshpande V, Mattoo H, et al. IgG4-related disease: clinical and laboratory features in one hundred and twenty-five patients. *Arthritis and Rheumatology* 2015; 67: 2466–75.

NOTES

Inhibin

Sources/clones

Biodesign (monoclonal E4), Biogenesis (monoclonal 16Ba), Santa Cruz (polyclonal), Serotec (R1, E4).

Fixation/preparation

Antibodies to inhibin may be applied to paraffin-embedded tissues fixed in formalin; however, microwave pretreatment in citrate buffer is essential for optimum immunostaining.

Background

Inhibin is a peptide hormone produced by ovarian granulosa cells, which selectively inhibits the release of follicle-stimulating hormone (FSH) from the pituitary gland, acting as a modulator of folliculogenesis. A peak of its serum levels is reached during the follicular phase of the menstrual cycle; being undetectable in the serum of menopausal women. It is produced and overexpressed by granulosa cell tumors, thus being an early marker for tumor growth. Hence, its usefulness pertains to being a marker of tumor recurrence before clinical manifestation. Several inhibin subunits can be detected by immunostaining in the granulosa cell layers of the human ovary and in neighboring theca cells. Clone R1 was raised against a synthetic peptide corresponding to the 1–32 peptide of the α-subunit of 32 kDa human inhibin and reacts specifically with this molecule (isotype IgG2b). Clone E4 was raised against a synthetic peptide corresponding to the 84–114 peptide sequence of the βA-subunit of 32 kDa human inhibin A and activin A (isotype 2b). E4 reacts with both the βA- and βB-subunits of human inhibin and activin.

Applications

Using monoclonal antibody to the human inhibin 32 kDa α-subunit, follicle epithelia in 6/6 samples of ovarian tissue (under 40 years), 6/6 adult granulosa cell tumors, and three late metastases from granulosa cell tumors in females showed positive immunoreaction. No staining was found in hemangiopericytomas, leiomyosarcoma, and malignant melanoma. This would be useful in distinguishing the sarcomatoid growth pattern of granulosa cell tumors from soft tissue tumors.

Inhibin immunostaining is also detected in stromal hyperthecosis, juvenile granulosa cell tumors, and Sertoli–Leydig cell tumors, proving that inhibin is a sensitive immunohistochemical marker of a wide range of gonadal stromal tumors. In Sertoli–Leydig cell tumors, inhibin stained more intensely the gonadal stromal component compared to the retiform areas, which stained more for keratin.

α-Inhibin is a good marker of syncytiotrophoblastic cells but does not stain cytotrophoblastic cells. It can therefore be employed for the identification of placental site nodule or of a trophoblastic tumor such as choriocarcinoma, placental site trophoblastic tumor, or epithelioid trophoblastic tumor.

Strong cytoplasmic staining of hepatocellular carcinoma, including pleomorphic and glandular variants, has been demonstrated. Focal weak luminal staining of glands of adenocarcinoma was also present. Hence, immunostaining with anti-inhibin antibody may be of value in the differentiation of hepatocellular carcinoma from adenocarcinoma involving the liver.

Together with calretinin, inhibin can be employed to identify adrenocortical tumors (Appendix 1.18). Inhibin was demonstrated in 73% of tumors and in combination with calretinin identified 94% of adrenocortical tumors, with no difference in staining patterns in normal adrenal cortex, adrenocortical adenomas, and adenocarcinomas.

Comments

Inhibin antibody is useful to confirm the diagnosis of both adult and juvenile granulosa cell tumors, especially tumors with unusual growth patterns and in metastatic sites. A cautionary note with this application is that uterine tumors resembling ovarian sex cord tumors have been shown to immunoexpress inhibin rarely (1/7 cases). It is also helpful in distinguishing hepatocellular carcinoma from adenocarcinomas in the liver. The demonstration of α-inhibin in granular cell tumors of the gallbladder and extra hepatic bile ducts adds to the list of inhibin-positive lesions that includes sex cord–stromal tumors (granulosa cells tumors, luteinized thecomas, Leydig cell tumors), placental and gestational trophoblastic lesions, and adrenal cortical tumors.

Selected reference

Flemming P, Wellman A, Maschek H, Lang H, Georgii A. Monoclonal antibodies against inhibin represent key markers of adult granulosa cell tumors of the ovary even in their metastases. A report of three cases with late metastasis, being previously misinterpreted as hemangiopericytoma. *American Journal of Surgical Pathology* 1995; 19: 927–33.

Islet1

Sources/clones

Abbiotec (1H9), Abcam (1B1), Abnova (1H9), GeneTex (1H9), LifeSpan BioSciences (1H9), Novus (1H9), Thermo Scientific Pierce (1H9).

Fixation/preparation

The antigen is preserved in formalin-fixed paraffin-embedded tissue.

Background

Islet1 is a 39 kDa transcription factor that binds to the enhancer region of the insulin gene and is necessary for mesenchymal and endocrine cell formation in the dorsal bud of the pancreas during embryogenesis. Outside of the gastrointestinal tract, it is also necessary in the development of cardiovascular progenitor cells and motor neuron development.

Applications

Islet1 is a nuclear stain, and expression is normally noted in the islet cells of the pancreas. It is useful diagnostically to assess the site of origin in cases of metastatic well-differentiated neuroendocrine tumors, as up to 13% of tumors may initially present as a metastasis. Determining site of origin is critically important, as pancreatic tumors may respond to chemotherapeutic agents that are less useful in tumors arising from the tubal gut. The initial study looking at expression in well-differentiated pancreatic neuroendocrine tumors (PancNETs) showed strong and diffuse staining in 58/84 (69%) of PancNETs. No differences were noted when the tumors were separated into syndromic vs. non-syndromic, although gastrinomas from the pancreas were more likely to be Islet1-negative. Expression appears to be retained when comparing primary tumors with their matched metastatic counterparts.

While Islet1 is relatively sensitive, it is not specific for tumors of pancreatic origin. Positive staining can be seen in well-differentiated neuroendocrine tumors of the duodenum, rectum, and appendix, but expression is rare in tumors from the ileum (which is often the main differential in liver metastases of unknown origin). High-grade neuroendocrine carcinomas, from sites within and outside of the gastrointestinal tract, tend to be strongly positive for Islet1. Other tumors, such as medullary thyroid carcinoma, carcinoid tumors of the lung, neuroblastoma, paraganglioma, and olfactory neuroblastomas, may also stain strongly.

At this time, it is most useful to use Islet1 in conjunction with a panel of immunostains including polyclonal PAX-8 (pPAX-8), CDX2, and TTF-1 to determine site of origin in well-differentiated tumors. pPAX-8 tends to stain a similar percentage of PancNETs as Islet1, while CDX2 and TTF-1 positivity is rare in these tumors. Islet1 is most useful in the rare pancreatic tumor that is positive for CDX2 and pPAX-8, or in pancreatic tumors that are pPAX-8-negative.

Selected references

Agaimy A, Erlenbach-Wünsch K, Konukiewitz B, et al. ISL1 expression is not restricted to pancreatic well-differentiated neuroendocrine neoplasms, but is also commonly found in well and poorly differentiated neuroendocrine neoplasms of extrapancreatic origin. *Modern Pathology* 2013; 26: 995–1003.

Ahlgren U, Pfaff SL, Jessell TM, Edlund T, Edlund H. Independent requirement for ISL1 in formation of pancreatic mesenchyme and islet cells. *Nature* 1997; 385: 257–60.

Bellizzi AM. Assigning site of origin in metastatic neuroendocrine neoplasms: a clinically significant application of diagnostic immunohistochemistry. *Advances in Anatomic Pathology* 2013; 20: 285–314.

Graham RP, Shrestha B, Caron BL, *et al.* Islet-1 is a sensitive but not entirely specific marker for pancreatic neuroendocrine neoplasms and their metastases. *American Journal of Surgical Pathology* 2013; 37: 399–404.

Hermann G, Konukiewitz B, Schmitt A, Perren A, Klöppel G. Hormonally defined pancreatic and duodenal neuroendocrine tumors differ in their transcription factor signatures: expression of ISL1, PDX1, NGN3, and CDX2. *Virchows Archiv* 2011; 459: 147–54.

Schmitt AM, Riniker F, Anlauf M, *et al.* Islet 1 (Isl1) expression is a reliable marker for pancreatic endocrine tumors and their metastases. *American Journal of Surgical Pathology* 2008; 32: 420–5.

Ki-67 (MIB1, Ki-S5)

Sources/clones

Accurate (MM1), Biogenex (Ki-67, MIB1), Boehringer Mannheim (Ki-67, Ki-S5), Cymbus Bioscience (Ki-67), Dako (Ki-67, polyclonal), Diagnostic Biosystems (Ki-67, polyclonal), Immunotech (MIB1), Novocastra (MM1), RDI (KI67), Serotec (KI67), Zymed (7B11).

Fixation/preparation

Monoclonal Ki-67 is immunoreactive in frozen sections but not in paraffin sections (although there are claims of reactivity following HIER, the results are not consistent). MIB1, Ki-S5, and polyclonal Ki-67 are all immunoreactive in routinely fixed paraffin-embedded tissues. Immunoreactivity is enhanced following HIER combined with proteolytic digestion.

Background

The Ki-67 antibody was generated against a Hodgkin disease cell line and was found to identify a nuclear antigen expressed in all non-G_0 phases of the cell cycle, i.e., all proliferating cells. The antigen recognized by Ki-67 is a 345–395 kDa non-histone protein complex that is highly susceptible to protease treatment. The gene encoding the Ki-67 protein is localized on chromosome 10 and organized in 15 exons. The center of the gene is formed by an extraordinary 6845 bp exon containing 16 successively repeated homologous segments of 366 bp, the "Ki-67 repeats," each containing a highly conserved new motif of 66 bp, the "Ki-67 motif." The deduced peptide sequence of this central exon is associated with high-turnover proteins such as other cell cycle-related proteins, oncogenes, and transcription factors. Like these transcription factors, the Ki-67 antigen plays a pivotal role in maintaining cell proliferation because Ki-67 protein antisense oligonucleotides significantly inhibit ^{3}H-thymidine uptake in human tumor cell lines in a dose-dependent manner.

There is a good correlation between the percentage of Ki-67+ cells in normal tissues and cell kinetic parameters such as ^{3}H-thymidine labeling indices, although generally Ki-67 immunostaining gives a higher proliferative index than the S-phase fraction, as defined by flow cytometric analysis or by ^{3}H-thymidine incorporation.

Several antibodies to the Ki-67 antigen are available which are immunoreactive in routinely fixed sections, namely, MIB1, Ki-S5, polyclonal Ki-67, and Ki-S1 (not commercially available to our knowledge). The proliferation indices obtained with all these antibodies correlated well with that obtained with monoclonal Ki-67 in frozen sections, indicating that they are suitable substitutes with the advantage of being immunoreactive in fixed paraffin-embedded sections. This was not the case with the antibodies to proliferating cell nuclear antigens PC10 and 19A2, both of which have been demonstrated to be fixation-dependent.

Applications

Numerous studies have compared the Ki-67 proliferation indices in frozen sections with other prognostic parameters such as tumor grade, hormone receptor status, and p53 expression. In general, Ki-67 indices have been shown to be of prognostic relevance. Similar studies have been performed in wax-embedded archival tissues with some of the antibodies, particularly MIB1, confirming their relevance as prognostic markers. Ki-67 counts have also been useful in distinguishing between benign and malignant liver proliferations and to predict progress of granulosa cell tumors, Barrett's dysplasia, and ovarian serous tumors. MIB1 has also been applied to brain tumors as a predictor of survival. Delays in fixation do not appear to affect Ki-67 counts (using a polyclonal antibody) in intracranial malignant tumors.

Comments

In many cells the Ki-67 antigen appears to be localized to the nucleoli or perinucleolar region, with lighter diffuse nuclear staining in both frozen and fixed sections. When assessing proliferation indices, notable intratumoral heterogeneity will be observed, and counts should be taken from the areas of highest proliferation, usually at the periphery of the tumor. MIB1 is the antibody of choice when assessing proliferation indices. Proliferating cell nuclear antigen (PCNA) produces a high background and is fixation-sensitive.

Membrane Ki-67 staining is seen in sclerozing pneumocytoma of lung and hyalinizing trabecular tumor of the thyroid; in both cases this is of diagnostic value.

Ki-67 quantification or counting methodology varies, and usually the so-called "hot-spot" areas are where the count is performed. Counting is done by mere eyeballing, but more accurate ways of counting are becoming routine, such as photocopying an image of the Ki-67 stain and the use of image analysis.

Selected reference

Brown DC, Gatter KC. Monoclonal antibody Ki-67: Its use in histopathology. *Histopathology* 1990; 17: 489–503.

Laminin

Sources/clones

Becton Dickinson (4C12.8), Biogenesis (2D8-39, 2D8-30, 2D8-33), Biogenex (LAMI), Dako (polyclonal, 4C7), Euro-Diagnostics (polyclonal), EY Laboratories (polyclonal), Immunotech (4C12), Monosan (polyclonal).

Fixation/preparation

Most available antibodies are immunoreactive in cryostat sections and fixed, embedded tissues but require antigen retrieval in the form of HIER or proteolytic digestion or both.

Background

Laminin, a glycoprotein of about 900 kDa, is secreted by fibroblasts, epithelial, myoepithelial, endothelial, and smooth muscle cells. Laminin and type IV collagen form the two principal components of basal lamina. There are three genetically distinct chains of laminin, α-, β-, and γ-chains, which are held together by disulfide bonds and by a triple-stranded coiled-coil structure. Ultrastructurally, the basal lamina is composed of a lamina lucida of low electron density, adjacent to the parenchymal cells, and a basal lamina densa of high electron density, adjacent to the connective tissue matrix. By rotary shadowing, laminin has a cross-like shape, consisting of three short arms of 200 kDa and one long arm of 400 kDa. Laminin is exclusively localized to the basal lamina, predominantly to the lamina lucida, and is invariably present in basal lamina surrounding muscle, nerve, fat, and decidua cells, and separating epithelial and endothelial cells from adjacent connective tissues. Laminins are potent modulators of numerous biological processes in development, including cell proliferation, migration, and differentiation. In adult tissues, laminins influence the maintenance of specific gene expression and are involved in various pathological situations, including fibrosis, carcinogenesis, and metastasis.

Applications

Laminin has been shown to play a role in cell adhesion and attachment to the basal lamina, both in vivo and in vitro. The basal lamina is generally extremely stable, but in certain pathological states it may undergo local dissolution. This process is likely to play a crucial role in the invasiveness and progression of malignant tumors. Loss or defective organization of the basal lamina matrix in malignant neoplasms may be the result of increased breakdown by tumor-derived degradative enzymes, decreased synthesis, or decreased or abnormal assembly of the secreted basal lamina components. In human breast carcinoma, there is a suggestion that overexpression of the nm23-H1 gene, a putative metastasis suppressor gene, leads to the formation of basal lamina and growth arrest. Antisera to type IV collagen and laminin, the major components of basal lamina, allow the study of the organization of the basal lamina in various benign and malignant tumors. Laminin immunostaining with the immunogold-silver technique in resin-embedded sections allows exquisite demonstration of the basal lamina in a variety of tissues. The majority of invasive carcinomas are recognized to synthesize varying amounts of basal lamina material, but the basal lamina surrounding the tumor nests are generally fragmented, and in many cases completely absent. Benign and in-situ lesions appear to be circumscribed by intact basal lamina.

Diagnostic applications of collagen type IV immunostaining have mostly centered on the demonstration of basal lamina in invasive tumors, particularly epithelial tumors, and their changes with tumor invasion and metastasis. In particular, the demonstration of an intact basal lamina has been used to distinguish benign glandular proliferations such as microglandular adenosis and sclerosing adenosis from well-differentiated carcinoma such as tubular carcinoma of the breast. Distinctive patterns of basal distribution have been demonstrated in various types of soft tissue tumors, adding to the diagnostic armamentarium for this group of neoplasms, which are often difficult to separate histologically and with existing immunological markers. While the presence of basal lamina cannot be used as an absolute discriminant for blood vessels and lymphatic spaces, the latter do not display the reduplication of the basal lamina characteristic of blood vessels and generally show thin and discontinuous staining of basal lamina. The distinctive staining observed around blood vessels has been employed as a marker when performing capillary density measurements. Laminin immunostaining together with collagen type IV has been employed to demonstrate frequent breaches in the basal lamina of the mucosa of patients with celiac disease, suggesting that interaction between gliadin and components of the extracellular matrix may have a role in the genesis of mucosal epithelial damage.

The presence of basal lamina as demonstrated with laminin immunostaining may be a clue to the identification of hepatocellular carcinoma, as non-malignant hepatocytes lack basal lamina.

Comments

The use of proteolytic digestion following HIER further enhances immunoreactivity. With the polyclonal antibodies we employ protease at 0.25 mg/ml for 2 minutes.

Selected references

Leong AS-Y, Vinyuvat S, Suthipintawong C, Leong FJ. Patterns of basal lamina immunostaining in soft-tissue and bony tumors. *Applied Immunohistochemistry* 1997; 5: 1–7.

Liotta LA. Tumor invasion and metastases: Role of the basement membrane. Warner-Lambert Parke-Davis Award Lecture. *American Journal of Pathology* 1984; 117: 339–48.

Mammaglobin

Sources/clones

Biocare (1A5), Cell Marque (31A5), Dako (304-1A5), Santa Cruz (E17, H47), Ventana (31A5).

Background

Mammaglobin, a member of the uteroglobin gene family, was identified in the 1990s, and at that time appeared to be expressed only in breast tissue. However, it has since been found to be expressed in tissues other than breast, including salivary gland.

Applications

Mammaglobin is useful in salivary gland neoplasms when considering a diagnosis of mammary analog secretory carcinoma (MASC) of the salivary gland. The morphology of this neoplasm is not entirely specific and overlaps with other salivary gland tumors, especially acinic cell carcinoma, mucoepidermoid carcinoma, and adenocarcinoma not otherwise specified. MASC is defined by *ETV6–NTRK* gene fusion, and identifying the rearrangement is confirmatory, but many laboratories do not have this test available. Mammaglobin has been shown to be highly sensitive for MASC, but immunostaining for mammaglobin can occur in a variety of salivary gland tumors that do not harbor the *ETV6* translocation. Mammaglobin staining has been reported in 60–67% of low-grade polymorphous adenocarcinoma, 11% of mucoepidermoid carcinomas, 13% of adenoid cystic carcinomas, and 67% of salivary duct carcinomas. Caution should therefore be exercised when using mammaglobin for diagnosing MASC in the absence of cytogenetic confirmation.

In the breast, mammaglobin messenger RNA expression has been reported in 70–80% of primary and metastatic breast tumor biopsies. Approximately 80% of breast cancers show mammaglobin expression by immunohistochemistry. However, recent studies have shown that only certain subtypes of breast cancer express mammaglobin (ductal and lobular) and in 50% of these staining for mammaglobin is weak and focal. In addition, triple-negative breast cancers including metaplastic and medullary carcinomas are negative for mammaglobin. Therefore, mammaglobin should be used in conjunction with other putative breast markers for determination of breast origin of metastatic carcinomas.

Selected references

Bishop JA, Yonescu R, Batista D, *et al*. Utility of mammaglobin immunohistochemistry as a proxy marker for the ETV6-NTRK3 translocation in the diagnosis of salivary mammary analogue secretory carcinoma. *Human Pathology* 2013; 44: 1982–8.

Leygue E, Snell L, Dotzlaw H, *et al*. Mammaglobin, a potential marker of breast cancer nodal metastasis. *Journal of Pathology* 1999; 189: 28–33.

Reyes C, Gomez-Fernandez C, Nadji M. Metaplastic and medullary mammary carcinomas do not express mammaglobin. *American Journal of Clinical Pathology* 2012; 137: 747–52.

Sasaki E, Tsunoda N, Hatanaka Y, *et al*. Breast-specific expression of MGB1/mammaglobin: an examination of 480 tumors from various organs and clinicopathological analysis of MGB1-positive breast cancers. *Modern Pathology* 2007; 20: 208–14.

NOTES

MART-1/Melan-A

Sources/clones

Biogenex (clone A103), Dako (clone A103), Novocastra (clone A103).

Fixation/preparation

The antibodies are suitable for immunohistochemical analysis of fresh frozen and formalin-fixed paraffin-embedded tissue. For best results on archival material, antigen heat-induced retrieval methods are essential.

Background

The *Melan-A* gene was cloned from the human melanoma cell line SK-Mel29. Independently, the same gene was found by another group using a different cell line and named *MART-1* (melanoma antigen recognized by T-cells). Both clones are recognized by most HLA-A_2-restricted tumor-specific tumor infiltrating lymphocytes harvested from patients with melanoma. MART-1 (clone M2-7C10) and Melan-A (clone A103) are two different antibody clones generated by separate groups but recognize the same antigen. The Melan-A/MART-1 protein comprises 118 amino acids with a molecular weight of 20–22 kDa. Although not fully characterized regarding subcellular localization, it is nevertheless thought to be associated with melanosomes and endoplasmic reticulum.

In normal tissue mRNA expression is limited to melanocytes in the skin and retina. Immunopositivity for Melan-A/MART-1 has been demonstrated in both primary and metastatic malignant melanoma with a range of positivity in 81–90% of tumors. These positive rates are slightly better than HMB-45 (75–80%). Unlike HMB-45, Melan-A/MART-1 is purported to yield a homogeneous cytoplasmic staining pattern in both melanomas and melanocytic nevi, with a stronger intensity and greater percentage of tumor cell immunopositivity. In contrast, HMB-45 stains mainly the intraepidermal and superficial dermal components of compound nevi. Melan-A/MART-1 has a limited role in the differential diagnosis of desmoplastic melanoma. In a study of 22 cases of HMB-45– melanomas including 8 desmoplastic melanomas, Melan-A was positive in 9, but not in any cases of desmoplastic melanoma. The epithelioid melanomas (primary and metastatic) show a better frequency of expression with these antibodies than spindle cell and desmoplastic melanomas.

Strong, diffuse granular staining of Melan-A has been demonstrated in adrenocortical adenomas and carcinomas (primary and metastatic) and Leydig/Sertoli–Leydig cell tumors of the ovary and testes. Clone A103 was shown to stain adrenal cortical tumors but not metastatic carcinomas to the adrenal, pheochromocytomas, or extra-adrenal carcinomas. Although regarded as being not specific, the recognition of steroid hormone-producing tumors was a consistent finding with Melan-A, but not with MART-1. This may reflect differences in the antigenic epitopes or purity of the two clones. Alternatively, cross-reactivity with a similar epitope of a different gene may explain the positive staining of steroid tumors with Melan-A. However, immunopositivity with both antibodies has been demonstrated in tumors of perivascular epithelioid cells (PEComas, e.g., angiomyolipoma, lymphangioleiomyomatosis, and "sugar" tumors of the lung), so that it has utility for both myoid and melanocytic differentiation.

Applications

The antibodies are useful for the detection of primary and metastatic melanomas, especially with an epithelioid morphology, but with limited value in spindle and desmoplastic melanomas. It should be noted that MART-1 has been better studied on cytologic material, while Melan-A has been more extensively studied on archival material.

In assessing metastatic tumors of unknown primary/origin, Melan-A is useful to distinguish adrenocortical carcinoma from renal cell and hepatocellular carcinomas. In such instances, other melanoma markers would be essential to rule out metastatic melanomas, reinforcing the importance of a panel of antibodies for immunohistological investigation. Melan-A is also a useful marker to distinguish adrenocortical tumors from other tumors in the adrenals and retroperitoneum (Appendix 1.18). Both antibodies have demonstrated usefulness in the confirmation of PEComas.

Selected reference

Busam KJ, Jungbluth AA. Melan-A, a new melanocytic differentiation marker. *Advances in Anatomic Pathology* 1999; 6: 182–7.

MDM-2 protein

Sources/clones

Accurate (19E3), Dako (SMP14), Novocastra (IB10, polyclonal), Oncogene (1F2).

Fixation/preparation

Several of the antibodies are immunoreactive in fixed paraffin-embedded tissue sections, besides fresh tissue and cell preparations.

Background

The MDM-2 protein encodes for a nuclear phosphoprotein that binds p53 and inhibits its ability to activate transcription by concealing the p53 activation domain. It has been suggested that MDM-2 overexpression might represent an alternative mechanism by which p53-mediated pathways are inactivated in human tumors, thus having a possible role in oncogenesis. MDM-2 overexpression as a result of gene amplification and/or increased mRNA expression can be detected by immunohistochemical analysis.

Applications

The ability to stain for MDM-2 protein in fixed tissue sections has stimulated a great deal of interest in its expression in various neoplasms. The correlation of MDM-2 protein levels with p53 may provide insights into oncogenesis and has the potential of providing prognostic information. Several studies have included the detection of p21/WAF1 protein together with MDM-2, as both these oncoproteins are downstream effectors of p53, p21 playing a major role in negatively regulating cell cycle progression, while MDM-2 inhibits the effects of p53.

Results of immunohistochemical analyses of MDM-2 and p53 protein are far from conclusive, although many support an inverse correlation between the two oncoproteins. Such studies have included uterine sarcoma, breast carcinoma, thymoma, osteogenic sarcoma, glioblastoma, lung carcinoma, oral carcinoma, malignant melanoma, thyroid carcinoma, and rhabdomyosarcoma.

Other studies support the role of MDM-2 protein in tumorigenesis in tumors such as oral squamous cell carcinoma, malignant fibrous histiocytoma of the jejunum, well-differentiated and dedifferentiated liposarcoma, non-small-cell carcinoma of the lung, adult medulloblastoma, carcinoma of the breast, oral ameloblastoma, and carcinoma of the urinary bladder. Interestingly, MDM-2 protein was found to be confined to follicular adenomas of the thyroid, whereas p53 protein was not immunoexpressed in such tumors.

MDM-2 has important applications in the workup of fatty tumors. There is nuclear positivity in atypical lipomatous tumors/well-differentiated liposarcoma. Other lipomatous tumors are generally negative.

Parosteal osteocarcoma and intimal sarcomas are also MDM-2-positive. Immunohistochemical staining often correlates with amplification demonstrated by FISH.

Comments

Immunostaining for MDM-2 has also been successfully conducted on cytological preparations.

Selected reference

Gelsleichter L, Gown AM, Zarbo RJ, et al. P53 and mdm-2 expression in malignant melanoma: an immunocytochemical study of expression of p53, mdm-2, and markers of cell proliferation in primary versus metastatic tumors. *Modern Pathology* 1995; 8: 530–5.

NOTES

Measles

Sources/clones

Biogenex (1.3, polyclonal), Chemicon (polyclonal), Sera Lab.

Fixation/preparation

This antibody is applicable to formalin-fixed paraffin-wax-embedded tissue. The number of positive cells is increased significantly with microwave pretreatment.

Background

Measles, an acute febrile eruption, has been one of the most common diseases of civilization. Despite the development of an effective vaccine, it remains a worldwide health problem.

The measles virion is composed of a central core of ribonucleic acid with a helically arranged protein coat surrounded by a lipoprotein envelope with spike-like structures. The virion is 120–200 nm in diameter and is classified as a morbillivirus in the paramyxovirus family.

Applications

Subacute sclerosing panencephalitis (SSPE) is a rare, fatal disease of children caused by a persistent measles virus infection of the central nervous system. Immunodetection of viral proteins using antibodies raised to measles is useful to confirm the diagnosis of SSPE in brain biopsies and postmortem CNS tissue.

Using microwave antigen retrieval systems, increased immunoreactivity is seen in neuronal processes, suggesting that this may represent virus spreading from cell to cell. Attempts to demonstrate the M-protein in the brain of an SSPE patient using immunohistochemistry have proved futile, even though nucleotide sequences coding for M protein were detected. This suggests diminished synthesis and/or rapid degradation of M protein in the SSPE brain.

Persistence of infection and ability to induce chronic inflammation have been used to argue for a role for measles in the etiology of Crohn's disease. Immunostaining using both measles virus-specific monoclonal and polyclonal antibodies was positive within endothelial cells in areas of granulomatous vasculitis. In-situ hybridization for measles virus genomic RNA also produced positive signals in a similar location, but also showed strongly positive cells in the secondary lymphoid follicles. By employing an immunogold method, ultrastructural studies have shown significantly higher levels of anti-measles antigen in Crohn's disease compared to ulcerative colitis, tuberculous lymphadenitis, and nongranulomatous areas of bowels with Crohn's disease, but no significant difference between Crohn's disease and SSPE. An epidemiological association between Crohn's disease and measles virus exposure in early life has been suggested in case–control studies. It is therefore suggested that Crohn's disease may be a chronic granulomatous vasculitis in reaction to a persistent infection with measles virus within the vascular endothelium. RT-PCR studies have suggested a link between measles virus and a new-variant inflammatory bowel disease (ileocolonic lymphonodular hyperplasia) in children.

Comments

Application of antibodies to measles virus would be useful in developing countries, where SSPE is more frequently seen. Both polyclonal and monoclonal antibodies give good immunoreactivity following microwave pretreatment.

Selected reference

Allen IV, McQuaid S, McMahon J, et al. The significance of measles virus antigen and genome distribution in the CNS in SSPE for mechanisms of viral spread and demyelination. *Journal of Neuropathology and Experimental Neurology* 1996; 55: 471–80.

NOTES

Mel-CAM (CD146)

Sources/clones

Alexis (polyclonal COM7A4), Biocytex (monoclonal F435H7).

Fixation/preparation

This antibody is applicable to formalin-fixed paraffin-embedded tissue. Antigen retrieval with citrate buffer is recommended.

Background

Melanoma cell adhesion molecule (Mel-CAM) is a cell adhesion molecule that belongs to the immunoglobulin supergene family. Mel-CAM was originally designated MUC18 and was discovered by differential screening of a cDNA library from a human melanoma cell line. Mel-CAM is a 113 kDa single chain molecule containing five immunoglobulin-like domains, a transmembrane stretch, and a short cytoplasmic tail with several potential phosphorylation sites. It functions by binding to an unidentified counter-receptor on the surface of adjacent cells. In addition to its action as a cell-to-cell adhesion molecule, the extracellular domain of Mel-CAM contains a potential proteoglycan-binding motif that may facilitate cell–extracellular matrix adhesion.

Mel-CAM expression has been detected in a variety of tissues, including hair follicles, cerebellar cortex, endothelium, and smooth muscle. Mel-CAM is expressed in more than 90% of cutaneous melanomas and has also been detected in angiosarcomas and leiomyosarcomas. Other neoplasms, including hematopoietic tumors, glial tumors, and a variety of carcinomas and sarcomas, have failed to demonstrate Mel-CAM immunoreactivity.

Mel-CAM has also been reported to be a specific cell surface marker for intermediate trophoblasts (ITs). In contrast, chorion-type intermediate trophoblasts, endometrial glandular and surface epithelium, and inflammatory cells in the implantation site were Mel-CAM immunonegative or only focally and weakly positive. Hence, Mel-CAM is a specific and sensitive marker for IT differentiation in normal placentas and implantation sites, and in gestational trophoblastic tumors. A double-staining technique with MIB-1 antibody to determine the proliferative index in Mel-CAM-defined IT was found to be useful in the differential diagnosis of exaggerated placental vs. placental site trophoblastic tumor and placental site trophoblastic tumor vs. choriocarcinoma.

Applications

Gestational trophoblastic tumors and tumor-like lesions can be confused with a variety of non-trophoblastic tumors. Since this distinction is important for management purposes, using an IT-specific marker like Mel-CAM would be useful in resolving the differential diagnosis (Appendix 1.34).

Selected references

Albelda SM, Muller WA, Buck CA, Newman PJ. Molecular and cellular properties of PECAM-1 (endoCAM/CD31): a novel vascular cell–cell adhesion molecule. *Journal of Cell Biology* 1991; 114: 1059–68.

Kuzu I, Bicknell R, Fletcher CDM, Gatter KC. Expression of adhesion molecules on the endothelium of normal tissue vessels and vascular tumors. *Laboratory Investigation* 1993; 69: 322–8.

NOTES

Mesothelin

Sources/clones

Mesothelin, CAK 1, Mab K1, 5B2 (Abcam, Novocastra, murine monoclonal [isotype IgG1]).

Background

Mesothelin, a 40 kDa glycosylphosphatidylinositol-linked cell-surface glycoprotein, was isolated by being reactive to a monoclonal antibody (Mab K1) originally found to be reactive against ovarian carcinoma and mesotheliomas. It is on the surface of mesothelial cells, mesotheliomas, and ovarian carcinoma, and plays a role in cellular adhesion.

Applications

Expressed in lung and mesothelial cells, with low levels of expression in heart, placenta, and kidney. It is expressed in epithelioid mesotheliomas, ovarian carcinomas, and some squamous cell carcinomas. Though initially thought to be specific for mesotheliomas and ovarian carcinomas, this antibody (5B2) has been reported to be positive in lung adenocarcinoma (39%), squamous cell carcinoma of lung (18%), esophagus (75%), and uterine cervix (25%), as well as in other adenocarcinomas (non-mucinous ovarian carcinoma 100%, peritoneum 100%, endometrium 67%, pancreas 91%, biliary tract 45%, stomach 50%, colon 31%) but not in carcinomas of breast, kidney, thyroid, adrenal, or prostate; nor in germ cell tumors, neuroendocrine tumors, or urothelial carcinoma.

Mesothelin is reported to be positive in desmoplastic small round cell tumors, and in the epithelial component of biphasic synovial sarcoma. Amongst non-mucinous ovarian carcinomas, mesothelin in expressed in serous, endometrioid, clear cell, and transitional carcinomas of the ovary, as well as in Brenner tumor of ovary (100%). Approximately 50% of mucinous carcinomas of ovary are reported variably positive for mesothelin. Mesothelin positivity with 5B2 antibody is reported in mature teratomas of the ovary (100%). Using the second-generation 5B2 antibody, sensitivity and specificity to identify epithelioid mesotheliomas is 75% and 71%, respectively. If the possibility of ovarian carcinoma is excluded, then the specificity of mesothelin for the diagnosis of epithelioid mesothelioma increases to 90%.

Comments

Useful in the differential diagnosis of clear cell carcinoma of ovary vs. endodermal sinus tumor or clear cell renal cell carcinoma, TCC of ovary vs. TCC of urinary bladder, cholangiocarcinomas vs. hepatomas, benign pancreatic ductal epithelium vs. pancreatic ductal adenocarcinoma.

Selected references

Chang K, Pastan I. Molecular cloning of mesothelin, a differentiation antigen present on mesothelium, mesotheliomas, and ovarian cancers. *Proceedings of the National Academy of Sciences of the USA* 1996; 93: 136–40.

Ordóñez NG. Value of mesothelin immunostaining in the diagnosis of mesothelioma. *Modern Pathology* 2003; 16: 192–7.

NOTES

Metallothioneins

Sources/clones

Dako (E9).

Fixation/preparation

Immunoreactive in fixed paraffin-embedded tissue sections as well as cell preparations and frozen sections. Immunoreactivity is enhanced following HIER.

Background

Metallothioneins (MTs) are low-molecular-weight, heavy-metal-binding proteins whose expression is induced by heavy metals as well as other factors such as stress, glucocorticoids, lymphokines, and xenobiotics. MTs have been described in most vertebrate and invertebrate species. Two major isoforms, MT-I and MT-II, are distributed in most adult mammalian tissues. Another isoform, MT-0, is also recognized, and genes for MT-III and MT-IV with restriction to brain neurons and stratified epithelium have been described. Interest in MTs has focused on their overexpression and susceptibility to carcinogenic and anticarcinogenic effects of cadmium, spontaneous mutagenesis and anti-cancer drugs, and tumor resistance to chemotherapeutic agents.

Applications

The ability to stain for MTs with immunohistochemical methods has produced a large amount of data concerning their expression at different stages of the development and progression of a wide variety of tumors. Briefly, overexpression of MTs has been associated with the type and grade of some tumors such as ductal breast carcinoma, skin carcinoma, cervical carcinoma, pancreatic carcinoma, prostatic carcinoma, melanoma, bladder carcinoma, renal cell carcinoma, small-cell carcinoma of the lung, and ovarian carcinoma. While overexpression of MTs appears to be mostly associated with locally invasive carcinomas of poor histological type and grade, reduced overall survival, and local recurrence of tumor (but not lymph node or distant metastases), this is not true of all tumors. In colonic, bladder, and fibroblastic skin tumors, overexpression of MTs is associated with lower-grade, better-differentiated tumors. In squamous cell carcinoma of the esophagus, overexpression of MT appears to predict tumors that benefit from chemotherapy. The reason for this apparent discrepancy is not clear. It has been suggested that current antibodies for immunostaining are unable to distinguish between MT-I and MT-II isoforms, or metal-bound and metal-free (apoMT) forms of the protein. Furthermore, they are also unable to detect overexpression of MT-0, MT-III, and MT-IV isoforms, accounting for the apparently conflicting observations. The use of MT expression to predict response to chemotherapy is another avenue that requires further study.

MT has been described as a marker of deep penetrating dermatofibroma, allowing its distinction from dermatofibrosarcoma protuberans, which was consistently negative by immunostaining. Increased immunoexpression of MT has been demonstrated in fibroblasts of all ulcerative lesions of ulcerative colitis and Crohn's disease, and a protective role for MT has been suggested. It was also immunoexpressed in a lower percentage of epithelial cells in these diseases.

Comments

MT staining is found in nucleus, cytoplasm, and cell membrane, and the proliferating edges of tumors show the most intense staining.

Selected references

Jasani B, Schmid KW. Significance of metallothionein overexpression in human tumors. *Histopathology* 1997; 31: 211–14.

Kagi JHR. Overview of methallothionein. Metallobiochemistry Part B: metallothionein and related molecules. *Methods in Enzymology* 1993; 205: 613–26.

Microphthalmia transcription factor (MiTF)

Sources/clones

Neomarker/Lab Vision (D5, monoclonal antibody recognizes only human MiTF; C5, recognizes both mouse and human MiTF, D5+C5).

Fixation/preparation

These antibodies are applicable to formalin-fixed paraffin-embedded tissues and require heat-induced antigen retrieval.

Background

The microphthalmia (*Mi*) gene is located on chromosome 3p and encodes a basic helix-loop-helix zipper protein. This DNA-binding protein regulates transcription of genes involved in melanin synthesis, such as tyrosinase. Studies in mice have shown that MiTF is essential for pigment synthesis, and embryogenesis and postnatal survival of melanocytes. In humans, MiTF comprises four isoforms that differ in their amino-termini and expression patterns. Isoforms A and B are present in retinal pigment epithelium, cervical cancer cells, and melanoma cells; isoform H is present in the retinal pigment epithelium and cervical cancer cells but not in melanoma cells; isoform M is present only in melanoma cells. Humans with heterozygous mutations of MitTF have Waardenburg syndrome 2a, which is characterized by the presence of a white forelock and deafness. Knockout mice with homozygous deletions of MiTF also show disruption of osteoclastogenesis, resulting in osteopetrosis.

100% of melanomas are positive with antibody D5, which recognizes both mouse and human MiTF. This high sensitivity and specificity for melanocytic differentiation was also duplicated for cutaneous nevi and in metastatic melanoma. These results compare favorably with HMB-45, Melan-A, and tyrosinase. However, the situation is less defined with the utility of MiTF in the diagnosis of desmoplastic malignant melanoma. Rates of immunopositivity in this tumor have ranged from 3% to 55%. This may be related to the size of the tumor, as MiTF expression appears to be less common in small dermal desmoplastic melanomas than in those that form a distinct mass.

MiTF immunoexpression has also been demonstrated in a rare group of neoplasms that display combined features of melanocytic and myoid differentiation, the perivascular epithelioid cell family of tumors or PEComas, e.g., angiomyolipoma and related tumors. The efficacy appears to approximate that of HMB-45 and Melan-A for the diagnosis of PEComas. An advantage of MiTF in small biopsies is that a greater number (>50%) of cells are positive. Other soft tissue neoplasms with melanocytic differentiation have also been demonstrated to show MiTF expression, namely, melanotic schwannomas, cellular blue nevi, and clear cell sarcomas.

Applications

MiTF appears to be the most sensitive marker for melanocytic nevi and typical epithelioid melanomas (Appendix 1.10). However, like other markers for melanoma including HMB-45 and Melan-A, it does not appear to show sensitivity for desmoplastic melanoma. MiTF has a definite role in soft tissue neoplasms with a melanocytic differentiation, e.g., PEComas, clear cell sarcoma, and melanotic schwannoma. As a nuclear marker, MiTF is largely free of the cytoplasmic artifacts that plague biotin-rich and/or peroxidase-rich tissues such as kidney and liver.

Selected reference

Busam KJ, Iversen K, Copian KC, Jungbluth AA. Analysis of microphthalmia transcription factor expression in normal tissues and tumors, and comparison of its expression with S-100 protein, gp100, and tyrosinase in desmoplastic malignant melanoma. *American Journal of Surgical Pathology* 2001; 25: 197–204.

Mitochondria

Sources/clones

Biogenex (113-1), Chemicon International (MAB 1273).

Fixation/preparation

Monoclonal antibody 113-1 is designed for the specific localization of mitochondria in formalin-fixed paraffin-embedded tissue sections, or 2% formaldehyde/acetone-fixed cell preparations. Antigen retrieval pretreatment is recommended prior to the immunohistochemical procedure.

Background

Monoclonal antibody clone 113-1 recognizes a 60 kDa non-glycosylated protein component of mitochondria in human cells. This marker may be useful in the identification of mitochondria in cells, tissues, and biochemical preparations. It produces a cytoplasmic granular "spaghetti-like" staining pattern in the cytoplasm of human cells.

Antimitochondrial antibody 113-1 has been shown to be a useful discriminatory adjunct in the complex differential diagnosis of granular renal cell tumors. Distinctive staining patterns were observed, with chromophobe RCC showing a peripheral accentuation of coarse cytoplasmic granules, a diffuse and fine granularity in renal oncocytomas, and an irregular cytoplasmic distribution of coarse granules in the granular variant of clear cell RCC. In addition, staining was most intense in the eosinophilic variant of papillary RCC with irregular cytoplasmic distribution of coarse granules.

In the salivary gland, immunohistochemistry using the antimitochondrial antibody proved to be a highly sensitive and specific method for light microscopic identification of mitochondria, and superior to routine H&E or PTAH stains for the detection of normal and metaplastic oncocytic cells. This was also useful in the demonstration of neoplastic cells rich in mitochondria: Warthin's tumor, benign oncocytoma and oncocytic carcinoma, and deciduoid mesothelioma, all of which show an intense, finely granular immunoreactivity in the cytoplasm.

Antimitochondrial antibody is also useful in the confirmation/identification of poorly differentiated oxyphilic (Hurthle cell) carcinomas of the thyroid, showing selective marking of oxyphilic, mitochondria-rich cells.

Oncocytic (mitochondria-rich) differentiation identifying a subset of meningiomas that behave aggressively may also be accomplished with the use of this antibody. Six so-called oncocytic meningiomas have all successfully shown an immunopositive reaction with antimitochondrial antibody.

Applications

Antimitochondrial antibody clearly has a role in the identification of oncocytic tumors on both paraffin sections and cell preparations. It is also applicable to the differential diagnosis of granular cell tumors of the kidney, with distinctive cytoplasmic immunopositive patterns delineating the various tumors. It is also helpful in the identification of oncocytic meningiomas (in conjunction with a panel including EMA and vimentin), which have a potential aggressive behavior.

Selected reference

BiogenexLaboratories. Monoclonal antibody to mitochondrial antigen (data sheet).

NOTES

MOC-31

Sources/clones

Dako (monoclonal, MOC-31).

Fixation/preparation

This antibody may be applied to both paraffin-embedded tissue sections and cytological material.

Background

MOC-31 is a monoclonal antibody generated with the use of neuramidase-treated cells from a small-cell lung carcinoma cell line (GLS-1). MOC-31 was clustered as an SCLC-cluster 2 antibody during the First International Workshop on Small-Cell Lung Cancer Antigens in 1987. The SCLC-cluster 2 antibodies detect a 38 kDa epithelial-associated transmembrane glycoprotein which is also named epithelial glycoprotein 2 or EGP-2, since it only occurs in epithelial cells. There is strong expression of EGP-2 in non-squamous carcinomas, and none in lymphomas, melanomas, and neuroblastomas. Hence, MOC-31 is a monoclonal antibody that recognizes a glycoprotein of unknown function present in the membrane of epithelial cells.

Reactivity is seen in 100% of pulmonary adenocarcinomas and 85% of non-pulmonary adenocarcinomas, but only in 5% of mesotheliomas. Reactivity in the latter was restricted to a few positive cells, in contrast to the adenocarcinomas, where it was strong and diffuse. Combining MOC-31 and HBME-1 has demonstrated diagnostic efficiency for the distinction between metastatic carcinoma and mesothelioma in the pleura. The range of specificity for MOC-31 is 80–97.7% (reduced to 12.5% with cytology samples), with sensitivity of 61.2–100%.

The role of MOC-31 has been expanded, and it has been shown to distinguish between hepatocellular carcinoma and adenocarcinoma (both metastatic and cholangiocarcinoma), being negative in primary hepatomas.

Applications

MOC-31 may be helpful as part of a panel of antibodies to distinguish between mesotheliomas and adenocarcinoma. There appears to be sufficient evidence to validate its inclusion in a panel to distinguish hepatomas from adenocarcinoma (both primary and secondary) in the liver.

Selected reference

Edwards C, Oates J. OV 632 and MOC 31 in the diagnosis of mesothelioma and adenocarcinoma: an assessment of their use in formalin fixed and paraffin wax embedded material. *Journal of Clinical Pathology* 1995; 48: 626–30.

NOTES

MSA (muscle-specific actin)

Sources/clones

Abcam (1A4), Biogenesis, Biogenex (HHF35), Dako (HHF35), Diagnostic Biosystems (HHF35), Enzo (HHF35), Sanbio (SA1C1), Zymed (ZMSA-5, ZCA34, ZSA-1).

Fixation/preparation

The antibody HHF35 is immunoreactive in fixed paraffin-embedded tissue sections and staining is enhanced following HIER.

Background

There are at least six different actin isotypes in mammals. They are four isotypes found exclusively in muscular tissues – α-skeletal, α-cardiac, and α- and γ- smooth muscle actins – and two other isotypes, β- and γ-cytoplasmic actin, found in most cell types, including non-muscle cells of the body. Early anti-actin antibodies were polyclonal and did not distinguish among various actin isotypes and were of low sensitivity and specificity. Various monoclonal antibodies have now been described, and the most widely used is clone HHF35, available commercially, which recognizes a common epitope of α-skeletal, α-cardiac, and α- and γ- smooth muscle actin isotypes. This antibody labels myoepithelial and smooth muscle cells as well as leiomyomas and leiomyosarcomas. Muscle-specific actins (MSAs) have also been described in pericytes, reactive myofibroblasts, and skeletal and cardiac muscle. Positive-staining cells have been reported in the deep ovarian cortical stroma and theca externa of secondary ovarian follicles, alveolar soft part sarcoma, epithelioid sarcoma, infantile digital fibromatosis, ovarian sclerosing stromal tumors, and Kaposi's sarcoma, representing either myofibroblasts or pericytes in these conditions. Glomus tumors stain positive for MSA, a finding that supports a smooth muscle derivation of these tumors, and the variable extent of MSA staining observed in malignant mesothelioma and malignant fibrous histiocytoma has been attributed to myofibroblastic differentiation in these tumors. Actin staining of unequivocal tumor cells has been reported in occasional cases of metastatic endometrial stromal sarcoma and malignant peripheral nerve sheath tumor, but it has not been ascertained if these findings represent aberrant actin expression of tumor cells or cross-reactivity of anti-actin antibodies. MSA has also been observed in the cells of the capsule of the liver, kidney, and spleen, and in decidual cells, some stromal cells of chorionic villi, and the so-called fibroblastic reticulum cells of lymph nodes and spleen.

Applications

The increased sensitivity and specificity of newer monoclonal antibodies allow the use of anti-MSA antibodies in the identification of pleomorphic spindle cell tumors. Because of varying sensitivities, it is best to employ MSA with other myogenic markers such as smooth muscle actin and desmin when examining tumors, which can potentially be confused with rhabdomyosarcoma (RMS), leiomyosarcoma (LMS), and myofibroblastic tumors. Much of the controversy as to which of these markers is the most sensitive for myogenic differentiation stems from the fact that the expression of the individual markers varies with the site of origin of the tumor. For example, most soft tissue and uterine LMS contain predominantly α-smooth muscle actin, but those from the gastrointestinal tract show only β- and γ-non-muscle actins and would thus be negative for HHF35. Myofibroblasts show heterogeneous immunophenotype and may be positive for vimentin only; for vimentin and α-smooth muscle actin; for vimentin and desmin; or for vimentin, desmin, and α-smooth muscle actin. Myofibroblastic proliferations such as nodular fasciitis may display characteristic peripheral/subplasmalemmal staining for muscle actin, yielding a "tram-track" appearance. Increased expression of MSA has been correlated with mesangial cell injury and proliferation in both rats and humans, and can be employed as a marker of mesangial cell injury, activation, and proliferation.

Comments

Zenker's fixative appears to cause a marked decrease in the intensity of MSA staining. False-positive reactivity with clones HHF35 and 1A4 has been reported in non-Hodgkin lymphoma, a problem attributed to contaminating antibodies, partial antibody degradation, or excess antibody concentration which may occur with ascitic fluid preparations of anti-MSA. The problem was not observed in tissue culture supernatant antibodies and was abolished by the addition of 50 mmol/L of EDTA to the prediluted antibody. MSA remains a well-used marker for contractile cells. Other myogenic markers include desmin, smooth muscle actin, and the actin-binding proteins calponin and h-caldesmon.

Selected references

Azumi N, Ben-Erza J, Battifora H. Immunophenotypic diagnosis of leiomyosarcomas and rhabdomyosarcomas with monoclonal antibodies to muscle specific actin and desmin in formalin-fixed tissue. *Modern Pathology* 1988; 1: 469–74.

Rangdaeng S, Truong LD. Comparative immunohistochemical staining for desmin and muscle specific actin: a study of 576 cases. *American Journal of Clinical Pathology* 1991; 96: 32–45.

MUM1

Sources/clones

Dako (clone MUM1p, mouse monoclonal IgG1).

Fixation/preparation

The antigen is preserved in formalin-fixed paraffin-embedded tissue.

Background

MUM1, or interferon response factor 4 (IRF4), is a nuclear transcription factor that is thought to be the master regulator of B-cell differentiation to plasma cells. MUM1-deficient mice are without functional plasma cells, and MUM1 has been shown to be required for immunoglobulin class switch recombination. As shown by RNA interference studies, MUM1 is required for myeloma tumor cell viability irrespective of the underlying oncogenic mechanism, and is therefore a putative target for therapeutic intervention. As an interferon response factor, MUM1 also plays a role in response to viral infections: for example, it is prominently expressed in Epstein–Barr virus (EBV)-infected B cells.

Applications

In normal B-cell differentiation, MUM1 is expressed in late germinal center B cells, enabling them to differentiate to marginal zone-type B cells or plasma cells. Importantly, a variety of gene expression profiling studies on diffuse large B-cell lymphoma (DLBCL) have shown unequivocally that MUM1 is an important marker of non-germinal center-type DLBCL/activated B-cell (ABC)-DLBCL. In the simple immunohistochemical algorithm, MUM1, along with CD10 and Bcl-6, is assessed to determine whether a de-novo DLBCL falls into the favorable-prognosis germinal center subtype, or the unfavorable-prognosis ABC subtype.

In addition to post-germinal center B cells and plasma cells, as well as neoplasms derived from these cells, MUM1 is expressed in other malignancies. It is perhaps the most sensitive marker of classic Hodgkin lymphoma, being strongly expressed in virtually 100% of Hodgkin/Reed–Sternberg (HRS) cells. It is expressed to a more variable extent in nodular lymphocyte-predominant Hodgkin lymphoma. A subset of follicular lymphomas, presumably those at the later stages of germinal center development, express MUM1. In contrast, "early" germinal center-type neoplasms, such as Burkitt lymphoma, typically lack MUM1 expression.

MUM1 expression is not limited to B cells. A subset of follicular helper T cells, particularly those that rosette the LP cells of nodular lymphocyte-predominant Hodgkin lymphoma, express MUM1. Similarly, a subset of follicular helper-derived T-cell lymphomas, including angioimmunoblastic T-cell lymphoma, will show some degree of MUM1 expression. Evaluation of MUM1 expression, which is localized to the nucleus, is therefore of use in the diagnostic arena as part of the overall immunohistochemical evaluation for DLBCL, Hodgkin lymphoma, and T-cell lymphoma.

Selected references

Falini B, Fizzotti M, Pucciarini A, *et al.* A monoclonal antibody (MUM1p) detects expression of the MUM1/IRF4 protein in a subset of germinal center B cells, plasma cells, and activated T cells. *Blood* 2000; 95: 2084–92.

Gualco G, Weiss LM, Bacchi CE. MUM1/IRF4: a review. *Applied Immunohistochemistry and Molecular Morphology* 2010; 18: 301–10.

Klein U, Casola S, Cattoretti G, *et al.* Transcription factor IRF4 controls plasma cell differentiation and class-switch recombination. *Nature Immunology* 2006; 7: 773–82.

Shaffer AL, Emre NC, Lamy L, *et al.* IRF4 addiction in multiple myeloma. *Nature* 2008; 454: 226–31.

NOTES

Mutated BRAF V600E

Sources/clones

Abnova (1 H 12), Millipore (EP152Y), SpringBio (VE1, pBR1), Venatana (VE1).

Fixation/preparation

- Formalin-fixed paraffin-embedded tissues are suitable.
- Deparaffinize slides using xylene or xylene alternative and graded alcohols.
- Suitable for automated slide staining system.

Background

V-raf murine sarcoma viral oncogene homolog B1 (*BRAF*) is a serine/threonine kinase which acts as an effector of ras. It regulates MAPkinase/ERK signaling. The RAF family of proteins includes three isoforms: ARAF, BRAF, and CRAF. While each isoform plays a role in the RAS–RAF pathway, *BRAF* is the main activator of MEK. The BRAF gene protein product plays an important role in regulating the MAP kinase/ERKs signaling pathway, which affects normal cell growth, differentiation, and survival.

Mutations in the *BRAF* gene allow BRAF to signal independently of upstream cues leading to a constitutively active BRAF. Continuous signaling via MEK and ERK will then lead to excessive cell proliferation and survival, independent of growth factors. Oncogenic BRAF signaling may lead to increased and uncontrolled cell proliferation and resistance to apoptosis. *BRAF* mutations are hence implicated in different types of cancers, including hairy cell leukemia, colorectal cancer, malignant melanoma, papillary thyroid carcinoma, and ovarian tumors.

The most common *BRAF* mutation is the V600E mutation, which results in an amino acid substitution at position 600 in the *BRAF* gene, from a valine (V) to a glutamic acid (E). This mutation occurs within the activation segment of the kinase domain. Antibodies directed against mutation V600E have shown excellent correlation with the presence of the mutation.

Applications

The *BRAF* mutation V600E is present in different types of human neoplasm. Most notably, it is seen in hairy cell leukemia, colorectal cancer, malignant melanoma, papillary thyroid carcinoma, and ovarian neoplasms. The *BRAF* V600E mutation is a well-known high-yield target for therapy. Several BRAF inhibitors have been developed and are been used for the treatment of tumors harboring the *BRAF* V600E mutation; the most notable example is the approval of the drug vemurafenib for the treatment of malignant melanoma. The antibodies currently on the market are excellent markers for the presence of the *BRAF* V600E mutation. These antibodies are useful in diminishing the diagnosis time.

Staining pattern

IHC expression in selected neoplasm	IHC staining pattern
Papillary thyroid carcinoma	Granular cytoplasmic
Non-small-cell lung carcinoma	Granular cytoplasmic
Melanoma	Granular cytoplasmic
Colorectal carcinoma	Granular cytoplasmic
Hairy cell leukemia	Granular cytoplasmic

Selected references

Andrulis, M., Penzel, R., Weichert, W., von Deimling, A., Capper, D. Application of a BRAF V600E mutation-specific antibody for the diagnosis of hairy cell leukemia. *American Journal of Surgical Pathology* 2012; 36: 1796–800.

Koperek O, Kornauth C, Capper D, *et al.* Immunohistochemical detection of the BRAF V600E-mutated protein in papillary thyroid carcinoma. *American Journal of Surgical Pathology* 2012; 36: 844–50.

Long GV, Wilmott JS, Capper D, *et al.* Immunohistochemistry is highly sensitive and specific for the detection of V600E BRAF mutation in melanoma. *American Journal of Surgical Pathology* 2013; 37: 61–5.

Preusser M, Capper D, Berghoff AS, *et al.* Expression of BRAF V600E mutant protein in epithelial ovarian tumors. *Applied Immunohistochemistry and Molecular Morphology* 2013; 21: 159–64.

Sinicrope FA, Smyrk, TC, Tougeron D, *et al.* Mutation-specific antibody detects mutant BRAFV600E protein expression in human colon carcinomas. *Cancer* 2013; 119: 2765–70.

Wan PT, Garnett MJ, Roe SM, *et al.* Mechanism of activation of the RAF-ERK signaling pathway by oncogenic mutations of B-RAF. *Cell* 2004; 116: 855–67.

Mutated IDH-1 (mIDH1-R132H, R132S, R132G)

Sources/clones

Dianova: mouse monoclonal (H09)
EMD Millipore: mouse monoclonal (HMab-1), mouse monoclonal R132S (SMab-1)
HistoBioTech: mouse monoclonal (H09)
IBL America: mouse monoclonal (HMab-1), mouse monoclonal R132S (SMab-1)
MBL International: mouse monoclonal (HMab-1), mouse monoclonal R132S (SMab-1), mouse monoclonal R132G (GMab-r1), anti-mutated IDH1/2 (MsMab-2)
Sigma Aldrich: mouse monoclonal (HMab-1)
Takara Bio: mouse monoclonal (HMab-1), mouse monoclonal R132S (SMab-1)
Wako: mouse monoclonal (HMab-1), mouse monoclonal R132S (SMab-1)

Fixation/preparation

All antibodies are proven to be immunoreactive in formalin-fixed paraffin-embedded tissue sections. HIER is required.

Background

Isocitrate dehydrogenase (IDH) is an enzyme involved in the Krebs cycle, with two predominant isoforms, IDH1 (cytoplasmic) and IDH2 (mitochondrial), encoded by the corresponding genes *IDH1* and *IDH2*. These two enzymes normally catalyze isocitrate to α-ketoglutarate, but mutated IDH1/2 acquires a novel enzymatic function that transforms α-ketoglutarate into the oncometabolite 2-hydroxyglutarate. This metabolic change is known to result in genome hypermethylation, histone methylation, and genetic instability.

Mutations in IDH1 were initially identified as one of the first oncogenic mutations in a metabolic enzyme, specifically involved in primary brain tumors of glial origin (gliomas). All mutations occur in amino acid 132, a highly conserved residue in the active enzymatic site. The most common change creates a substitution from an arginine to a histidine, and it is known as R132H. Much less common are other R132 mutations and mutations in *IDH2*, which occur in a similar hotspot, amino acid 172. Subsequently, *IDH1/2* mutations have been identified in other neoplasms, including acute myeloid leukemias, chondroid tumors, and osteosarcoma, and rarely in prostatic adenocarcinoma and cholangiocarcinoma.

Applications

Approximately 70% of diffuse infiltrating gliomas, including astrocytomas and oligodendrogliomas WHO grades II and III, contain the R132H mutation in *IDH1*. In addition, this same mutation is present in approximately 10–15% of WHO grade IV glioblastomas (largely thought to represent so-called secondary glioblastomas), in which the presence of the mutation conveys a more favorable prognosis than its absence.

Mouse monoclonal anti-human antibody mIDH1-R132H was developed to specifically recognize this point mutation in immunohistochemistry, and has demonstrated high sensitivity and specificity when compared with direct sequencing. Monoclonal antibodies specific to other IDH1 mutations as well as IDH2 mutations are available, but given the predominance of R132H they are of limited use in everyday practice.

Comments

Mutated IDH1 immunohistochemistry is useful in the differentiation of low-grade infiltrating astrocytomas from reactive gliotic processes in addition to being recommended in the characterization of diffuse gliomas. Diffuse cytoplasmic staining of tumor cells is the most common finding in positive cases. Red blood cells, foci of necrosis, and areas rich in plasma and fibrin can demonstrate weak non-specific staining.

Selected references

Byers R, Hornick JL, Tholouli E, Kutok J, Rodig SJ. Detection of IDH1 R132H mutation in acute myeloid leukemia by mutation-specific immunohistochemistry. *Applied Immunohistochemistry and Molecular Morphology* 2012; 20: 37–40.

Kato Y. Specific monoclonal antibodies against IDH1/2 mutations as diagnostic tools for gliomas. *Brain Tumor Pathology* 2015; 32: 3–11.

Liu X, Kato Y, Kaneko MK, *et al.* Isocitrate dehydrogenase 2 mutation is a frequent event in osteosarcoma detected by a multi-specific monoclonal antibody MsMab-1. *Cancer Medicine* 2013; 2: 803–14.

Mauzo SH, Lee M, Petros J, *et al.* Immunohistochemical demonstration of isocitrate dehydrogenase 1 (IDH1) mutation in a small subset of prostatic carcinomas. *Applied Immunohistochemistry and Molecular Morphology* 2014; 22: 284–7.

Preusser M, Capper D, Hartmann C; Euro-CNS Research Committee. IDH testing in diagnostic neuropathology: review and practical guideline article invited by the Euro-CNS Research Committee. *Clinical Neuropathology* 2011; 30: 217–30.

Takano S, Tian W, Matsuda M, *et al.* Detection of IDH1 mutation in human gliomas: comparison of immunohistochemistry and sequencing. *Brain Tumor Pathology* 2011; 28: 115–23.

Mycobacterial antigen

Sources/clones

Dako (polyclonal rabbit anti-BCG).

Fixation/preparation

These antibodies are applicable to formalin-fixed paraffin-embedded tissue sections.

Background

The identification of mycobacteria in tissue sections and smears is the most rapid method of detection compared with culture and polymerase chain reaction (PCR). This is underscored by the fact that mycobacterial infections carry a significant morbidity and mortality, emphasizing the need for rapid identification in tissue sections. The yield of acid-fast stains for the detection of mycobacteria may be less than one organism per tissue section, and acid-fast stains require relatively intact organisms with retained capsular integrity.

The polyclonal rabbit anti-BCG (Bacillus Calmette–Guérin) was raised against an attenuated strain used to immunize against *Mycobacterium tuberculosis* infections, containing a substantial number of shared antigens with other mycobacterial species. Hence, this antibody is capable of detecting antigen in debris and fragmented organisms that retain their antigenicity and immunoreactivity. Using immunohistochemistry, it has been demonstrated that fragments and wall components of BCG persist in inoculation sites long after acid-fast stains can no longer detect bacilli. In cases of culture-proven infection in which acid-fast stains were negative, immunoreactivity with anti-BCG showed clumps of mycobacterial debris, cells, and cell fragments in caseating granulomata. In histiocytic granulomata of mycobacterial infections, the cytoplasm of epithelioid cells contained both organisms and debris. Furthermore, this immunostaining reaction was evident at low-power (scanning) magnification.

However, immunohistochemical detection of mycobacterial antigen has a limited utility in cases where many of the organisms are viable and abundant; having no advantage over established procedures (acid-fast stains) in these circumstances.

Applications

Anti-BCG has a role in detecting mycobacterial organisms/antigens in fixed paraffin-embedded sections, especially in cases in which acid-fast stains are negative and a high index of suspicion exists on morphological interpretation. Further, the cross-reactivity of polyclonal anti-BCG with a variety of mycobacterial species allows for the detection of organisms in a wide range of clinical settings. Immunohistochemical staining with the Dako antibody compared to mycobacterial culture is reported to show a sensitivity of 50%, specificity of 75%, positive predictive value of 60%, and negative predictive value of 70%.

Selected reference

Carabias E, Palenque E, Serrano R, *et al.* Evaluation of an immunohistochemical test with polyclonal antibodies raised against mycobacteria used in formalin-fixed tissue compared with mycobacterial specific culture. *APMIS* 1998; 106: 385–8.

NOTES

Myeloperoxidase

Sources/clones

Accurate (CLB-MPO-1/1), Axcel/Accurate (MPO-7, polyclonal), Biodesign (polyclonal), Dako (MPO-7, polyclonal), Research Diagnostics (CLB-MPO-1/1).

Fixation/preparation

May be applied to formalin-fixed paraffin-embedded tissue sections. This antibody may also be used to label acetone-fixed cryostat sections and fixed cell smears. The rabbit polyclonal antibody reacts with myeloperoxidase in a variety of fixatives including Zenker's acetic acid solution, B5 solution, and formalin. Pretreatment with trypsin is essential before immunostaining. HIER does not appear to enhance immunoreactivity but is not deleterious. The monoclonal antibodies do not work on formalin-fixed tissues and should only be used on frozen sections.

Background

Myeloperoxidase is the major constituent of primary granules of myeloid cells. It therefore serves as a reliable marker for myeloid cells, including early (immature) and mature forms. The appearance of myeloperoxidase precedes neutrophil elastase during myeloid cell differentiation. Further, myeloperoxidase antibody does not react with lymphoid or epithelial cells. The myeloperoxidase immunogen was isolated from human granulocytes.

Other immunohistochemical markers for myeloid cells, e.g., lysozyme, CD15, MAC387, and CD68, despite being sensitive, lack specificity in that they also stain histiocytes and other cell types including epithelium. CD43 and CD45RO also stain myeloid cells frequently, but demonstrate T cells and histiocytes as well.

Applications

Immunostaining for myeloperoxidase on paraffin sections is helpful in confirming the myeloid nature of the primitive cells that infiltrate marrow tissue. Positive reaction excludes lymphoblastic leukemia and malignant lymphoma and is therefore crucial for patient management. Skin infiltrates with acute myeloid leukemia, which may be subtle, benefit from the application of antimyeloperoxidase antibody to highlight the neoplastic population.

Granulocytic sarcoma presenting as a tumor mass may occur in isolation or in association with myeloid disorders. In the absence of a history of a hematological malignancy, an erroneous diagnosis of lymphoma may lead to inappropriate treatment being instituted. Hence a high index of suspicion and the use of antibodies (including myeloperoxidase) for the demonstration of the myeloid nature of the cellular proliferation avoids a misdiagnosis. Myeloperoxidase immunostaining is the most sensitive marker for demonstrating neoplastic myeloid cells, being positive in all cases, and in granulocytic sarcoma. Chloroacetate esterase and lysozyme were positive in only 70% and 85% of cases, respectively. Lysozyme may show a strong reaction in some cases of granulocytic sarcoma, complicating acute myelomonocytic leukemia. The advantage of myeloperoxidase is the reduced background staining. Other markers of myeloid cells include CD43, CD15, and histochemical staining for chloroacetate–esterase.

Comments

Anti-myeloperoxidase should be included in the immunohistochemical panel for lymphoma investigation. Any "lymphoma" that cannot be classified with confidence should raise the suspicion of a granulocytic sarcoma. Furthermore, tumor cells marking with only T-cell markers CD43 or CD45RO, but not the specific T-marker CD3, or alternatively that stain only for histiocytic markers such as CD68 or CD15, should raise the alarm for a possible granulocytic sarcoma. Myeloperoxidase is not only specific but by far the most sensitive of the myeloid markers.

Selected references

Mason DY, Taylor CR. The distribution of muramidase (lysozyme) in human tissues. *Journal of Clinical Pathology* 1975; 28: 124–32.

Pinkus GS, Pinkus JL. Myeloperoxidase: a specific marker for myeloid cells in paraffin sections. *Modern Pathology* 1991; 4: 733–41.

MyoD1

Sources/clones
Accurate/Novocastra (5.8A), Dako (5.8A).

Fixation/preparation
Anti-MyoD1 can be used on formalin-fixed paraffin-embedded tissue sections. Deparaffinized tissue sections require heat pretreatment in citrate buffer prior to immunohistochemical staining. Sialinized slides are recommended to improve adherence of tissue sections to glass slides. Ideally, this antibody requires fresh frozen tissue for optimum results.

Background
The differentiation of skeletal muscle at the molecular level requires activation and transcription of genes encoding muscle-specific proteins and enzymes such as desmin and creatine kinase. These activities are controlled by a set of genes including *MyoD1*, *myogenin*, *MYF5* and *MYF6*. It is thought that *MyoD1* activation is an early event that commits the cell to skeletal muscle lineage. Transfection of the *MyoD1* gene into non-muscle cells has been shown to induce conversion of fibroblasts into myoblasts. Similarly, muscle-specific genes in tumor cell lines may be activated by forced expression of exogenously introduced MyoD1. The *MyoD1* gene has been localized to the short arm of chromosome 11. The activation of the *MyoD1* gene, as reflected in the detection of mRNA or protein product, represents a stage of skeletal muscle differentiation that is earlier than that of currently available immunohistochemical markers, such as desmin and myoglobin.

The MyoD1 protein is a 45 kDa nuclear phosphoprotein (5.8A reacts with an epitope between amino acid residues 170 and 209), with nuclear expression restricted to skeletal muscle tissue. Monoclonal anti-MyoD1 strongly stains nuclei of myoblasts in developing skeletal muscle, while the majority of adult skeletal muscle has been found to be negative, including a wide variety of normal tissue. However, weak cytoplasmic staining has been observed in non-muscle tissue, including glandular epithelium.

Applications
MyoD1 nuclear immunostaining has been demonstrated in the majority of rhabdomyosarcomas of various histological subtypes (Appendix 1.27). In fact it has been shown that the MyoD1 expression in rhabdomyosarcomas is inversely related to the degree of cellular differentiation of tumor cells. This phenomenon is useful to distinguish embryonal rhabdomyosarcomas from other small blue round cell tumors of childhood, i.e., Ewing's sarcoma/peripheral primitive neuroectodermal tumor, neuroblastoma, and childhood lymphomas. Wilms tumors and ectomesenchymoma with rhabdomyosarcomatous foci also show nuclear expression of MyoD1 (Appendix 1.3). It has also been shown that the sensitivity and specificity of the MyoD1 antibody in the differential diagnosis of adult pleomorphic soft tissue sarcomas approaches that of pediatric rhabdomyosarcomas. The demonstration of MyoD1 protein in four cases of alveolar soft part sarcoma was initially used as evidence for its rhabdomyosarcomatous differentiation; however, subsequent studies have not confirmed the presence of this regulatory protein in the tumor. Other evidence of myogenic differentiation in alveolar soft part sarcoma include the demonstration of desmin and/or myoglobin.

Comments
A note of caution worthy of mention is that granular cytoplasmic immunoreactivity for MyoD1 has been demonstrated in most neuroblastomas, and in occasional Ewing's sarcomas/PNETs and alveolar soft part sarcomas. Only nuclear staining should be considered as evidence of

skeletal myogenic differentiation, although our own experience has been that nuclear expression occurs in the primitive skeletal tumors, while tumors with cytoplasmic/myogenic differentiation have demonstrated cytoplasmic immunopositivity. The cytoplasmic immunostaining with anti-MyoD1 (clone 5.8A) has been suggested to represent cross-reactivity with an unknown cytoplasmic antigen. Cytoplasmic and nonspecific background staining and reactivity for non-myoid tissues can hinder the practical utility in paraffin-embedded sections. Staining seems to be more consistent in alveolar rhabdomyosarcomas, especially in tumor cells lining fibrous septae and perivascular areas, and embryonal rhabodomyosarcomas showing more variable staining. MyoD1 is generally expressed in small, primitive tumor cells, and larger cells exhibiting morphologic evidence of skeletal muscle differentiation fail to stain for the protein.

With regards to the sensitivity of MyoD1 in fixed tissue, only 35% of rhabdomyosarcomas are positive in paraffin sections, compared to 60% positivity in frozen sections.

Selected references

Cessna MH, Zhou H, Perkins SL, *et al.* Are myogenin and myoD1 expression specific for rhabdomyosarcoma? A study of 150 cases, wioth emphasis on spindle cell mimics. *American Journal of Surgical Pathology* 2001; 25: 1150–7.

Wesche WA, Fletcher CDM, Dias E, *et al.* Immunohistochemistry of MyoD1 in adult pleomorphic soft tissue sarcomas. *American Journal of Surgical Pathology* 1995; 19: 261–9.

Myogenin

Sources/clones

Dako (F5D), Pharmingen (5FD), Santa Cruz (polyclonal).

Fixation/preparation

F5D is immunoreactive in fixed paraffin-embedded tissue sections, and HIER enhances immunoreactivity.

Background

Myogenin belongs to a family of regulatory proteins essential for muscle development. Studies in mice indicate that myogenin is not required for the initial aspects of myogenesis, including myotome formation and the appearance of myoblasts, but late stages of embryogenesis are more dependent on myogenin. Expression levels in fetal skeletal muscle have been found to be 20-fold higher than that of adult rat skeletal muscle. Chickens appear to show the same pattern of myoblast development, with fetal myoblasts expressing both MyoD and myogenin within the first day of culture whereas adult myoblasts are essentially negative for both proteins at the same period of culture and subsequently express first MyoD and myogenin before expressing sarcomeric myosin. Expression of myogenin is restricted to cells of skeletal muscle origin and appears to be inversely related to the degree of cellular differentiation, making it a potentially useful marker for skeletal muscle differentiation in the identification and typing of anaplastic round cell tumors in childhood (Appendix 1.3, 1.11).

Applications

F5D recognizes an epitope located in the amino acid region 138–158 of the myogenin protein and has been found to label nuclei of myoblasts of human fetus, but no reactivity was observed in adult skeletal muscle. The antibody to F5D labels nuclei of the majority of human rhabdomyosarcomas and Wilms tumors. The extent of staining for myogenin has been reported to be inversely related to the degree of cellular differentiation in rhabdomyosarcoma tumor cells. Strong immunostaining for myogenin is significantly associated with tumors of the alveolar subclass of rhabdomyosarcoma. Although all rhabdomyosarcomas show staining for myogenin, the alveolar variant shows the strongest nuclear staining even in cases with subtle alveolar architecture, in which myogenin highlights and enhances visualization of the alveolar pattern. Embryonal rhabdomyosarcomas, in contrast, shows greater variability in staining pattern and intensity. No reactivity has been reported with Ewing's sarcoma/peripheral primitive neuroectodermal tumor, neuroblastoma, adult skeletal muscle tumors, nodular fasciitis, malignant fibrous histiocytoma, malignant peripheral nerve sheath tumor, leiomyosarcoma, or alveolar soft part sarcoma. Focal nuclear staining is rarely seen in desmoid, synovial sarcoma, infantile fibromatosis, and infantile fibrosarcoma. In contrast to myogenin, MyoD1 staining is much less useful in the identification of rhabdomyosarcoma because of cytoplasmic and nonspecific background staining and reactivity of non-myoid tissues (Appendix 1.27).

Comments

Only nuclear staining should be regarded as positive. Clone F5D shows strong reactivity in paraffin sections following HIER. Myogenin has proven to be a better and more sensitive marker of skeletal muscle differentiation in poorly differentiated rhabdomyosarcoma than MyoD1, given that the latter displays nonspecific cross-reactivity with an unknown cytoplasmic antigen in non-muscle cells and tumors. Pleomorphic rhabdomyosarcoma also stain for myogenin. The absence of immunoexpression of myogenin in alveolar soft part sarcoma casts doubts on its alleged skeletal muscle lineage.

Selected reference

Flope AL. MyoD1 and myogenin expression in human neoplasia: a review and update. *Advances in Anatomic Pathology* 2002; 9: 198–203.

Myoglobin

Sources/clones

Accurate (M-2-167, M-3-416), American Research Products (1B4, 1F6, 4G8, 8H5), Axcel/Accurate (polyclonal), Biogenesis (DA2, polyclonal), Biogenex (MG-1, polyclonal), Chemicon (polyclonal), Dako (polyclonal), Sera Lab (polyclonal), Sigma Chemical (MG-1), Zymed (Z001).

Fixation/preparation

Myoglobin is resistant to formalin fixation. Immunoreactivity is not significantly enhanced by proteolytic digestion and is not responsive to HIER.

Background

Myoglobin, a 17.8 kDa protein, is the oxygen carrier hemoprotein, a specific marker for striated muscle cells. It is also present in cardiac muscle. The antibodies do not cross-react with hemoglobin. Cross-reactivity with myoglobins of other mammalian species may occur with some antibodies.

Applications

Anti-myoglobin has been used to indicate early myocardium necrosis and skeletal muscle trauma and necrosis. Myoglobin was one of the earliest markers of striated muscle differentiation, but its expression appears to be linked to the differentiation of rhabdomyosarcoma cells, so that a sizeable number of such tumors, particularly the poorly differentiated ones, exhibit no staining. In our experience, morphologically recognizable rhabdomyoblasts express myoglobin, whereas poorly differentiated tumors fail to stain so that this marker is not helpful when it is actually required. Its application as a marker of early ischemic myocardium appears to be less reliable than cytoskeletal proteins such as vinculin, desmin, and α-actinin. Myoglobin immunostaining has been employed in the study of ragged-red fiber of patients with mitochondrial encephalomyopathy.

Staining for myoglobin can also be performed in renal biopsies of patients with myoglobin-containing casts due to conditions such as necrotizing myopathy or rhabdomyolysis.

Comments

Myoglobin is obviously not a dependable marker of striated muscle differentiation, especially in poorly differentiated rhabdomyosarcoma. Other markers such as desmin, muscle-specific actin, and MyoD1 should be employed for the identification of striated muscle differentiation. The use of myoglobin as a marker of skeletal muscle tumors has been surplanted by myogenin and, to a lesser extent, MyoD1. The protein released from necrotic muscle may be phagocytosed by macrophages, which should not be mistaken for rhabdomyoblasts.

Selected references

Kunishige M, Mitsui T, Akaike M, et al. Localisation and amount of myoglobin and myoglobin mRNA in ragged-red fiber of patients with mitochondrial encephalomyopathy. *Muscle and Nerve* 1996; 19: 175–82.

Zhang JM, Riddick L. Cytoskeleton immunohistochemical study of early ischemic myocardium. *Forensic Science International* 1996; 80: 229–38.

NOTES

Napsin-A

Sources/clones

Abcam (KCG1.1), Novocastra (IP64), Novus Biologicals (Napsin-A, TMU-AD02/6A1), 4B2; Mouse or rabbit monoclonal or polyclonal (IgG).

Fixation/preparation

Formalin-fixed paraffin-embedded tissue, antigen retrieval (+).

Background

Napsin, an aspartic proteinase belonging to the class of endopeptidases, was originally discovered in two isoforms (napsin-A and napsin-B), of which napsin-A was noted to be the functional isoform predominantly found in human kidney and lung. Napsin-A is a 38 kDa single-chain protein. Type II pneumocytes, alveolar macrophages, subset of type I pneumocytes, respiratory epithelium of terminal and respiratory bronchioles, plasma cells, cells of distal convoluted tubule, collecting duct, loop of Henle, and subset of lymphocytes stain positive for this marker immunohistochemically.

Applications

Napsin-A positivity is reported in primary lung adenocarcinomas (80–85%), large cell carcinoma of lung (30%), sarcomatoid carcinoma (20%) sclerosing hemangioma (100%), papillary renal cell carcinoma (79%), clear cell renal cell carcinoma (34%), chromophobe renal cell carcinoma (3%), papillary thyroid carcinoma with tall cell morphology (5%), as well as in anaplastic (15%), poorly differentiated (13%), and micropapillary (100%) pattern thyroid carcinomas. Napsin-A expression has also been reported in clear cell carcinoma of endometrium, as well as in clear cell and endometrioid adenocarcinomas of ovary and metastatic adenoid cystic carcinoma to lung.

Comments

Napsin-A is known to be a good immunostain to differentiate primary lung adenocarcinoma from metastatic adenocarcinoma to lung. Pulmonary adenocarcinoma with enteric differentiation is negative for napsin-A, which is also not a reliable marker to determine the site of origin in mucin-producing adenocarcinomas. Napsin is a specific marker for lung adenocarcinomas and can be used in a panel of immunostains to differentiate from squamous cell carcinoma and other neuroendocrine tumors of lung.

Selected references

Hirano T, Gong Y, Yoshida K, et al. Usefulness of TA02 (napsin A) to distinguish primary lung adenocarcinoma from metastatic lung adenocarcinoma. *Lung Cancer* 2003; 41: 155–62.

Schauer-Vukasinovic V, Bur D, Kling D, Grüninger F, Giller T. Human napsin A: expression, immunochemical detection, and tissue localization. *FEBS Letters* 1999; 462: 135–9.

Suzuki A, Shijubo N, Yamada G, et al. Napsin A is useful to distinguish primary lung adenocarcinoma from adenocarcinomas of other organs. *Pathology, Research and Practice* 2005; 201: 579–86.

NOTES

Neurofilaments

Sources/clones

Neurofilament triplet proteins

Antibodies are available from Accurate (A286), Biogenex (2F11, NF01), Dako (2F11, NR4), Diagnostic, Enzo, EY Labs, Labsystems, Sera Lab (BIO-51H, 2F11).

Neurofilament 70 kDa

Antibodies are available from Accurate, Biodesign (NR4, DP5-1-12), Biogenesis (NF01), Boehringer Mannheim (N52), Calbiochem, Chemicon, Cymbus Bioscience (NR4), Immunotech (DP5-1-12), Novocastra, Oncogene (NR4), Sera Lab (NR4), Serotec (DP5-1-12), Sigma (NR4, N52), Zymed (RMS12).

Neurofilament 150 kDa

Antibodies are available from Accurate (NN18, RNF403), American Research (NF403), Amersham, Biodesign (DP43.16), Biogenesis (BIO-46H, polyclonal), Boehringer Mannheim (BF10, NN18), Chemicon, Cymbus Bioscience (BF10), Immunotech (DP43.16), Medac, Milab (NF403), Novocastra (BF10), Oncogene (NN-18), RDI (BF10), Saxon (403), Sera Lab (NN18), Sigma (NN18), Zymed (RM0270, RM0281, FNP7).

Neurofilament 200 kDa

Antibodies are available from Accurate (N52.1.7), American Research (NF402), Amersham, Biodesign (RT97), Biogenesis (BIO-66H), Boehringer Mannheim (RT97, NE14), Calbiochem, Chemicon, Cymbus Bioscience (RT97), ICN (402), Immunotech (DP12.10), Medac, Milab, Novocastra (RT97), Oncogene (NE-14), Pierce (NE14), RDI (RT97), Saxon (402), Sera Lab (NE 14), Serotec, Sigma (NE14), Zymed (RM024, TA51).

Fixation/preparation

Most antibodies available are immunoreactive in routine processed tissues, but the neurofilament triplet proteins are fixation-dependent and immunostaining is enhanced following HIER.

Background

Neurofilaments (NFs) differ from other intermediate filaments (IFs) in that they are composed of three different subunits of distinct but related proteins of 70, 150, and 200 kDa, whereas other IFs range from 40 to 70 kDa in molecular weight. The antigenic determinants of each of the subunits may be unique or shared, and each NF protein is a separate gene product. NFs are found in neurons and the neuronal processes of the central and peripheral nervous tissue. It is likely that nearly all neurons can constitutively express all three NF genes, and reports of absence of subunits of NF in certain neurons probably reflect technical limitations, as the proteins are fixation-dependent. It is likely that neurofilaments play an important role in the health of the neuron, with evidence that overexpression of NF 200 kDa results in severe neurological disorder while elimination of this IF appears to impart resistance to some neurotoxic agents.

Applications

The antibodies to NFs stain all neurons and axonal processes of the central and peripheral nervous system. The only exception seems to be the olfactory sensory neurons, which contain only vimentin IFs and are unique in that they die and are replenished throughout the lifespan of the mammal. The immunostaining of NF is employed for the study of neuronal distribution and innervation in normal and abnormal tissues, and neuronal differentiation in neoplasms. The detection of NF helps identify neurons and axonal processes in cases of suspected Hirschsprung's disease. NFs are found in a variety of tumors including neuroblastoma, ganglioglioma, medulloblastoma, retinoblastoma, and pineal parenchymal tumors (Appendix 1.7, 1.37), in neuroendocrine and neuroepithelial tumors such as Merkel cell carcinoma, carcinoid, esthesioneuroblastoma, ganglioneuroblastoma, ganglioneuroma, neuroblastoma, oat cell carcinoma, paraganglioma, pheochromocytoma, and in teratomas with neuronal differentiation. NF may also be expressed in primitive/peripheral neuroectodermal tumors (PNETs). Anti-NF is useful in the separation of neuroblastoma and PNET from other small round cell tumors in childhood, which include rhabdomyosarcoma, lymphoblastic leukemia and small-cell osteogenic sarcoma (Appendix 1.3). Immunohistochemical analysis for neural differentiation in Ewing's sarcoma/PNET of bone and soft tissues has shown good concordance with ultrastructural findings.

Comments

As all neurons express all three subunits of NF, antibodies to the triplet protein should be employed in diagnostic workups for intracranial tumors and small round cell tumors in childhood.

Selected reference

Gotow T. Neurofilaments in health and disease. *Medical Electron Microscopy* 2000; 33: 173–99.

Neutrophil elastase

Sources/clones

Axcel/Accurate (MP57), Biogenesis (AHN-10), Calbiochem (polyclonal), Chemicon (AHN-10), Dako (NP57).

Fixation/preparation

NP57 may be used on both formalin-fixed paraffin-embedded sections and frozen sections. If other fixatives are used, e.g., acetone or methanol, there is a tendency for the antigen to diffuse from the myeloid cell cytoplasm and to localize in the cell nucleus.

Background

Neutrophil elastase is a neutral protease, which plays a major role in the killing of microorganisms and in the initiation of tissue injury during inflammatory reactions. The enzyme is present in the primary (azurophilic) granules of myeloid cells. Neutrophil elastase consists of three isoenzymes with similar molecular weights (approximately 30 kDa). Monoclonal anti-neutrophil elastase (NP57) was raised against human neutrophil granule proteins. This antibody labels neutrophils in routinely processed histological specimens and also reacts (although more weakly) with a minor population of normal blood monocytes. Other cell types, including epithelial cells, are NP57-negative.

Applications

75% of neoplastic cells in bone marrow specimens of acute myeloid leukemia were NP57-positive. The number of positive cells varied from few (5–10%) to virtually all. In routinely processed biopsy specimens from lymphoid organs with extramedullary hematopoiesis or infiltrates of chronic myeloid leukemia, NP57 was confined to neutrophils and their precursors. Other studies have demonstrated NP57 positivity in 53% of acute myeloid leukemia and 54% of extramedullary myeloid cell tumors. These percentages appear to be slightly lower than that obtained when staining for myeloperoxidase. This probably indicates that elastase is synthesized later during myeloid maturation than myeloperoxidase. Leukemias of lymphoid origin are not stained.

Comments

The detection of elastase with monoclonal NP57 forms a useful supplement to other immunohistochemical markers for myeloid disorders. However, a study that compared a variety of markers for myeloid precursors in granulocytic sarcoma concluded that CD43, lysozyme, myeloperoxidase, and CD15 were the most sensitive markers staining a large proportion of the cells of the majority of well-differentiated tumors and a smaller proportion of poorly differentiated/blastic tumors. Neutrophil elastase was the least sensitive of the markers of myeloid differentiation, including chloroacetate esterase histochemical staining.

Selected references

Ohlsson K, Olsson I. The neutral proteases of human granulocytes. Isolation and partial characterization of granulocyte elastases. *European Journal of Biochemistry* 1974; 42: 519–27.

Pulford KAF, Erber WN, Crick JA, *et al*. Monoclonal antibody against human neutrophil elastase for the study of normal and leukaemic myeloid cells. *Journal of Clinical Pathology* 1988; 41: 853–60.

NOTES

nm23/*NME1*

Sources/clones

Accurate (NM301), Accurate/Novocastra (37.6), Dako (polyclonal), Novocastra (nm23-301, polyclonal), Oncogene (NM301, polyclonal), Pharmingen (NM301).

Fixation/preparation

Some of the available antibodies are immunoreactive in fixed paraffin-embedded sections. HIER is required.

Background

The nm23 gene family was originally identified in a murine melanoma cell line, and nm23-H1 was found to be transcribed at a 10-fold higher rate in cells of lower metastatic potential. Two highly homologous human genes have subsequently been identified – *nmE1* and *nmE2*, located on chromosomes 17q, and coding for the 18.5 and 17 kDa proteins nm23-H1 and nm23-H2 respectively. nm23 is mainly cytoplasmic, but nuclear and membrane localization has also been seen.

Applications

The nm23 gene product was believed initially to play a role in suppressing tumor metastasis. This may be too simplistic a view, with both metastasis suppression and disease progression being linked to elevated gene expression in different tumors. Isotype-specific studies on breast neoplasms have indicated that it is nm23-H1 and not nm23-H2 that correlates with metastases. A recent report found statistical correlation between nm23-H1 and tenascin immunoexpression, and between nm23-H1 immunoexpression and lymph node metastases. Somatic allelic deletions of nm23-H1 have been reported in some human neoplasms such as breast, kidney, colon, and lung cancer, in some cases associated with an increased incidence of metastases. The loss of nm23 function appears to correlate with phenotypic markers of metastatic potential in some human tumors.

However, there is no strong evidence of direct involvement of nm23 in metastasis, and a bystander effect rather than a causative role for nm23 cannot be ruled out, the reduced nm23 level being a reflection of a more dedifferentiated state of the tumor. nm23 expression correlates inversely with metastatic potential in in-vitro and experimental animal systems, with transfection of the nm23 gene into melanoma K1735 cells resulting in a reduction of tumor metastases.

Initially in esophageal carcinoma there was failure to express p53 and nm23, which may be related to an unfavorable prognosis in patients with advanced esophageal carcinoma. Similarly, there is reduced staining of nm23-H1 in laryngeal squamous cell carcinoma compared with laryngeal polyps. In contrast, progression of ovarian carcinoma is accompanied by overexpression of nm23 protein. While some studies suggest that overexpression of nm23-H1 is an early event in the development of prostatic adenocarcinoma, others show elevated levels of nm23-H1 and H2 in benign prostatic hyperplasia and postulate a role in the suppression of malignancy.

In pituitary adenoma, strong expression of nm23-H2 is associated with noninvasive adenomas, and may restrain tumor aggression. Expression in uveal melanoma appears to be inversely proportional to the depth of scleral invasion. However, in melanoma of the skin there are conflicting studies. Reduced nm23-H1 immunohistological expression has been found to be associated with melanomas that have high metastatic potential and poorer prognosis, but other studies have found that nm23 does not have a direct correlation with metastatic potential.

In transitional cell carcinoma of the bladder and FIGO stage IB cervical carcinoma, nm23 protein immunoreactivity is not an independent prognostic factor. Staining for nm23 has little value in testicular seminoma, where expression of neither nm23-H1 nor nm23-H2 proteins is associated with the metastatic or invasive status of the tumor.

Expression of nm23 protein (and c-ras products) was significantly decreased in complete hydatidiform moles that progressed to gestational trophoblastic tumors compared to those that remitted spontaneously after evacuation. The decreased expression of nm23 protein and increased expression of c-*erb*B-2 protein were strong predictors for the malignant transformation of complete mole. Similar studies have shown nm23 to be a significant factor for predicting a favorable prognosis in non-small-cell carcinoma of the lung, and laryngeal squamous cell carcinoma.

Comments

Polyclonal antiserum to nm23 produces strong cytoplasmic staining after HIER.

Selected references

Graham AN, Maxwell P, Mulholland K, *et al*. Increased nm23 immunoreactivity is associated with selective inhibition of systemic tumour cell dissemination. *Journal of Clinical Pathology* 2002; 55: 184–9.

Urano T, Furukawa K, Shiku H. Expression of nm23/NDP kinase proteins on the cell surface. *Oncogene* 1993; 8: 1371–6.

NUT

Sources/clones

Abcam: rabbit polyclonal
Abnova Corporation: rabbit polyclonal
Atlas Antibodies: rabbit polyclonal
Cell Signaling Technology: rabbit monoclonal (C52B1)
Novus Biologicals: mouse monoclonal (1G6), rabbit polyclonal

Fixation/preparation

These antibodies react with formalin-fixed paraffin-embedded tissue. Heat-mediated antigen retrieval with citrate buffer pH 6 is recommended.

Background

NUT midline carcinoma family member 1, *NUTM1*, previously known as "nuclear protein in testes", was first identified as a novel gene involved in a t(15;19) translocation, characteristic of a highly aggressive carcinoma known as NUT midline carcinoma. In the majority of cases the fusion partner in chromosome 19 is *BRD4*, with *BRD3* and other variants being much less frequent. *NUTM1* is predicted to encode a nuclear protein normally expressed in germ cells of the testes and ovary. The oncogenic mechanism of the fusion protein is associated with chromatin dysregulation, leading to global transcriptional repression and blockade of differentiation.

Applications

Genetically defined by this translocation, NUT midline carcinoma is a rare and extremely aggressive subtype of poorly differentiated squamous cell carcinoma arising in midline structures, most frequently in the mediastinum and head and neck regions. The demonstration of nuclear reactivity to NUT protein in tumor cells with immunohistochemistry is a highly sensitive and specific surrogate marker for the presence of the underlying t(15;19) translocation, and thus determines the diagnosis. Ancillary studies to characterize the fusion oncogene, such as FISH, are not required.

Current recommendations suggest immunohistochemical testing for NUT expression in all poorly differentiated carcinomas without glandular differentiation arising in the chest, head, and neck.

Selected references

Bishop JA, Westra WH. NUT midline carcinomas of the sinonasal tract. *American Journal of Surgical Pathology* 2012; 36: 1216–21.

French CA, Miyoshi I, Kubonishi I, *et al*. BRD4-NUT fusion oncogene: a novel mechanism in aggressive carcinoma. *Cancer Research* 2003; 63: 304–7.

Haack H, Johnson LA, Fry CJ, *et al*. Diagnosis of NUT midline carcinoma using a NUT-specific monoclonal antibody. *American Journal of Surgical Pathology* 2009; 33: 984–91.

Stelow EB, Bellizzi AM, Taneja K, *et al*. NUT rearrangement in undifferentiated carcinomas of the upper aerodigestive tract. *American Journal of Surgical Pathology* 2008; 32: 828–34.

NOTES

OCT2

Sources/clones

Lyca (clone Oct-207, mouse monoclonal IgG 2B).

Fixation/preparation

The antigen is preserved in formalin-fixed paraffin-embedded tissue.

Background

The OCT2 transcription factor is a member of the POU (Pit-Oct-Unc) family of transcription factors. OCT2 derives its name from its ability to bind eight-nucleotide (octamer) recognition sites in the immunoglobulin genes, thus regulating their expression. While OCT2 typically has a positive effect on gene expression of B cells, it has a negative effect on gene expression in neuronal cells, the other major tissue type in which it is expressed. A POU homeodomain is the DNA binding site in OCT2, and it is flanked by two transcriptional activation domains. OCT2 is required for B-cell maturation, and knockout mice die shortly after birth due to an absence of functional B cells.

Applications

In hematolymphoid cell populations, OCT2 should be considered a B-cell-associated antigen rather than a B-cell-specific antigen, as low-level OCT2 expression has been described in benign monocytes/macrophages, and in some non-B-lymphoid neoplasms, including T-lymphoid neoplasms. In normal B-lymphoid cells, OCT2 expression is acquired in immature B lymphoblasts and is uniformly expressed in mature B cells and plasma cells. Because it is a transcription factor, OCT2 immunoreactivity is almost entirely nuclear, although when OCT2 is highly expressed there may be low-level cytoplasmic immunoreactivity.

Perhaps the most common use of OCT2 immunohistochemistry in diagnostic hematopathology is the distinction of classic Hodgkin lymphoma (CHL) from large B-cell non-Hodgkin lymphoma (B-NHL) or nodular lymphocyte-predominant Hodgkin lymphoma (NLPHL). OCT2 expression is retained in the large majority of immature and mature B-lymphoid neoplasms and plasma cell neoplasms, including NLPHL, while the neoplastic cells of CHL either fail to express OCT2 or are only very weakly positive. In the rare CHL cases showing retained OCT2 expression, another major B-cell-associated transcription factor, BOB-1 (see separate chapter in this volume), is invariably negative. A third transcription factor, PU.1, is also absent in virtually all cases of CHL. The singularly high level of OCT2 expression in the LP cells of NLPHL can help distinguish NLPHL from a more aggressive mimic, T-cell/histiocyte-rich large B-cell lymphoma.

A second potential use of OCT2 immunohistochemistry is in the diagnosis of presumed B-NHL in which typical B-lineage markers (e.g., CD19, CD20, CD22, CD79a, and/or PAX-5) are absent or equivocal. In such cases, uniform OCT2 expression can help support the possibility of B-lineage. For example, OCT2 immunohistochemistry can be helpful in plasmablastic lymphomas, including primary effusion lymphomas, which are notorious for loss of B-lymphoid-associated antigens. Importantly, because of the occasional reports of OCT2 expression in large T-cell lymphomas, one should try to find additional evidence of B-lymphoid lineage in such cases, e.g., demonstration of cytoplasmic light chain restriction by immunohistochemistry or flow cytometry, or detection of a clonal immunoglobulin gene rearrangement by PCR.

Selected references

Gibson SE, Dong HY, Advani AS, Hsi ED. Expression of the B cell-associated transcription factors PAX5, OCT-2, and BOB.1 in acute myeloid leukemia: associations with B-cell antigen expression and myelomonocytic maturation. *American Journal of Clinical Pathology* 2006; 126: 916–24.

Marafioti T, Ascani S, Pulford K, *et al*. Expression of B-lymphocyte-associated transcription factors in human T-cell neoplasms. *American Journal of Pathology* 2003; 162: 861–71.

Nasr MR, Rosenthal N, Syrbu S. Expression profiling of transcription factors in B- or T-acute lymphoblastic leukemia/lymphoma and Burkitt lymphoma: usefulness of PAX5 immunostaining as pan-Pre-B-cell marker. *American Journal of Clinical Pathology* 2010; 133: 41–8.

OCT4

Sources/clones

OCT4: Clone POU5F1, Santa Cruz Biotechnology
OCT3/4: Clone C-10, Santa Cruz Biotechnology

Fixation/preparation

Standardized for formalin-fixed paraffin-embedded tissue. Nuclear staining.

Background

OCT4, also known as OCT3 or POU5F1, is a transcription factor that is required for the maintenance of pluripotency of primordial germ cells and embryonic stem cells. OCT4 is downregulated when embryonic stem cells are triggered for differentiation. In-vivo mutagenesis has shown that loss of OCT4 in the blastocyst stage causes the cells of the inner cell mass to differentiate into trophoectoderm cells. An understanding of the role of OCT4, its target genes and dimerization ability, has provided insights into the early steps regulating mammalian embryogenesis. Additionally, OCT4 may also play a role in maintaining the viability of mammalian germline, thus functioning as a "stem-cell survival" factor. OCT4 has been extensively studied for its expression in germ cell tumors from different sites using both polyclonal and monoclonal antibodies directed against the COOH terminus of the protein. In addition to its diagnostic utility in germ cell tumors, OCT4 is associated with prognosis in esophageal squamous cell carcinoma and non-small-cell lung cancers.

Applications

1. **OCT4 in the differential diagnosis of intratubular germ cell neoplasia unclassified (IGCNU)**

   OCT4 expression is seen only in early stages of differentiation, i.e., the gonocyte/PGC stage, with progressive reduction of its immunohistochemical expression in normal spermatogenic cells in the second and third trimesters of fetal development. Only sporadic immunostaining for OCT4 is seen in the late stages of embryonal development. OCT4 therefore has become an extremely useful tool in detecting IGCNU. Strong nuclear staining is seen in 90–100% of atypical cells. The sensitivity of OCT4 in detecting IGCNU is similar to that of PLAP (placental-like alkaline phosphatase) with the added advantage of minimal background and a greater intensity.

   It is important to distinguish IGCNU from reactive germ cells, and from other forms of atypical germ cell proliferations. While IGCNU uniformly progresses to invasive germ cell tumor, the natural history of other forms of atypical proliferations is unknown. This is particularly important in the setting of testicular biopsies of patients who are being worked up for infertility, cryptorchidism, and disorders of sex development.

2. **OCT4 in the differential diagnosis of germ cell tumors (GCTs)**

   The majority of primary testicular tumors are of germ cell origin. Accurate subtyping is critical in determining the treatment strategy. Best practice recommendations by the International Society of Urological Pathology have likened the role of OCT4 to a "gatekeeper" function in the subtyping of testicular germ cell tumors. On the basis of nuclear reactivity for OCT4, GCTs may be divided into two groups: an OCT4+ group (embryonal carcinoma and seminoma) and an OCT4– group comprising yolk sac tumor, spermatocytic seminoma, and choriocarcinoma. In the OCT4+ group, embryonal carcinoma and seminoma can be differentiated by additional staining with CD30, which is positive in 93–100% of embryonal carcinomas.

OCT4 is virtually 100% sensitive for embryonal carcinoma and seminoma. While the majority of other neoplasms of non-testicular origin are negative, rare cases of non-small-cell carcinoma of the lung, clear cell carcinoma of the kidney, and large B-cell lymphomas have been reported to be positive. Rare post-chemotherapy embryonal carcinomas can also be negative.

3. **OCT4 in the differential diagnosis of germ cell tumor and metastatic carcinoma**

   Metastases of high-grade carcinoma to testis, or metastasis from a testicular germ cell tumor – usually embryonal carcinoma, seminoma, or yolk sac tumors – may be diagnostically challenging, especially in the context of a limited biopsy specimen. In such cases a panel including OCT4, SALL4, glypican-3 (GPC3), EMA, and CD30 is helpful. SALL4 and OCT4 positivity with a negative EMA points to a seminoma or embryonal carcinoma; additional positivity for CD30 will suggest embryonal carcinoma.

   SALL4 positivity and OCT4 negativity, with a positive GPC3, negative EMA, and negative CD30, suggests yolk sac tumor.

   SALL4, OCT4, GPC3, and CD30 negativity, with a positive EMA, suggests a high-grade carcinoma.

4. **OCT4 in the differential diagnosis of germ cell tumor and sex cord–stromal tumors**

   Light microscopy is usually sufficient to identify sex cord–stromal tumors without the need to perform an extensive panel of stains. Occasionally Sertoli cell tumors have been described to have a diffuse infiltrative pattern of growth with associated lymphocytes. This pattern may bring seminoma into the differential diagnosis. Some Sertoli cell tumors have been described to have a cord-like growth pattern suggestive of yolk sac tumor. A recommended panel includes SALL4, OCT4, GPC3, α-inhibin, and calretinin.

5. **OCT4 and the differential diagnosis of germ cell tumor and lymphoma**

   Seminoma is most likely to be misinterpreted as a lymphoma. Occasionally it may be hard to distinguish large-cell lymphomas from embryonal carcinomas. An efficient and concise panel for differentiating large-cell lymphoma from GCT should consist of SALL4, CD45, CD20, and CD3. SALL4 positivity will suggest a germ cell tumor. When SALL4 is not available, OCT4, GPC3, AE1/AE3, CD45, CD20, and CD3 can be used. OCT4 positivity suggests embryonal carcinoma or seminoma.

   Tumors negative for SALL4 and OCT4 can be further assessed for lymphoid markers.

6. **OCT4 in the differential diagnosis of choriocarcinoma and seminoma with syncytiotrophoblast cells**

   Rare cases of seminoma may develop syncytiotrophoblast cells with associated microhemorrhages. This combination may raise concern for choriocarcinoma. While seminoma is uniformly positive for OCT4, trophoblastic cells are negative. A positive OCT4 will support a diagnosis of seminoma, while a negative OCT4 will support trophoblastic cells.

Selected references

Cheng L, Sung MT, Cossu-Rocca P, et al. OCT4: biological functions and clinical applications as a marker of germ cell neoplasia. *Journal of Pathology* 2007; 211: 1–9.

de Jong J, Stoop H, Dohle GR, et al. Diagnostic value of OCT3/4 for pre-invasive and invasive testicular germ cell tumours. *Journal of Pathology* 2005; 206: 242–9.

Jones TD, Ulbright TM, Eble JN, Baldridge LA, Cheng L. OCT4 staining in testicular tumors: a sensitive and specific marker for seminoma and embryonal carcinoma. *American Journal of Surgical Pathology* 2004; 28: 935–40.

Jones TD, Ulbright TM, Eble JN, Cheng L. OCT4: a sensitive and specific biomarker for intratubular germ cell neoplasia of the testis. *Clinical Cancer Research* 2004; 10: 8544–7.

Looijenga LH, Stoop H, de Leeuw HP, et al. POU5F1 (OCT3/4) identifies cells with pluripotent potential in human germ cell tumors. *Cancer Research* 2003; 63: 2244–50.

Sung MT, Jones TD, Beck SD, Foster RS, Cheng L. OCT4 is superior to CD30 in the diagnosis of metastatic embryonal carcinomas after chemotherapy. *Human Pathology* 2006; 37: 662–7.

OLIG2 (oligodendrocyte transcription factor 2)

Sources/clones

Biorbyt: mouse monoclonal (1G11, 64), rabbit polyclonal
EMD Millipore: rabbit polyclonal
Life Technologies: rabbit polyclonal
R&D Systems: mouse monoclonal (257224)
Sino Biological: rabbit polyclonal, rabbit monoclonal (064)
Thermo Scientific: mouse monoclonal (1G11), rabbit polyclonal

Fixation/preparation

Most of these antibodies are validated in formalin-fixed paraffin-embedded tissue. Please refer to vendor instructions for specific antigen retrieval requirements.

Background

OLIG2 (oligodendrocyte transcription factor 2) is a member of the basic helix-loop-helix transcription factor family encoded by the gene *OLIG2*, with expression largely restricted to the central nervous system. Normal adult oligodendrocytes demonstrate strong nuclear expression. As a transcription factor, OLIG2 is required for oligodendrocyte and motor neuron differentiation, and appears to be involved in sustaining cellular replication in early development and glioma formation.

Infiltrating gliomas are classified into astrocytomas, oligodendrogliomas, and mixed oligoastrocytomas, based on their histologic similarities with astrocytes, oligodendrocytes, or their progenitors. Occasionally the morphological differentiation is controversial, particularly when considering mixed gliomas. Oligodendroglial neoplasms, however, are known to portend a somewhat better prognosis and response to treatment than astrocytic tumors of the same grade, making the differentiation a relevant issue and prompting the search for lineage differentiation markers.

Initial studies by in-situ hybridization demonstrated that OLIG2 was upregulated in oligodendroglial neoplasms and not in other primary brain tumors, suggesting this protein as a potential specific oligodendroglial marker, while at the same time establishing the definite lineage of oligodendrogliomas as derived from oligodendroglial progenitors. Subsequent work, however, showed that although OLIG2 expression was more common in oligodendrogliomas, it is not restricted to these tumors, since it can also be seen in tumors of astrocytic lineage, including glioblastomas and astrocytomas.

Applications

OLIG2 can be used as a general marker for gliomas, as it is expressed in tumor nuclei in all glioma subtypes including pediatric diffuse infiltrating pontine gliomas, glioneuronal tumors, and pilocytic astrocytoma. Strong expression, however, suggests oligodendroglial differentiation in the right histomorphological setting, and is correlated with the presence of whole arm co-deletion of 1p and 19q, the molecular hallmark and determinant of good prognosis in oligodendrogliomas. In glioblastomas, high expression of OLIG2 may be associated with the proneural molecular subtype.

Selected references

Ligon KL, Alberta JA, Kho AT, *et al.* The oligodendroglial lineage marker OLIG2 is universally expressed in diffuse gliomas. *Journal of Neuropathology and Experimental Neurology* 2004; 63: 499–509.

Marie Y, Sanson M, Mokhtari K, *et al.* OLIG2 as a specific marker of oligodendroglial tumour cells. *Lancet* 2001; 358: 298–300.

Popova SN, Bergqvist M, Dimberg A, *et al*. Subtyping of gliomas of various WHO grades by the application of immunohistochemistry. *Histopathology* 2014; 64: 365–79.

Yokoo H, Nobusawa S, Takebayashi H, *et al*. Anti-human Olig2 antibody as a useful immunohistochemical marker of normal oligodendrocytes and gliomas. *American Journal of Pathology* 2004; 164: 1717–25.

Osteopontin

Sources/clones

National Institute for Dental Research (OPN LF7, rabbit polyclonal antibody), Santa Cruz (OPN (K-20): SC-10591, goat polyclonal antibody).

Fixation/preparation

OPN LF7 is applicable to formalin-fixed paraffin-embedded tissue sections.

Background

Osteopontin (OPN, also designated bone sialoprotein 1, urinary stone protein, spp-1, eta-1, nephropontin, uropontin) is an extracellular matrix cell adhesion phosphoglycoprotein. OPN is produced predominantly by osteoblasts but is also synthesized by brain and kidney cells. OPN is deposited into unmineralized matrix at the cement lines before calcification, and between collagen fibrils of fully matured tissue. OPNs isolated from or secreted by various tissues have molecular weights between 44 and 75 kDa, due to post-translational modifications. OPN exists in multiple forms, such as glycosylated, phosphorylated, and cleaved mature forms of approximately 66–68 kDa molecular weight, suggestive of diverse functions in various tissues.

OPN functions as a substrate for transglutaminase and is involved in cell adhesion. OPN (K-20) is an affinity-purified goat polyclonal antibody raised against a peptide mapping near the carboxyl terminus of osteopontin of human origin.

While OPN was originally extracted from bone extracellular matrix stroma, it has also been detected in normal epithelia of various organs with luminal epithelial surfaces. OPN has been detected in breast, endometrial, and renal adenocarcinomas, where it has been postulated to function in the adhesive interaction of cancer cells with the extracellular matrix, influencing biological behavior. A study of primary ovarian tumors and their metastases from 30 patients demonstrated weak or absent immunoexpression in the majority of ovarian adenocarcinomas and their metastases. In contrast, the majority of borderline ovarian tumors were OPN immunopositive, suggesting a potential importance in the pathogenesis of ovarian BOTs. Lung, gastrointestinal, prostate, bladder, and other human carcinomas do not express OPN. OPN was detected in the cytoplasm of infiltrating leukocytes, granulation tissue cells, fibroblasts, and mast cells in the peritoneum of patients with peritoneal calcification following long-term continuous peritoneal dialysis, and was also found in all calcified vessels in patients with calciphylaxis or calcific uremic arteriopathy.

Applications

OPN currently has no diagnostic applications. It may have a role in the genesis of some cancers, as has been suggested with hepatocellular carcinoma and squamous cell carcinoma of the lung.

Selected references

Brown LF, Papadopoulos-Sergiou A, Berse B, et al. Osteopontin expression and distribution in human carcinomas. *American Journal of Pathology* 1994; 145: 610–23.

Butler WT. The nature and significance of osteopontin. *Connective Tissue Research* 1989; 23: 123–36.

Butler WT. Structural and functional domains of osteopontin. *Annals of the New York Academy of Sciences* 1995; 760: 6–11.

Denhardt T, Guo X. Osteopontin: a protein with diverse functions. *FASEB Journal* 1993; 7: 475–82.

NOTES

p16

Sources/clones

Biogenex (INK4), Santa Cruz (C20), Ventana (E6H4).

Fixation/preparation

Antibody clones are immunoreactive in fixed paraffin-embedded sections.

Background

p16 is a cyclin-dependent kinase-4 inhibitor that is expressed in a limited range of normal tissues and tumors. The major diagnostic applications of p16 immunohistochemistry have been in pathology of the gynecologic tract. p16 overexpression is usually both cytoplasmic and nuclear, although sometimes only cytoplasmic staining is present.

Applications

Infection with high-risk human papillomavirus (HPV) causes inactivation of the retinoblastoma (*RB*) gene by the HPV E7 protein. Normally Rb inhibits transcription of p16, resulting in accumulation of p16 protein. Diffuse p16 positivity in the cervix can be regarded as a surrogate marker of the presence of high-risk HPV infection. In normal cervical squamous epithelium p16 expression is absent or focally positive. In reactive changes and metaplastic lesions, p16 is generally negative whereas in low-grade squamous intraepithelial lesions (CIN1) it can be negative or it can be expressed, usually confined to the lower third of the epithelium. In high-grade squamous intraepithelial lesions (CIN2/3), p16 is expressed strongly and diffusely and can be used to distinguish high-grade CIN from atrophy, immature squamous metaplasia, and transitional metaplasia.

Normal endocervical glands are p16-negative or weakly positive, in contrast with most neoplastic glandular lesions, which exhibit p16 positivity as a result of association with high-risk HPV infection. p16 is useful in distinguishing endocervical adenocarcinoma in situ (AIS) from microglandular hyperplasia, tuboendometrial metaplasia, and endometriosis. The patchy p16 positivity of endometriosis and tuboendometrial metaplasia differs from the diffuse positivity seen in AIS. There are some subtypes of endocervical adenocarcinomas that are not HPV-driven, such as adenoma malignum. However, 30% of adenoma malignum cases can express p16, through a mechanism that does not involve HPV infection.

On small biopsies, distinguishing between tumors of endocervical and endometrial origin can be challenging. In this situation p16 is a useful marker, which will be diffusely positive in endocervical adenocarcinoma and negative or focally positive in endometrial adenocarcinoma. Of note, the benign squamoid elements in the endometrioid adenocarcinomas are usually p16-positive.

Since cervical small-cell carcinoma is also driven by high-risk HPV infection, these tumors will be p16-positive.

In the uterus, a high proportion of serous carcinomas are p16-positive, and most endometrial endometrioid carcinomas are negative or focally positive for p16.

In uterine smooth muscle tumors, gene expression studies have shown p16 expression in uterine leiomyosarcomas. A few studies have shown p16 staining to be diffuse and stronger in leiomyosarcomas when compared to leiomyomas, with no difference in staining pattern between STUMPs and leiomyomas.

In the vulva, p16 may be used to distinguish HPV-associated vulvar intraepithelial neoplasia (VIN) (p16+, usual type VIN) from differentiated VIN which is not associated with HPV infection and is p16-negative.

In the ovary, serous carcinomas appear to express p16 more commonly than other subtypes, and p16 is usually negative in benign and borderline tumors. Cervical metastases to the ovary are known to mimic primary mucinous or endometrioid ovarian carcinomas, and in this instance p16 expression is suggestive of a metastasis from a cervical adenocarcinoma.

Selected references

Ansari-Lari MA, Staebler A, Zaino RJ, Shah KV, Ronnett BM. Distinction of endocervical and endometrial adenocarcinomas: immunohistochemical p16 expression correlated with human papillomavirus (HPV) DNA detection. *American Journal of Surgical Pathology* 2004; 28: 160–7.

Armes JE, Lourie R, De Silva M, *et al.* Abnormalities of the RB1 pathway in ovarian serous papillary carcinoma as determined by overexpression of the p16^{INK4A} protein. *International Journal of Gynecological Pathology* 2005; 24: 363–8.

Bodner-Adler B, Bodner K, Czerwenka K, *et al.* Expression of p16 protein in patients with uterine smooth muscle tumors: an immunohistochemical analysis. *Gynecologic Oncology* 2005; 96: 62–6.

Dray M, Russell P, Dalrymple C, *et al.* p16^{INK4a} as a complementary marker of high-grade intraepithelial lesions of the uterine cervix. I: Experience with squamous lesions in 189 consecutive cervical biopsies. *Pathology* 2005; 37: 112–24.

Kalof AN, Evans MF, Simmons-Arnold L, Beatty BG, Cooper K. p16^{INK4A} immunoexpression and HPV in situ hybridization signal patterns: potential markers of high-grade cervical intraepithelial neoplasia. *American Journal of Surgical Pathology* 2005; 29: 674–9.

Klaes R, Friedrich T, Spitkovsky D, *et al.* Overexpression of p16^{INK4A} as a specific marker for dysplastic and neoplastic epithelial cells of the cervix uteri. *International Journal of Cancer* 2001; 92: 276–84.

Qiao X, Bhuiya TA, Spitzer M. Differentiating high-grade cervical intraepithelial lesion from atrophy in postmenopausal women using Ki-67, cyclin E, and p16 immunohistochemical analysis. *Journal of Lower Genital Tract Disease* 2005; 9: 100–7.

Sano T, Oyama T, Kashiwabara K, Fukuda T, Nakajima T. Expression status of p16 protein is associated with human papillomavirus oncogenic potential in cervical and genital lesions. *American Journal of Pathology* 1998; 153: 1741–8.

p27^{kip1}

Sources/clones

Lab Vision Corp (DCS70), Pharmingen (G173-524), Transduction Laboratory.

Fixation/preparation

The anti-p27 antibody is immunoreactive in fixed paraffin-embedded sections, but only following HIER in citrate buffer at neutral pH.

Background

The p27^{kip1} (p27) gene encodes an inhibitor of cyclin-dependent kinase (CDK) activity. Two families of proteins that generally inhibit cell cycle progression regulate the activity of CDK complexes. These are the INK4 group of p16, p15, p18, and p19, which may have suppressor functions and whose activities are dependent on a normal retinoblastoma protein and show maximal expression during S-phase, and the group of CDK inhibitors that includes p21/WAF1/CIP1, p27^{kip1}, and p57^{kip2}. Overexpression of the latter group inhibits kinase activities of several cyclins and causes cell cycle arrest.

Applications

Several studies have revealed a marked decrease in the percentage of cells expressing p27 in benign and malignant neoplasms compared to normal tissues, with an inverse relationship to Ki-67 antigen, a marker of cell proliferation. Studies with transgenic knockout mice deficient in p27 have shown that p27 protein inhibits proliferation in tissues such as the thymus, pituitary, and spleen, leading to hyperplasias of these organs. The exact role of p27 abnormalities in tumor development remains uncertain. Mutations are relatively uncommon in the p27 gene, and other mechanisms such as translational control with decreased p27 or downregulation of p27 by specific mitogens may occur during tumor development. The observation that p27 levels are markedly decreased in highly malignant tumors such as anaplastic thyroid carcinomas compared with normal thyroid and benign adenomas suggests that loss of p27 expression may be associated with tumor progression.

Evaluation of p27 protein has the potential of predicting the biological behavior of various neoplasms and can be employed to study cell cycle regulation during tumor progression. Data have shown loss or low immunoexpression of p57 with poor prognosis or lymph node metastasis in patients with astrocytoma, cervical carcinoma, rectal carcinoma, papillary thyroid carcinoma, renal cell carcinoma, and gastric carcinoma. The results in breast carcinoma have been conflicting, and describe decreased immunoexpression to be associated with lymph node metastasis in one study in men, and high levels in tumors with nodal metastasis in another study of women. Parodoxical overexpression of p27 has been described in endometrioid adenocarcinoma of the uterus with lymph node metastasis, myometrial invasion, and advanced-stage disease.

Comments

The antibody from Transduction Laboratory, Lexington, KY, is immunoreactive in routine-fixed paraffin-embedded tissues. The antigen is located in the nucleus.

Selected references

Hengst L, Reed SI. Translational control of p27^{kip1} accumulation during the cell cycle. *Science* 1996; 271: 1861–4.

Lloyd RV, Jin L, Qian X, Kulig E. Aberrant p27^{kip1} expression in endocrine and other tumors. *American Journal of Pathology* 1997; 150: 401–7.

Toyoshima H, Hunter T. p27, a novel inhibitor of Gl cyclin-Cdk protein kinase activity is related to p21. *Cell* 1994; 78: 67–74.

p40

Sources/clones

Anti-p40 (1:3000): Calbiochem
BC28: Abcam
Mouse monoclonal, rabbit polyclonal

Fixation/preparation

Formalin-fixed paraffin-embedded tissue, antigen retrieval (+).

Background

DeltaNp63 (p40) is a truncated p63 variant (a member of the *p53* gene family), which was originally found to label keratinocytes as well as kidney/adrenal, spleen, and thymus; but not heart, testis, brain, or liver. DeltaNp63 was also noted to be an inhibitor of p53.

Applications

Antibody p40 was noted to label normal thymic cortical and medullary epithelial cells and thymomas, normal placentas, hydatidiform moles, invasive moles, choriocarcinoma and epithelial trophoblastic tumors (but not placental site trophoblastic tumors), lung squamous cell carcinomas, preinvasive and invasive esophageal squamous cell carcinomas, urothelial carcinomas, adamantinoma-like Ewing family tumors of soft tissue, craniopharyngioma, esthesioneuroblastoma, sinonasal undifferentiated carcinomas, adenoid cystic carcinomas, pleomorphic adenomas, mucoepidermoid carcinoma, NUT midline carcinomas, small-cell carcinomas of sinonasal tract and primitive neuroectodermal tumors, cutaneous squamous cell carcinoma, myoepithelial cells in breast diseases, sclerosing hemangioma of lung, malignant phyllodes tumor, sarcomatoid carcinoma.

Comments

It is a specific marker for squamous differentiation. In lung cancer, p40 is a useful immunostain to differentiate squamous cell carcinoma from adenocarcinoma as well as from small-cell carcinoma.

Selected references

Alomari AK, Glusac EJ, McNiff JM. p40 is a more specific marker than p63 for cutaneous poorly differentiated squamous cell carcinoma. *Journal of Cutaneous Pathology* 2014; 41: 839–45.

Bishop JA, Teruya-Feldstein J, Westra WH, et al. p40 (Δ Np63) is superior to p63 for the diagnosis of pulmonary squamous cell carcinoma. *Modern Pathology* 2012; 25: 405–15.

Geddert H, Kiel S, Heep HJ, Gabbert HE, Sarbia M. The role of p63 and deltaNp63 (p40) protein expression and gene amplification in esophageal carcinogenesis. *Human Pathology* 2003; 34: 850–6.

Kim SK, Jung WH, Koo JS. p40 (Δ Np63) expression in breast disease and its correlation with p63 immunohistochemistry. *International Journal of Clinical and Experimental Pathology* 2014; 7: 1032–41.

Righi L, Graziano P, Fornari A, et al. Immunohistochemical subtyping of nonsmall cell lung cancer not otherwise specified in fine-needle aspiration cytology: a retrospective study of 103 cases with surgical correlation. *Cancer* 2011; 117: 3416–23.

Tilson MP, Bishop JA. Utility of p40 in the differential diagnosis of small round blue cell tumors of the sinonasal tract. *Head and Neck Pathology* 2014; 8: 141–5.

Zhang HJ, Xue WC, Siu MK, et al. P63 expression in gestational trophoblastic disease: correlation with proliferation and apoptotic dynamics. *International Journal of Gynecological Pathology* 2009; 28: 172–8.

NOTES

p53

Sources/clones

Antibodies to both wild-type and mutant p53 are available from Accurate, Biodesign (Pab1801, 53-12), Bioprobe (BP53-12), BioSource, Chemicon, Cymbus Bioscience, Dako (DO-7), Immunotech, Medac (CM-1), Novocastra, Oncogene (Pab1801, Pab421, Pab122), Oncor, Pharmingen (G59-12), Serotec (Pab1801, BP53-12), and Signet.

Antibodies to mutant p53

Biogenesis, Chemicon, Oncogene (Pab240).

Antibodies to wild-type p53

Biodesign (Pab246), Oncogene (Pab1620), Serotec (Pab246).

Fixation/preparation

Fresh or frozen tissues; clones Pab1801 and DO-7 effective in formalin-fixed tissue and with best results following microwave epitope retrieval.

Background

In the current constellation of oncogenes and recessive tumor suppressor genes, the p53 molecule represents one of the most common genetic changes associated with human cancer, being implicated in a wide range of malignancies. The *p53* gene displays several unusual features, the most important of which is the ability to act as either a dominant oncogene or a recessive tumor suppressor gene. A combination of genetic events that affect both alleles of the gene results in the loss of expression of wild-type (WT) *p53*. This may occur as a complete loss of one allele of the gene as a result of a large chromosomal deletion combined with a point missense mutation on the other allele. Mutation leads to the loss of DNA binding and transcriptional regulatory activities of the p53 phosphoprotein with a corresponding loss of its growth suppressive activity and its role as "the guardian of the genome." The mutated protein has abnormal conformation, impaired DNA binding, and a prolonged or stabilized half-life, the last of which results in immunohistochemically stainable levels within nuclei in nearly all tumors showing *p53* gene mutation. While a loss of transformation-suppression activity and a gain of transforming potential often accompany mutation of *p53*, not all p53 mutants are equal in terms of their biological activity. Mutations at different hotspots manifest different and distinct phenotypes, and there is geographic variation in the sites of mutations thought to reflect the effects of different environmental and regional carcinogens and cofactors.

The *p53* gene is located on the short arm of human chromosome 17, and the majority of mutations in the gene are clustered in the most highly conserved domains spanned by 4–9 axons. An important relationship exists between DNA damage hotspots and the capacity to repair the DNA, as mutation abolishes the arrest or delay seen in the normal cellular response to DNA damage. Although the WT *p53* gene product is not essential for progress of cells through the cell cycle, it does negatively regulate cell growth or division. By binding to specific DNA sequences, the p53 WT product is able to inhibit adjacent gene transcription and serves to prevent uncontrolled cellular proliferation. Thus loss of WT p53 activity induces a release from G_1–S cell cycle checkpoint control following DNA damage, increasing genomic instability and promoting gene amplification. Binding of WT p53 to a variety of viral proteins such as protein E6, a product of the human papillomavirus, simian virus 40T antigen, and the Epstein–Barr nuclear antigen, as well as to cellular proteins such as heat shock protein 70 and MDM-2 replication protein, may result in an inactivated complex and a loss of transformation suppression activity.

Applications

Immunohistochemical detection of nuclear p53 protein is based on the increase in concentration of the protein to detectable levels, secondary to an increased synthesis and a lower degradation with longer half-life. In general, there is good agreement between the frequency of positive immunostaining and the frequency of tumors with mutations detected by direct DNA sequencing. However, there are discrepancies between these findings and analysis at the protein level. There is also a danger in assuming positive staining to be an indication of an underlying mutation, as p53 protein can be stabilized by other means such as sequestration of normal nuclear protein in the cytoplasm with inactivation of its tumor suppressor function or by binding with the cellular proteins previously mentioned. Also, the use of anti-p53 antibodies that do not react with all mutant forms and other events may lead to failure to detect p53 in neoplasms. The analysis of p53 in neoplastic and pre-neoplastic states is a powerful tool which provides molecular information on the oncogenic process, and the ability to stain for abnormal forms of the protein in tissue sections, particularly those fixed in formalin, allows an important avenue of investigation. Furthermore, there is evidence to suggest that the expression of abnormal p53 may be a prognostic parameter in phyllodes tumor of the breast, high-risk breast cancer patients undergoing high-dose chemotherapy, and thyroid neoplasms.

Comments

Immunostaining of p53 can be affected by degradation of antigen during tissue processing, and it is important to recognize the fixation conditions and the nature of the antibody employed. Monoclonal antibody Pab1801 (Biogenesis, Medac) recognizes most of the mutant and wild-types of p53, but 1801 is not suitable for paraffin-embedded tissues. Our own experience is largely with DO-7 (Medac, Dako) which identifies both wild-type and mutant protein in formalin-fixed paraffin-embedded sections and best results are obtained after microwave epitope retrieval.

Selected references

Batsakis JG, El-Naggar AK. p53: 15 years after discovery. *Advances in Anatomic Pathology* 1995; 2: 71–88.

Chang F, Syrjanen S, Tervahauta A, Syrjanen K. Tumorigenesis associated with the p53 tumour suppressor gene. *British Journal of Cancer* 1993; 68: 653–61.

p63

Sources/clones

Dak-p63: Dako
4A4: Biocare, Dako, Santa Cruz, Zeta Corporation
7JUL: Leica/Novocastra

Fixation/preparation

Formalin-fixed paraffin-embedded (FFPE) tissues are suitable. Antigen retrieval is critical. Suitable for automated slide staining.

Background

The *p63* gene (chromosome 3q27-19) is part of the p53 tumor suppressor family and has structural similarity to both p53 and p73. During embryogenesis, it is responsible for epithelial development. Germline mutations lead to cleft lip and palate syndrome, ectrodactyly, ectodermal dysplasia, and limb–mammary syndrome – a group of disorders resulting in variable ectodermal abnormalities.

p63 expression is nuclear in location and seen in normal squamous epithelium including that of skin, esophagus, uterine ectocervix, tonsil, bladder, or other sites that exhibit squamous metaplasia. p63 is expressed in basal epithelial and/or myoepithelial cells of several organs including breast, skin, uterine cervix, urogenital tract, and prostate. It is also expressed in thymic epithelial cells and cytotrophoblastic cells.

Applications

Useful for identification of squamous carcinomas, urothelial carcinoma, a proportion of anaplastic large-cell lymphoma, mucoepidermoid carcinoma, adenoid cystic carcinoma, metaplastic carcinoma of the breast, sarcomatoid carcinoma, giant cell tumor of bone. Key applications in daily practice include the identification of squamous differentiation, baso-myoepithelial cells in the breast (DCIS vs. invasive carcinoma) and prostate (atypical glands vs. invasive carcinoma).

Cytoplasmic p63 staining has been reported in tumors with skeletal muscle differentiation.

Selected references

Di Como CJ, Urist MJ, Babayan I, *et al.* p63 expression profiles in human normal and tumor tissues. *Clinical Cancer Research* 2002; 8: 494–501.

Martin SE, Temm CJ, Goheen MP, *et al.* Cytoplasmic p63 immunohistochemistry is a useful marker for muscle differentiation: an immunohistochemical and immunoelectron microscopic study. *Modern Pathology* 2011; 24: 1320–6.

Weinstein MH, Signoretti S, Loda M. Diagnostic utility of immunohistochemical staining for p63, a sensitive marker of prostatic basal cells. *Modern Pathology* 2002; 15: 1302–8.

NOTES

Pancreatic hormones: insulin, somatostatin, vasoactive intestinal polypeptide, gastrin, glucagon, pancreatic polypeptide

Pancreatic endocrine tumors have been associated with several distinct clinical syndromes, such as hypoglycemia, glucagonoma syndrome, Zollinger–Ellison syndrome, and WDHA (watery diarrhea, hypokalemia, and achlorhydria) syndrome. Routine histological examination usually fails to predict the behavior and endocrine manifestations of these neoplasms. Immunohistochemistry permits the specific demonstration of various pancreatic hormones in tissue sections.

Sources/clones

Insulin

Accurate (K36AC10), Axcel/Accurate (polyclonal), Biodesign (MAb1, E2-E3, polyclonal), Biogenesis (E6E5, D4B8, IN05, C7C9, polyclonal), Biogenex (AE9D6, polyclonal), Caltag Laboratories (polyclonal), Cymbus Bioscience (Mab1), Dako (polyclonal), EY Labs, Fitzgerald (M91284, M91285, M322212, M322213, polyclonal), Immunotech (E2E3), Novocastra (polyclonal), Research Diagnostics (Mab1), Sanbio/Monosan (N-05, polyclonal), Sigma Chemical (K36AC10), Zymed (Z005, Z006, polyclonal).

Somatostatin

Accurate (YC7, BM17), Axcel/Accurate (polyclonal), Biogenesis (170.3, polyclonal), Biogenex (polyclonal), Caltag Laboratories (polyclonal), Dako (polyclonal), Fitzgerald (polyclonal), Novocastra (polyclonal), Pharmingen (YC7), Sanbio/Monosan (polyclonal), Zymed (polyclonal).

Vasoactive intestinal polypeptide (VIP)

Accurate, Biodesign (polyclonal), Biogenesis (VIP-001), Biogenex (polyclonal), Immunotech (103.10), Serotec, Zymed (polyclonal).

Gastrin

Axcel/Accurate (polyclonal), Biodesign (polyclonal), Biogenesis (polyclonal), Biogenex (polyclonal), Caltag Laboratories (polyclonal), Dako (polyclonal), Fitzgerald (M28046, M28047, polyclonal), Immunotech (4C7A1), Novocastra, Sanbio/Monosan (polyclonal), Zymed (polyclonal).

Glucagon

Accurate/Sigma Chemical (K79bB10), Axcel/Accurate (polyclonal), Biodesign (polyclonal), Biogenesis (polyclonal), Biogenex (polyclonal), Caltag Laboratories (polyclonal), Dako (polyclonal), Fitzgerald (polyclonal), Immunotech (polyclonal), Sanbio/Monosan (polyclonal), Zymed (polyclonal).

Pancreatic polypeptide (PP)

Axcel/Accurate (polyclonal), Becton Dickinson, Biodesign (polyclonal), Biogenesis (polyclonal), Biogenex (polyclonal), Dako (polyclonal), Eli Lilly (polyclonal), Zymed (polyclonal).

Fixation/preparation

These antibodies are applicable to formalin-fixed paraffin-embedded tissue as well as frozen sections. No pretreatment or antigen unmasking is necessary for any of the antibodies.

Background

The antigens used as immunogens to raise rabbit antibodies against the pancreatic hormones were as follows: insulin – porcine pancreatic insulin; somatostatin – synthetic peptide somatostatin-14; VIP – natural porcine VIP, conjugated to glutaraldehyde as carrier protein; gastrin – synthetic human gastrin-17 non-sulfated form conjugated to bovine serum albumin; glucagon – porcine glucagon.

Although there are at least eight different cell types identified in the pancreatic islets, only the resident four major cell types (A, B, D, and PP cells) and G and VIP cells (in neoplastic conditions) will be considered here. In the normal adult islet, insulin-containing B cells account for 60–80% of endocrine cells and occupy the central portion of the islets. Glucagon-containing A cells constitute 20–30%, and somatostatin-containing D cells 5–11%. A and D cells are mostly present in the periphery of the islets and are also scattered within the islets along capillaries. Physiologically, glucagon increases hepatic glucose production and opposes hepatic glucose storage; insulin increases peripheral glucose uptake and opposes glucagon-mediated hepatic glucose production. Hence, the delicate balance of these two hormones maintains blood glucose homeostasis. Somatostatin has inhibitory actions on both A and B cells through a "paracrine" effect, thereby regulating the balance of A- and B-cell functions. PP cells are the least numerous and are present both within and outside the islets. The function of pancreatic polypeptide is not fully understood. PP cells have a variable distribution in the pancreas, with PP-cell-rich islets being occasionally present in the posterior lobe of the pancreatic head. Hence, caution should be exercised when evaluating hyperplastic changes of PP cells.

Although the presence of gastrin in D-cells has been disputed, studies indicate that gastrin is not present in normal adult islets. VIP has been localized in human islets, but the exact cellular origin is not fully understood. In the rat, diabetes mellitus induced by streptozotocin resulted in a reduction of the number of insulin-positive cells in the islet of Langerhans while that of VIP and neuropeptide-Y increased significantly after the onset of diabetes. Both these hormones evoked large and significant increases in insulin release from pancreatic tissue fragments of normal rats.

In the gastroduodenal segment, gastrin has been immunolocalized to the G cells of the gastric antrum, while somatostatin has been found in endocrine cells and nerves of the intestinal wall digestive mucosa.

Applications

Endocrine tumors of the gastrointestinal tract and pancreas may demonstrate a wide variety of histomorphological patterns: (1) solid (nodular solid nests with peripheral invading cords), (2) solid and glandular (with focal glandular formation), (3) gyriform (trabecular or ribbon-like structures forming anastomosing pattern), and (4) glandular (tubular or acinar structures). With the availability of antibodies to the secretory products, specific designation of these neoplasms has led to terms such as insulinoma, glucagonoma, gastrinoma, somatostatinoma, and VIPoma. However, small tumors found incidentally at autopsy may be clinically silent and do not necessarily cause clinical symptoms. Further, many pancreatic endocrine tumors are multihormonal. Hence, the designation of pancreatic endocrine tumor followed by the description of the hormone(s) demonstrated in situ (e.g., insulin-producing) whenever this can be ascertained is the preferred terminology. Pancreatic endocrine tumors that do not cause clinically apparent endocrine syndromes are usually labeled as nonfunctioning tumors. However, with the acceptance of hormone production as a sign of function, the number of nonfunctioning tumors decreases with application of immunohistochemical staining procedures using antibodies to specific hormones.

In general, most insulin-producing tumors associated with hypoglycemia are benign. Conversely, endocrinologically active gastrin-producing tumors, glucagon-producing tumors, VIP-producing tumors, and somatostatin-producing tumors are often malignant. However, there are no definite morphologic criteria to predict hormonal activity or behavior. Metastasis is the only sign of malignancy. Therefore, all pancreatic endocrine tumors should be regarded as potentially malignant, even though metastasis may not be apparent at the time of initial surgery.

The common clinical syndromes and their causative hormones are as follows: hypoglycemia (insulin), Zollinger–Ellison syndrome (gastrin), glucagonoma syndrome (glucagon), WDHA syndrome (Verner–Morrison syndrome) (vasoactive intestinal pancreatic polypeptide), and somatostatinoma syndrome (somatostatin). The first two syndromes are relatively frequent, but the remaining three are either infrequent or rare. Occasionally, pancreatic endocrine tumors fail to demonstrate immunoreaction in the presence of clinical syndromes. Explanations for this aberrant phenomenon include abnormal (although biologically active) peptides that may not react with specific anti-hormone antibodies, fixation artifact, or alternatively rapid turnover in tumor cells resulting in only minute amounts being stored.

Tumors from some patients with WDHA syndrome have been found to secrete PP. PP also appears to be the most commonly found hormone in silent/nonfunctioning tumors. While the physiologic function of PP is not yet fully understood, PP cells are nevertheless a component often demonstrated in multihormonal tumors. The frequency of multihormone production by islet cell tumors has been stated to be as high as 50%. These tumors usually cause only one clinical syndrome, and a combination of syndromes is extremely rare. In fact, the predominant cell type in a tumor does not necessarily cause the corresponding syndrome. Any combination of cell types is possible in pancreatic endocrine tumors, the most striking example being the high frequency of PP cells in tumors secreting VIP and causing the WDHA syndrome. The most likely explanation for the common presence of several cell types in pancreatic endocrine tumors is that they derive from a multipotential stem cell that may differentiate in various directions.

Antibodies to pancreatic hormones may also be applied to the diagnosis of islet cell hyperplasia seen in the non-neoplastic pancreas of patients with islet cell tumors and primary G-cell hyperplasia (gastrin-producing) in the antrum of the stomach. The latter is clinically indistinguishable from Zollinger–Ellison syndrome due to gastrinoma. The demonstration of an increase in number and size of the p-cell mass in the ductuloinsular complexes in neonatal hyperinsulinemic hypoglycemia is another application of pancreatic hormone immunohistochemistry. An immunohistochemical study of 100 pancreatic tumors in 28 patients with multiple endocrine neoplasia type I demonstrated a predominant hormonal secretion in 83 tumors (with 50–90% of the same cell type), including 37 glucagon, 27 insulin, 11 PP, 1 gastrin, and 1 VIP cell tumors.

Duodenal (periampullary) somatostatin-rich carcinoid tumors (psammomatous somatostatinoma) need to be distinguished from adenocarcinoma, because the prognosis is better in the former even though lymph node metastases may occur with carcinoids. Other neuroendocrine tumors of the duodenum that require immunohistochemistry for their recognition include gastrinomas (most common), gangliocytic paraganglioma, serotonin-/calcitonin-/ pancreatic polypeptide-producing tumors, and poorly differentiated neuroendocrine carcinomas. A characteristic feature of MEN-associated gastrinoma is their frequent multicentricity.

Gastrointestinal carcinoid tumors have also benefited from the development of immunohistochemical technology: gastrin, VIP, PP, and glucagon have been demonstrated in cases of carcinoid syndrome. In children, WDHA syndromes have been reported in association with VIP-secreting ganglioneuromas and ganglioneuroblastomas. Two-thirds of the ampullary tumors expressed somatostatin, while over half of the duodenal carcinoid tumors expressed gastrin. Another study also confirmed the gastrin expression in duodenal carcinoids (75% immunopositive), with only 20% of ampullary carcinoids expressing gastrin. Somatostatin, pancreatic polypeptide, and gastrin have also been demonstrated in carcinoid tumors of the extrahepatic bile ducts, albeit in less than a third of cases.

Increased neuroproliferation in the appendix is associated with an increase in VIP, substance P, and growth-associated protein-43 in adults with acute right lower quadrant abdominal pain. It has also been demonstrated in children by immunostaining. Increased neuroproliferation was demonstrated in the appendiceal lamina propria and muscularis of children who presented with abdominal pain compared with appendices removed incidentally. The VIP immunoexpression in these children was higher or similar to those appendices that showed histological inflammatory changes.

Comments

Immunohistochemistry has contributed extensively to the understanding of the morphofunctional relationship of pancreatic (and related) endocrine tumors. Apart from the cellular localization of secretory products in these tumors, prediction of biological behavior has also been possible. Positive control tissue for this panel of pancreatic hormones includes normal pancreas (insulin, glucagon, somatostatin, and PP), gastric antrum (gastrin), and colon (VIP).

Selected reference

Bouchard S, Russo P, Radu AP, Adzick NS. Expression of neuropeptides in normal and abnormal appendices. *Journal of Pediatric Surgery* 2001; 36: 1222–6.

NOTES

Parafibromin (CDC73)

Sources/clones

Abbiotec (rabbit polyclonal), Abcam (rabbit polyclonal), Antibodies-online (rabbit polyclonal), Aviva Systems Biology (rabbit polyclonal), Bethyl Laboratories (rabbit polyclonal), Biorbyt (rabbit polyclonal), Bioss Inc (rabbit polyclonal), Creative Biomart (rabbit polyclonal), GeneTex (rabbit polyclonal N1C1), LifeSpan BioSciences (rabbit polyclonal), NovaTeIn Bio (rabbit polyclonal), ProteinTech Group (rabbit polyclonal), Santa Cruz Biotechnology (mouse monoclonal (2H1)), Thermo Scientific (rabbit polyclonal), United States Biological (rabbit polyclonal).

Fixation/preparation

Most of these antibodies react in formalin-fixed paraffin-embedded tissue. Please refer to vendor instructions for specific antigen retrieval requirements.

Background

Parafibromin is a nuclear protein encoded by the endocrine tumor suppressor gene *CDC73* (cell division cycle 73). The protein is part of the PAF complex, which associates with the RNA polymerase II subunit POLR2A, crucial for histone modification. It is thus involved in transcriptional and likely post-transcriptional control pathways and may be involved in cell cycle progression through the regulation of cyclin D1/*PRAD1* expression. Germline inactivating mutations in this gene are responsible for isolated familial hyperparathyroidism and hyperparathyroidism with jaw tumor syndrome (HPT-JT), which is associated with parathyroid carcinoma in approximately 15% of cases.

Applications

Parathyroid carcinoma is a rare malignancy, accounting for less than 1% of all cases of primary hyperparathyroidism. Clinically, the diagnosis is determined by the presence of local invasion, which frequently creates difficulty in surgical resection, and distant metastasis. Histological features can be quite similar to those seen in parathyroid adenomas, making the morphological diagnosis of parathyroid carcinoma a particularly challenging endeavor. Histologically, a definitive diagnosis of malignancy should be considered in cases with unequivocal extratumoral vascular invasion, capsular invasion with growth into adjacent tissues beyond the gland, or distant metastases.

In addition to parathyroid carcinomas arising in hereditary syndromes, sporadic parathyroid carcinomas also display mutations in *CDC73* leading to loss of parafibromin. In fact, most parathyroid carcinomas will exhibit loss of parafibromin proven by immunohistochemistry. Therefore, staining can be useful in cases of histologically atypical parathyroid adenomas (i.e., with fibrous bands, increased mitotic activity and prominent nuclear atypia), in which loss of parafibromin is associated with worse clinical behavior, despite absence of definitive criteria for malignancy.

Selected reference

Cetani F, Banti C, Pardi E, *et al.* CDC73 mutational status and loss of parafibromin in the outcome of parathyroid cancer. *Endocrine Connections* 2013; 2: 186–95.

NOTES

Parathyroid hormone

Sources/clones

Binding Site (polyclonal), Biodesign (polyclonal), Biogenesis (polyclonal), Biogenex (polyclonal), Dako (polyclonal), Fitzgerald (polyclonal), Novocastra (polyclonal).

Fixation/preparation

This antibody is applicable to formalin-fixed paraffin-embedded tissue, frozen sections, and cytologic preparations. Although not always required, enzyme pretreatment before immunodetection may improve results on paraffin-embedded sections.

Background

The parathormone gene, closely linked to that of β-globin, is located on the short arm of chromosome 11 in humans (as are the genes for calcitonin and insulin). The initial form in which parathormone is synthesized within the cell is a single-chain polypeptide of 115 amino acid residues, preproparathyroid hormone. This is cleaved within the cell to form a proparathyroid hormone, from which a further 6 amino acids are split, leaving the 84-amino acid chain of parathormone. The rate of parathormone secretion is directly responsive to the level of calcium in the serum, and indeed the cytoplasm, of parathyroid cells, as has been shown by studies both in vivo and in vitro. In-vitro studies of osteoclast turnover suggest that both PTH and PTH-related protein exert both pro- and anti-apoptotic effects in mesenchymal cells.

Applications

Surgical pathologists are familiar with the ability of parathyroid proliferations to assume a variety of histological guises, making it difficult to categorize any given lesion as hyperplastic, adenomatous, or carcinomatous in nature. This is usually resolved with the macroscopic appearance of the remaining parathyroid glands as assessed by the surgeon. The role of the surgical pathologist is to identify the lesion as parathyroid in nature and to assess whether it is normocellular or hypercellular. Although this is easily accomplished in the majority of instances, rare examples of parathyroid hyperplasia/adenoma showing a follicular/trabecular arrangement may cause concern over the alternative diagnosis of a thyroid adenoma. This becomes more pertinent when the parathyroid lesion abuts into the thyroid gland or lies within the thyroid capsule. Immunodetection for thyroglobulin and parathyroid hormone (PTH) is especially useful to resolve the problem. Nevertheless, caution should be exercised, since parathyroid cells often discharge their hormonal product almost as soon as it is packaged in the cytoplasm, resulting in false-negative PTH immunostaining, although the cells are biologically synthetic.

PTH antibody is also useful to distinguish cell parathyroid hyperplasia/neoplasms from thyroid and metastatic neoplasms, although the pathologist is typically aware of the preoperative hypercalcemic status. Occasionally, when the surgeon does not supply this information, PTH immunohistochemistry is essential. Even more problematic are situations in which clear cell parathyroid carcinomas are non-secretory, without an abnormality in mineral metabolism. In such situations, metastatic renal cell carcinoma or metastatic clear cell carcinoma of the lung is evident, warranting PTH immunohistochemistry to arrive at the correct diagnosis. The other instance in which PTH antibodies are useful is in the consideration of parathyroid carcinomas located primarily in the anterior mediastinum (intrathymically). In this situation distinction from primary thymic metastatic carcinomas, non-Hodgkin lymphoma, and germ cell tumors is necessary.

Comments

The diagnosis of the majority of parathyroid proliferations may be accomplished with an adequate history, biochemistry profile, and histomorphological assessment. However, rare instances in which the tumors have an abnormal location or clear cell morphology, or where they are non-secretory, may result in erroneous diagnoses, warranting PTH immunohistochemistry. Normal parathyroid glands are adequate for positive control tissue.

Selected references

Aldinger KA, Hickey RC, Ibanez ML, Samaan NA. Parathyroid carcinoma: a clinical study of seven cases of functioning and two cases of nonfunctioning parathyroid cancer. *Cancer* 1982; 49: 388–97.

Brown EM. PTH secretion in vivo and in vitro: regulation by calcium and other secretagogues. *Mineral and Electrolyte Metabolism* 1982; 8: 130–50.

Chen HL, Demiralp B, Schneider A, *et al.* Parathyroid hormone and parathyroid hormone-related protein exert both pro- and anti-apoptotic effects in mesenchymal cells. *Journal of Biological Chemistry* 2002; 277: 19, 374–81.

Parathyroid hormone-related protein (PTHrP)

Sources/clones

Biogenesis (polyclonal), Calbiochem (212-10.7), Fitzgerald (polyclonal).

Fixation/preparation

Applicable to both frozen sections and formalin-fixed paraffin-embedded tissue sections.

Background

Humoral hypercalcemia of malignancy (HHM) is a syndrome characterized by low levels of parathyroid hormone (PTH), few or absent bone metastases, and hypophosphatemia. Parathyroid hormone-related protein (PTHrP) has been isolated from tumors with HHM and shown to be responsible for the PTH-like effects and disruption of calcium homeostasis. The amino acid sequence of PTHrP bears homology to PTH from amino acid 1 to 13, but is unique thereafter. Although functioning via PTH receptor, PTHrP is the product of a separate gene located on the short arm of chromosome 12. Antibody to PTHrP (Ab-1) reacts with amino acid residues 38–64 of human PTHrP and shows no cross-reactivity with human PTH.

In addition to being produced by malignant tumors, PTHrP is found in normal keratinocytes, lactating mammary tissue, placenta, parathyroid glands, the central nervous system, and a number of other sites, suggesting that it may have a widespread physiologic role. PTHrP is thought to act in an autocrine and paracrine manner in various tissues to modulate other functions in addition to regulating calcium mobilization.

Through studies of osteoblast turnover in vitro it was suggested that PTHrP and the PTH-1 receptor might play an important role in exerting both pro- and anti-apoptotic effects in mesenchymal cells.

Immunostaining for PTHrP suggests that production of the peptide by stromal cells and giant cells may be involved in the formation of osteoclast-like cells in giant cell tumor of tendon sheath by acting in an autocrine/paracrine fashion.

Applications

Most squamous cell carcinomas from a variety of sites synthesize PTHrP irrespective of the calcium status of the patient. Using a polyclonal antibody to PTHrP (1–130), 93% of invasive squamous cell carcinomas were found to be immunopositive. Interestingly, the strongest immunoreactivity for PTHrP in the squamous carcinomas was in areas of invasion and with desmoplasia. Adenocarcinomas (smaller percentage than squamous cancers) of breast, lung, and kidney, hepatocellular carcinoma, mesothelioma, neuroendocrine tumors, and T-cell leukemias are other neoplasms that may express PTHrP. The presence of PTHrP and its receptor has been demonstrated in normal breast epithelium and breast carcinomas, suggesting that most breast tumors are able to respond to PTHrP.

Cholangiocarcinomas may be immunopositive for PTHrP (and chromogranin A), while all hepatocellular carcinomas are negative. Mixed primary liver tumors contain PTHrP immunoreactivity only in areas of cholangiocellular differentiation. Moreover, all metastatic adenocarcinomas (especially from the gastrointestinal tract) are negative except for 2/5 metastatic breast carcinomas.

Using polyclonal antibodies against synthetic PTHrP peptides, immunopositivity has been demonstrated in primary parathyroid adenomata and hyperplastic glands from patients with chronic renal failure, while primary hyperplastic glands are negative.

Comments

The frequency of expression of PTHrP is so great and widespread that it may be useful as a tumor marker in the histological diagnosis of certain cancers, e.g., squamous cell carcinoma of the lung. The protein has been shown to be a potential marker of pancreatic adenocarcinoma, and the co-expression of PTHrP and PTH/PTHrP receptor in chondrosarcomas may be of value in differentiating between benign and malignant cartilaginous lesions. Furthermore, the role of PTHrP in distinguishing between primary hepatocellular carcinoma and cholangiocarcinoma in the liver appears to be fairly reliable. Reactive bile ductules or squamous epithelium of epidermis are recommended control tissues. PTHrP has also been demonstrated in uterine tumors resembling ovarian sex cord tumors, multiple myeloma, endometrium, and salivary glands.

Selected references

Bouvet M, Nardin SR, Burton DW, *et al.* Parathyroid hormone-related protein as a novel tumor marker in pancreatic adenocarcinoma. *Pancreas* 2002; 24: 284–90.

Burtis WJ, Brady TG, Orloff JJ, *et al.* Immunochemical characterization of circulating parathyroid hormone-related protein in patients with humoral hypercalcemia of cancer. *New England Journal of Medicine* 1990; 322: 1106–12.

PAX-2 (paired box gene 2)

Sources/clones
Cell Marque (polyclonal), Invitrogen (polyclonal), Santa Cruz (60P, B24).

Fixation/preparation
Antibody clones to PAX-2 are immunoreactive in fixed paraffin-embedded sections.

Background
PAX-2 is a transcriptional protein that, together with PAX-8, plays a role in development of the urogenital system. It is expressed in Wolffian and Müllerian ducts during early embryologic stages.

Applications
PAX-2 is expressed in a spectrum of urologic neoplasms including renal cell carcinomas, papillary renal cell carcinomas, chromophobe carcinomas, and oncocytoma, but not in urothelial renal carcinomas. In addition, it has been shown to be expressed in Wilms tumor and nephrogenic adenomas. PAX-2 is a diagnostically useful marker for both primary and metastatic renal neoplasms, especially in small core needle biopsies. PAX-2 is also normally expressed in epithelium of rete testis to ejaculatory duct, and neoplasms arising from these cells (carcinoma rete testis, Wolffian adnexal tumor of the seminal vesicle, and endometrioid carcinoma of the seminal vesicle) will express PAX-2. In contrast, it is not expressed in prostatic adenocarcinomas.

PAX-2 has been reported in some normal Müllerian tissues including endometrium, fallopian tube mucosa, endocervix, foci of endosalpingiosis and endometriosis. In addition, it is present in mesonephric remnants and mesonephric hyperplasia. In Müllerian epithelial neoplasms, PAX-2 expression is seen in approximately 55% of serous tumors from ovary, uterus, and peritoneum; 25% of endometrioid adenocarcinomas; 19% of clear cell tumors; 11% of undifferentiated tumors; and 10% of mucinous tumors. When compared with PAX-8, although both stain the same tumors, PAX-2 staining is usually less intense and in fewer cells, indicating that PAX-2 sensitivity for epithelial tumors is lower than that of PAX-8.

In the cervix PAX-2 is not expressed in minimal deviation adenocarcinoma, and it is useful to distinguish this entity from mesonephric hyperplasia and lobular endocervical hyperplasia, both of which will be positive for PAX-2. In addition, endocervical adenocarcinoma in situ is negative for PAX-2, in contrast to endocervical tubal metaplasia or cervical endometriosis. A strong, diffuse nuclear PAX-2 expression in cervical glandular epithelium suggests a benign diagnosis.

Selected references
Daniel L, Lechevallier E, Giorgi R, et al. Pax-2 expression in adult renal tumors. *Human Pathology* 2001; 32: 282–7.

Dressler GR, Douglass EC. Pax-2 is a DNA-binding protein expressed in embryonic kidney and Wilms tumor. *Proceedings of the National Academy of Sciences of the USA* 1992; 89: 1179–83.

Ordóñez NG. Value of PAX2 immunostaining in tumor diagnosis: a review and update. *Advances in Anatomic Pathology* 2012; 19: 401–9.

Ozcan A, Liles N, Coffey D, Shen SS, Truong LD. PAX2 and PAX8 expression in primary and metastatic mullerian epithelial tumors: a comprehensive comparison. *American Journal of Surgical Pathology* 2011; 35: 1837–47.

Rabban JT, Mcalhany S, Lerwill MF, Grenert JP, Zaloudek CJ. PAX2 distinguishes benign mesonephric and mullerian glandular lesions of the cervix from endocervical adenocarcinoma, including minimal deviation adenocarcinoma. *American Journal of Surgical Pathology* 2010; 34: 137–46.

NOTES

PAX-5

Sources/clones

Cell Marque (clone 24, mouse monoclonal IgG1).

Fixation/preparation

The antigen is preserved in formalin-fixed paraffin-embedded tissue.

Background

PAX-5, also known as B-cell-specific activator protein (BSAP), is a nuclear transcription factor thought to play a critical role in the commitment of the common lymphoid progenitor to the B-cell lineage. PAX genes code for a family of nine transcription factors that have important roles in regulating cell proliferation, migration, and differentiation during embryonic development and organogenesis. PAX-5 expression is thought to trigger B-cell development by transcriptionally activating target genes such as *CD19*, which in turn drive B-cell differentiation. PAX-5 is expressed through almost all of B-cell differentiation, including the entire range of immature B-cell stages in the bone marrow, and the full range of mature B cells in peripheral lymphoid tissues, the blood, and bone marrow. As B cells terminally differentiate the plasma cells, PAX-5 is normally downregulated by the coordinate activity of several proteins involved in plasmacytic differentiation, primarily BLIMP and APRIL. PAX-5 is thought to act in concert with a second transcription factor, E2A, and mouse knockout experiments suggest that both are required for B-cell differentiation in mammals. Because of PAX-5's ubiquitous expression in immature and mature B cells, it represents an excellent marker for the entire range of B-cell differentiation prior to the plasma cell stage.

Applications

In normal bone marrow, PAX-5 is uniformly and strongly expressed in all immature and mature B cells, but not in plasma cells. Similarly, in peripheral lymphoid tissue, PAX-5 is uniformly expressed in B-cell follicles, including both primary and secondary follicles. It tends to be somewhat more highly expressed in naïve/mantle zone-type B cells compared to germinal center B cells. To the extent a marginal zone is visible, as in splenic white pulp, PAX-5 expression will be seen among marginal zone B cells. As in normal tissue, PAX-5 is ubiquitously expressed in neoplastic immature B cells (B-lymphoblastic leukemia/lymphoma) and in virtually all mature B-cell non-Hodgkin lymphomas. PAX-5 is uniformly expressed in the neoplastic cells of nodular lymphocyte-predominant Hodgkin lymphoma (LP cells), although typically at lower levels than in normal germinal center-derived B cells. Roughly 90% of classic Hodgkin lymphomas (CHL) are thought to show PAX-5 expression in the Hodgkin/Reed–Sternberg (HRS) cells, always at low level, and sometimes on only a small portion of the HRS cells. Rare cases of CHL are thought to include PAX-5– HRS cells, although in such cases exclusion of other potential entities, such as anaplastic large-cell lymphoma of T-lineage, would be required before diagnosis is rendered.

While normal plasma cells lack PAX-5 expression, the neoplastic plasma cells in several B-lymphoid malignancies will show PAX-5 expression. In B-cell lymphomas with significant plasmacytic differentiation, most notably lymphoplasmacytic lymphoma (LPL) and marginal zone lymphoma (MZL), both the neoplastic B cells and plasma cells typically express PAX-5. In contrast, true plasma cell neoplasms, including plasma cell myeloma and extramedullary plasmacytoma, lack PAX-5 expression in the large majority of cases. The one exception is plasma cell neoplasms containing t(11;14), which frequently do aberrantly retain PAX-5 expression.

Importantly, rare non-hematopoietic neoplasms are known to express PAX-5. The most important such neoplasm is Merkel cell carcinoma (MCC). Not only is MCC reported to express PAX-5 in 80–90% of cases, it also expresses nuclear terminal deoxynucleotidyltransferase (TdT) in a majority of cases, making MCC a significant diagnostic pitfall in the diagnosis of cutaneous B-LBL.

Other non-hematopoietic neoplasms known to express PAX-5 include neuroendocrine tumors of the lung, especially small-cell carcinoma (80%), where PAX-5 was been shown to upregulate c-MET, atypical carcinoids (65%), and large-cell neuroendocrine carcinomas (75%). While the veracity of these staining patterns using clone 24 of the antibody is not in doubt, it should be noted that another study has demonstrated cross-reactivity with PAX-2 in transfected cells and Wilms tumor via Western blotting and qRT-PCR, respectively, which illustrates a potential pitfall of using PAX-5 for identification of tumors outside of the hematopoietic lineage.

Selected references

Baker SJ, Reddy EP. B cell differentiation: role of E2A and Pax5/BSAP transcription factors. *Oncogene* 1995; 11: 413–26.

Desouki MM, Post GR, Cherry D, Lazarchick J. PAX-5: a valuable immunohistochemical marker in the differential diagnosis of lymphoid neoplasms. *Clinical Medicine and Research* 2010; 8: 84–8.

Morgenstern DA, Hasan F, Gibson S, *et al.* PAX5 expression in nonhematopoietic tissues: reappraisal of previous studies. *American Journal of Clinical Pathology* 2010; 133: 407–15.

O'Brien P, Morin P, Ouellette RJ, Robichaud GA. The Pax-5 gene: a pluripotent regulator of B-cell differentiation and cancer disease. *Cancer Research* 2011; 71: 7345–50.

PAX-8

Sources/clones

Cell Marque (MRQ-50, polyclonal), ProteinTech (polyclonal), Santa Cruz (PAX8R1), Ventana (MRQ-50).

Fixation/preparation

The antibodies are immunoreactive in fixed paraffin-embedded tissues.

Background

PAX-8 is a member of the paired box gene family that encodes a transcription factor that is predominantly expressed in the glandular epithelium of the thyroid gland, kidney, and Müllerian tract.

Applications

Antibodies against PAX-8 are used in various situations to identify malignancies that arise from various epithelia. In the normal thyroid gland, PAX-8 is expressed in follicular cells and focally expressed in C cells. In tumors, approximately 90% of thyroid neoplasms are immunoreactive for PAX-8, and sensitivity is greatest for follicular adenomas, follicular carcinomas, and papillary carcinomas. Sensitivity decreases in poorly differentiated (insular and anaplastic) thyroid carcinomas, to 75% and 60% respectively.

In normal kidney, PAX-8 is expressed in the nuclei of epithelial cells of the proximal and distal tubules, Henle loops, collecting ducts and parietal epithelial cells in Bowman's capsule. In renal tumors PAX-8 is identified in clear cell, papillary, chromophobe, and Wilms tumors, nephrogenic adenomas, and translocation (Xp11.2) renal cell carcinomas. It has also been reported in metastatic clear cell carcinomas regardless of their degree of differentiation. Conventional urothelial carcinomas of the urinary bladder are PAX-8-negative, but a subset of renal pelvis urothelial carcinomas and clear cell adenocarcinomas of the bladder can express PAX-8.

In the normal female tract it is expressed in epithelial cells of endocervix and endometrium, in non-ciliated cells in fallopian tube, and in epithelial ovarian inclusion cysts. PAX-8 expression is useful in distinguishing serous ovarian carcinoma from breast carcinoma, malignant mesothelioma, and primary adnexal tumors. Multiple studies have shown that all ovarian clear cell and serous (low and high grade) from peritoneum, ovary, and fallopian tube are immunoreactive for PAX-8. In mucinous ovarian carcinomas, PAX-8 positivity supports a primary ovarian tumor rather than a metastasis from the gastrointestinal tract, but the sensitivity of this marker in this situation is low (40%). Therefore, PAX-8 negativity in a mucinous ovarian tumor does not entirely exclude an ovarian primary. Endometrioid adenocarcinomas of ovarian and uterine origin are usually PAX-8-positive (92% and 98% respectively), as well as clear cell and serous endometrial carcinomas. In the cervix, PAX-8 is expressed in invasive and in-situ endocervical adenocarcinomas, as in conventional in-situ and invasive carcinomas of the cervix.

Selected references

Albadine R, Schultz L, Illei P, et al. PAX8 (+)/p63 (−) immunostaining pattern in renal collecting duct carcinoma (CDC): a useful immunoprofile in the differential diagnosis of CDC versus urothelial carcinoma of upper urinary tract. *American Journal of Surgical Pathology* 2010; 34: 965–9.

Argani P, Hicks J, De Marzo AM, et al. Xp11 translocation renal cell carcinoma (RCC): extended immunohistochemical profile emphasizing novel RCC markers. *American Journal of Surgical Pathology* 2010; 34: 1295–303.

Bowen NJ, Logani S, Dickerson EB, *et al.* Emerging roles for PAX8 in ovarian cancer and endosalpingeal development. *Gynecologic Oncology* 2007; 104: 331–7.

Chu PG, Chung L, Weiss LM, Lau SK. Determining the site of origin of mucinous adenocarcinoma: an immunohistochemical study of 175 cases. *American Journal of Surgical Pathology* 2011; 35: 1830–6.

Danialan R, Assaad M, Burghardt J, *et al.* The utility of PAX8 and IMP3 immunohistochemical stains in the differential diagnosis of benign, premalignant, and malignant endocervical glandular lesions. *Gynecologic Oncology* 2013; 130: 383–8.

Laury AR, Hornick JL, Perets R, *et al.* PAX8 reliably distinguishes ovarian serous tumors from malignant mesothelioma. *American Journal of Surgical Pathology* 2010; 34: 627–35.

Nonaka D, Tang Y, Chiriboga L, Rivera M, Ghossein R. Diagnostic utility of thyroid transcription factors Pax8 and TTF-2 (FoxE1) in thyroid epithelial neoplasms. *Modern Pathology* 2008; 21: 192–200.

Sangoi AR, Fjiwara M, West RB, *et al.* Immunohistochemical distinction of primary adrenal cortical lesions from metastatic clear cell renal cell carcinoma: a study of 248 cases. *American Journal of Surgical Pathology* 2011; 35: 678–86.

PD-1

Sources/clones

Abcam (NAT105, mouse monoclonal), MyBioSource (mouse monoclonal), Thermo Scientific (rabbit polyclonal).

Fixation/preparation

The antigen is preserved in formalin-fixed paraffin-embedded tissue.

Background

Programmed death 1 (PD-1) (CD279) is an inhibitory cell receptor that belongs to the CD28/CTLA-4 family of receptors and binds two ligands: PD-L1 (also known as B7-H1 or CD274) and PD-L2 (also known as B7-DC or CD273). While PD-1 expression is induced on activated T cells, B cells, and myeloid cells, the function of PD-1 has been best characterized in T cells, where it inhibits T-cell receptor (TCR) signaling. Upon engagement with PD-L1 or PD-L2, PD-1 suppresses the activation and function of T cells through the recruitment of SHP-2, which dephosphorylates and inactivates ZAP-70, an important integrator of TCR-mediated signaling. Interfering with the PD-1/PD-L1 pathway during the early stage of immune activation can result in improved T-cell responses and has been used as a treatment modality in advanced cancer patients.

Applications

PD-1 is normally expressed by germinal center-associated helper T cells (follicular helper T cells), a CD4+ T-cell subset that typically resides in the germinal center and helps coordinate immunologic reactions in this location. Activated T cells outside of lymph node germinal centers and in other tissues can also transiently express PD-1, but sustained non-germinal center PD-1 expression is associated with T-cell dysfunction. In reactive nodal lymphoid proliferations, immunohistochemical staining for PD-1 will highlight a small subset of T cells within the germinal centers, as would be expected for germinal center helper T cells, and only occasional interfollicular T cells. In reactive lymphoid proliferations in the skin, a small subset of the T cells may also express weak PD-1. The pattern of staining seen with PD-1 is typically both surface and cytoplasmic immunoreactivity.

PD-1 immunohistochemical staining has clinical applications in the diagnostic workup of both Hodgkin and non-Hodgkin lymphomas. Nodular lymphocyte-predominant Hodgkin lymphoma (NLPHL) is clinically and immunophenotypically distinct from classic Hodgkin lymphoma (CHL) and is characterized by scattered large neoplastic B cells (so called "popcorn" or LP cells) surrounded by small lymphocytes. Classically, the neoplastic cells are ringed by small T cells, which exhibit the immunophenotype of follicular helper T cells. These T-cell rosettes are considered to be a diagnostic feature of NLPHL (when present) and express strong PD-1 as well as CD57. PD-1+ T-cell rosettes are not entirely specific for NLPHL as the Reed–Sternberg cells in CHL can reportedly also be surrounded by varying numbers of PD-1+ T cells.

Angioimmunoblastic T-cell lymphoma (AITL) is a peripheral T-cell lymphoma characterized by numerous high endothelial venules, expanded follicular dendritic cell meshworks, and a proliferation of neoplastic small/intermediate-sized T lymphocytes with clear/pale cytoplasm and distinct cell membranes. The neoplastic T cells are derived from follicular helper T cells and consequently express CD10, Bcl-6, CXCL13, and PD-1. Uniform and/or strong expression of PD-1 is unusual in other T-cell lymphoproliferative disorders, but has been reported in a subset of peripheral T-cell lymphoma not otherwise specified (PTCL-NOS), which lack the characteristic clinical and histologic features of AITL. PD-1 expression has also been reported in a small subset of ALK+ and ALK− anaplastic large-cell lymphomas. Similarly, some authors have suggested a provisional category of "primary cutaneous follicular helper T-cell lymphoma" for cases with cutaneous involvement by a T-cell population with a TFH phenotype (including expression of PD-1), in which the patients lack significant adenopathy at the onset of disease or the clinical signs/symptoms suggestive of AITL. However, PD-1 expression is most commonly seen in AITL, is expressed by few B cells (unlike CD10 and Bcl-6), and is a useful diagnostic feature.

The atypical cells in primary cutaneous CD4+ small/medium-sized pleomorphic T-cell lymphoma characteristically express PD-1, Bcl-6, and CXCL13, without CD10; and PD-1 usually highlights the greatest proportion of the cells of interest. Other primary cutaneous T-cell lymphoproliferative disorders/T-cell lymphomas are largely negative for PD-1. A small subset of mycosis fungoides cases is reportedly positive for PD-1; however, no significant PD-1 expression has been reported in cutaneous anaplastic large-cell lymphoma, lymphomatoid papulosis, or aggressive CD8+ epidermotropic cytotoxic cutaneous T-cell lymphoma.

PD-1 immunoreactivity can be seen in chronic lymphocytic leukemia/small lymphocytic lymphoma (CLL/SLL); however, this immunophenotypic finding is not reliable enough for primary histopathologic diagnosis of CLL/SLL. PD-1 expression is generally not present on neoplastic cells in other B-cell NHLs. Similarly, the neoplastic B cells in cutaneous B-cell lymphomas rarely express PD-1. Of note, increased numbers of PD-1+ "tumor-infiltrating" T cells have been described in primary cutaneous follicle center lymphomas, follicular lymphoma, and CHL, with varying prognostic implications.

PD-1 expression has also been investigated in several reactive lymphadenopathies. In HIV-associated lymphadenopathy, the number of PD-1+ cells within germinal centers is reportedly low, with increased marginalization of the PD-1+ cells beneath the mantle zones. Increased numbers of PD-1+ T cells are also seen within the paracortex of lymph nodes in patients with Castleman's disease.

Selected references

Carreras J, Lopez-Guillermo A, Roncador G, et al. High numbers of tumor-infiltrating programmed cell death 1-positive regulatory lymphocytes are associated with improved overall survival in follicular lymphoma. *Journal of Clinical Oncology* 2009; 27: 1470–6.

Cetinozman F, Koens L, Jansen PM, Willemze R. Programmed death-1 expression in cutaneous B-cell lymphoma. *Journal of Cutaneous Pathology* 2014; 41: 14–21.

Dorfman DM, Brown JA, Shahsafaei A, Freeman GJ. Programmed Death-1 (PD-1) is a marker of germinal center-associated T cells and angioimmunoblastic T cell lymphoma. *American Journal of Surgical Pathology* 2006; 30: 802–10.

Muenst S, Dirnhofer S, Tzankov A. Distribution of PD-1+ lymphocytes in reactive lymphadenopathies. *Pathobiology* 2010; 77: 24–27.

Muenst S, Hoeller S, Willi N, Dirnhofera S, Tzankov A. Diagnostic and prognostic utility of PD-1 in B cell lymphomas. *Disease Markers* 2010; 29: 47–53.

Nam-Cha SH, Roncador G, Sanchez-Verde L, et al. PD-1, a follicular T-cell marker useful for recognizing nodular lymphocyte-predominant Hodgkin lymphoma. *American Journal of Surgical Pathology* 2008; 32: 1252–7.

P-glycoprotein (P-170), multidrug resistance (MDR)

Sources/clones

Accurate (MRPrl), Biodesign (JSB-1), Coulter (UIC1), Dako (C494, 4E3, C219), Immunotech (MRK-16, UIC2), Monosan (JSB-1, MRPmó, LRP-56), Novocastra, Oncogene, Sanbio (MRPrl), Sera Lab (JSB-1), Signet (C219, C494, JSB-1), Zymed (JSB-1).

Fixation/preparation

Most of the available antibodies are immunoreactive in frozen sections, and some react in fixed paraffin-embedded sections, enhanced by HIER treatment.

Background

P-glycoprotein (P-170) is a transmembrane protein of 170 kDa molecular weight. It has been associated with both intrinsic and acquired resistance to certain chemotherapeutic agents, particularly anthracyclines and vinca alkaloids. It is an energy-dependent pump which functions in drug efflux, reducing intracellular accumulation of chemotherapeutic agents, thus conferring the so-called multidrug resistance (MDR) phenomenon on cells expressing increased levels of this protein. One of the most perplexing problems encountered in chemotherapy is the resistance of certain tumors to all chemotherapeutic regimens, while other tumors, which are initially chemosensitive to a particular agent, show resistance to treatment over time and with disease progression. Furthermore, tumor cells which are resistant to one drug often show cross-resistance to a wide variety of other, structurally unrelated drugs. For example, tumor cells resistant to adriamycin can show cross-resistance to diverse drugs to which they have never been exposed, including vinca alkaloids and mitomycin C, but not to other drugs such as alkylating agents. This is known as the MDR phenomenon. A family of so-called MDR genes encodes the P-glycoprotein, apparently with only the protein encoded by the *MDR1* gene inducing the MDR phenotype.

There is extensive evidence from in-vitro studies, especially with non-human cell lines, that overexpression of P-glycoprotein results in reduced accumulation of drug within the cell. Mice have been generated with knockout of *MDR1*, and these animals show abnormalities of transport at the blood–brain barrier and are more sensitive to drugs.

Applications

Molecular and immunohistochemical studies of P-glycoprotein reveal that it is overexpressed in a number of intrinsically resistant tumors such as carcinomas of the liver, pancreas, colon, adrenal cortex, and kidney, and appears to vary according to the differentiation of the cells. Interestingly, in these cases, high levels of the protein have also been demonstrated in the normal tissues from which the tumors are derived. The physiologic function of P-glycoprotein can be deduced from its normal tissue distribution in that high levels of expression are seen in endothelial cells of the blood–brain barrier and in renal proximal tubules, both cell types having the primary function of moving toxic molecules across cell membranes.

P-glycoprotein expression has been found significantly more frequently in soft tissue sarcomas, neuroblastomas, and hepatoblastomas, and generally in disseminated tumors but not in malignant brain tumors and nephroblastoma. Tumors responsive to chemotherapy generally show low levels of P-glycoprotein expression, and solid tumors that are most responsive to systemic chemotherapy, such as seminomas and embryonal carcinomas, rarely display detectable levels of the protein. Tumors from patients previously treated with chemotherapy show frequent elevation of P-glycoprotein, suggesting that the MDR phenotype is induced by exposure to chemotherapy. The detection of elevated levels of P-glycoprotein expression has the potential to identify tumors likely to be resistant to conventional chemotherapy and may provide a rationale for the use of alternative treatments for such patients. Immunohistological evaluation appears to be the method of choice for the assessment of P-glycoprotein, largely because it allows morphological correlation and discrimination from that in non-tumor cells. However, the published results are conflicting, with immunoexpression of P-glycoprotein and other MDR-related proteins not changing significantly after chemotherapy. It has been shown that there is no significant correlation between P-glycoprotein expression in tumor cells and clinical course, stage, and grade of nephroblastoma. However, positivity in tumor capillary endothelial cells correlates significantly with unfavorable outcome, suggesting that chemoresistance depended on an active blood–tumor barrier.

Comments

Only two *MDR* genes are know to be present in man, namely *MDR1* and *MDR3*, but only the MDR1 gene product confers the MDR phenotype. One of the most widely used antibodies to P-glycoprotein is clone C219 that reacts with both the MDR1 and MDR3 gene products. Several other antibodies specific to the MDR1 gene product have now been described. They include HYB-241 and HYB-612, and C494. While earlier studies were conducted on frozen sections, HIER has improved the immunoreactivity in fixed paraffin-embedded sections. Renal proximal tubules are used as the standard positive control because of the high levels of expression of P-glycoprotein in the epithelial cells. The antigen is localized to the cell membrane and shows specific polarization in some cell types, e.g., the apical and basolateral membranes of pulmonary epithelium and the trabecular structures resembling canalicular membrane, or in the luminal membrane in hepatocellular carcinoma cells.

Selected references

Cordon-Cardo C, O'Brien JP, Boccia J, *et al.* Expression of the multidrug resistance gene product (P-glycoprotein) in human normal and tumor tissues. *Journal of Histochemistry and Cytochemistry* 1990; 38: 1277–87.

Lopes JM, Bruland OS, Bjekehagen B, *et al.* Synovial sarcoma: Immunohistochemical expression of P-glycoprotein and glutathione S transferase-pi and clinical drug resistance. *Pathology Research and Practice* 1997; 193: 21–36.

Scheffer GL, Pijnenborg AC, Smit EF, *et al.* Multidrug resistance related molecules in human and murine lung. *Journal of Clinical Pathology* 2002; 55: 332–9.

Phosphohistone H3 (pHH3)

Sources/clones

Cell Marque (369A), Cell Signaling Technology (9701), Millipore (06-570), Ventana (760-4591).

Fixation/preparation

The antibody can be used in formalin-fixed paraffin-embedded tissue. Pretreatment of deparaffinized tissue sections with HIER is required.

Background

Histone H3, a core histone protein, and other histone proteins form the major protein constituents of eukaryotic chromatin. In mammalian cells, phosphorylation of the serine 10 residue of histone H3, a rare event during interphase, reaches a maximum for chromatin condensation during mitosis. No phosphorylation of histone H3 has been noted during apoptosis or karyorrhexis. Additionally, in comparison to the Ki-67 immunostain, which stains cells in all phases of the cell cycle (except G_0), studies have shown that the antibody directed against phosphohistone H3 (pHH3) is a more sensitive and effective marker for identifying mitotic activity.

Applications

Studies have shown that the pHH3 immunostain helps focus attention on the most mitotically active areas of a tumor, allows for easy and objective differentiation of mitotic from apoptotic nuclei, and consequently reduces intra- and interobserver variability. Its role in facilitating the rapid reliable grading of meningiomas, astrocytomas, melanomas, and well-differentiated neuroendocrine tumors of the pancreas has been well studied.

Selected references

Juan G, Traganos F, James WM, *et al.* Histone H3 phosphorylation and expression of cyclins A and B1 measured in individual cells during their progression through G2 and mitosis. *Cytometry* 1998; 32: 71–7.

Ribalta T, McCutcheon IE, Aldape KD, *et al.* The mitosis-specific antibody anti-phosphohistone-H3 (PHH3) facilitates rapid reliable grading of meningiomas according to WHO 2000 criteria. *American Journal of Surgical Pathology* 2004; 28: 1532–6.

Shibata K, Ajiro K. Cell cycle-dependent suppressive effect of histone H1 on mitosis-specific H3 phosphorylation. *Journal of Biological Chemistry* 1993; 268: 18, 431–4.

Tetzlaff MT, Curry JL, Ivan D, *et al.* Immunodetection of phosphohistone H3 as a surrogate of mitotic figure count and clinical outcome in cutaneous melanoma. *Modern Pathology* 2013; 26: 1153–60.

Voss SM, Riley MP, Lokhandwala PM, Wang M, Yang Z. Mitotic count by phosphohistone H3 immunohistochemical staining predicts survival and improves interobserver reproducibility in well-differentiated neuroendocrine tumors of the pancreas. *American Journal of Surgical Pathology* 2015; 39: 13–24.

NOTES

PIT1 (*POU1F1*)

Sources/clones

Abcam (2C11, mouse monoclonal), Abnova Corporation (rabbit polyclonal), Acris Antibodies GmbH (rabbit polyclonal), Antibodies-online (rabbit polyclonal), Atlas Antibodies (rabbit polyclonal), GeneTex (rabbit polyclonal), Genway Biotech (rabbit polyclonal), Novus Biologicals (rabbit polyclonal), Thermo Scientific (rabbit polyclonal).

Fixation/preparation

Most of these antibodies are validated in formalin-fixed paraffin-embedded tissue. Please refer to vendor instructions for specific antigen retrieval requirements.

Background

PIT1, a member of the POU (Pit-Oct-Unc) family of transcription factors, is a pituitary-specific transcription factor responsible for pituitary development and hormone expression in mammals. PIT1 contains two protein domains, which are both necessary for DNA binding on genes encoding growth hormone, thyroid-stimulating hormone β-subunit, and prolactin. Thus, PIT1 is involved in the specification of the somatotrope, thyrotrope, and lactotrope phenotypes in the developing anterior pituitary and in tumors derived from this lineage, giving them the designation of "PIT1 family". Defects in *POU1F1*, the gene that encodes PIT1, are the cause of pituitary hormone deficiency combined type 1 (CPHD1), characterized by impaired production of growth hormone (GH) and one or more of the other five anterior pituitary hormones.

Applications

Pituitary adenomas require appropriate and precise histopathological classification for adequate patient treatment and follow-up. PIT1 immunohistochemistry can help to identify so-called null-cell adenomas that do not express any hormone by immunostaining as belonging to the PIT1 family of tumors, and thus not really meeting the criteria for null-cell adenoma (defined as negative for all hormones and transcription factors). Silent subtype 3 adenomas are rare tumors with no biochemical evidence of hormonal hypersecretion that may variably label with several adenohypophyseal hormones and belong to the PIT1 family. These tumors are more likely to recur, and demonstrate an aggressive local behavior.

Selected references

Kobayashi I, Oka H, Naritaka H, *et al.* Expression of Pit-1 and growth hormone-releasing hormone receptor mRNA in human pituitary adenomas: difference among functioning, silent, and other nonfunctioning adenomas. *Endocrine Pathology* 2002; 13: 83–98.

Mete O, Asa SL. Therapeutic implications of accurate classification of pituitary adenomas. *Seminars in Diagnostic Pathology* 2013; 30: 158–64.

Puy LA, Asa SL. The ontogeny of Pit-1 expression in the human fetal pituitary gland. *Neuroendocrinology* 1996; 63: 349–55.

NOTES

Pituitary hormones: ACTH, FSH, hGH, LH, PRL, TSH

Sources/clones

Anti-adrenocorticotropin (ACTH)

Axcel/Accurate (polyclonal), Biodesign (polyclonal), Biogenesis (polyclonal), Biogenex (polyclonal), Caltag Laboratories (polyclonal), Chemicon (polyclonal), Dako (02A3, polyclonal), Fitzgerald (polyclonal), Milab (polyclonal), Novocastra, Sanbio/Monosan (polyclonal), Sera Lab, Serotec (A1H5, A5B12), Sigma (polyclonal), Zymed (polyclonal).

Anti-follicle-stimulating hormone (FSH)

Axcel/Accurate (polyclonal), Biodesign (301, 1801, 29, 701, 702, 706, 709, SI, polyclonal), Biogenesis (754, 143, BIO-FSHb-00, polyclonal), Biogenex (78/74 1 F11, polyclonal), Dako (polyclonal), Fitzgerald (polyclonal, M27301, M210201, M26092, M94166, M94163, M94164).

Anti-human growth hormone (hGH)

Accurate (12), Biodesign (901, 902, polyclonal), Biogenesis (2F10, Rt, polyclonal), Biogenex (54/9 2A2, polyclonal), Dako (polyclonal), Fitzgerald (M94168, M94169, M32222, polyclonal), Novocastra (polyclonal), Sera Lab (polyclonal) Serotec (B008, E1, G1), Sigma Chemical (GHC2), Zymed (ZMGH2, polyclonal).

Anti-human luteinizing hormone (LH)

American Research Products (1561–18), Axcel/Accurate (polyclonal), Biodesign (2004, 6101, 6102, 6103, [6206, 6207, 62], polyclonal), Biogenesis (ICIO, 3D7, 4E3, Gil, polyclonal), Biogenex (3LH 5B6YH4, polyclonal), Cymbus Bioscience (6101), Dako (polyclonal), Fitzgerald (polyclonal), Serotec (INNbLH1), Zymed (ZMLH2, ZSL11).

Anti-prolactin (PRL)

Axcel/Accurate (polyclonal), Biodesign (164.22.12, [6201–6204, 62], [ME.121, ME.1], S2, [2605, 2606]), Biogenesis (1D5, 626/02, 633/1, polyclonal), Dako (polyclonal), Fitzgerald (M94192, M94193, M94194, M31031, M31032, M31033, M310110, M310111, M310112, polyclonal), Immunotech (164.22.16), Zymed (ZMPL1).

Anti-human thyroid-stimulating hormone (TSH)

American Research Products (25TH7G12), Axcel/Accurate (polyclonal), Biodesign (9001-90010), Biogenesis (TSH-03, polyclonal), Biogenex (5404, polyclonal), Dako (polyclonal), Fitzgerald (polyclonal), Novocastra (QB2.6, polyclonal), Sera Lab (JOS2.2, polyclonal), Zymed (ZMTS2, ZMTS4).

Fixation/preparation

All of the antibodies against the pituitary hormones are applicable to formalin-fixed paraffin-embedded sections. Although not essential, enzyme antigen retrieval pretreatment with Target Unmasking Fluid (TUF, Signet) or trypsin may improve immunoreaction on paraffin-embedded and frozen sections.

Background

In all instances antibodies against the pituitary hormones were raised using purified extract from human pituitary glands as immunogen. The adenohypophysis comprises approximately 75% of the normal pituitary gland. It consists of the pars distalis, pars intermedia, and pars tuberalis. The pars distalis is roughly divided into a midline zone (PAS-positive mucosubstance containing ACTH [15–20%], FSH/LH [10%], and TSH [5%] cells) and two lateral portions that stain positively with acidic dyes (PBX 15–20% and GH

Table 1 Normal cellular composition of the pituitary gland: morphological, functional and immunohistochemical characteristics

Cell	Product	Location/percentage	Immunohistochemistry
Somatotroph	GH 21 kDa polypeptide	Lateral 50%	GH
Lactotroph	PRL 23.5 kDa polypeptide	Posterolateral 15–20%	PRL
Corticotroph	ACTH 4.5 kDa polypeptide	Midline 15–20%	ACTH
Gonadotroph	FSH 35 kDa and LH 28.2 kDa glycoproteins	Generalized 10%	FSH and LH
Thyrotroph	TSH 28 kDa glycoprotein	Anterior midline 5%	TSH

Modified from Scheithauer BW. Surgical pathology of the pituitary: the adenomas. Part 1. *Pathology Annual* 1984; **19**: 317–69.

Table 2 Functional classification of pituitary hormones

Adenoma type	H&E	PAS	Immunohistochemistry
Prolactin	C, A	−	PRL
Growth hormone cell	A, C	−	GH
Mixed GH and prolactin cell	A, C	−	GH and PRL
Mammosomatotroph cell	A	−	GH, strong +PRL, week +
Acidophil stem cell	C	−	PRL+, GH (variable)
Corticotroph cell	B, C	−	ACTH
Gonadotroph cell	B, C	+	Both or either FSH, LH
Thyrotroph cell	B, C	+	±TSH
Null-cell	C	−	None
Null-cell, oncocytic	A	−	None

Modified from Scheithauer BW. Surgical pathology of the pituitary: the adenomas. Part 1. *Pathology Annual* 1984; **19**: 317–69.

50%). It should be noted that cells are not strictly limited in their geographic distribution. Trichrome stains such as the PAS–orange-G method serve to highlight the PAS+ basophils and the orange-G+ acidophils. Since this reactivity correlates only crudely with hormonal function, it is necessary to resort to immunohistochemical characterization for proper identification. The cells are arranged in cords, and are encircled by well-formed basement membrane. These cells lie in the immediate proximity of a capillary to facilitate the secretory process. The general, histochemical, and immunohistochemical characteristics of normal adenohypophyseal cells are summarized in Table 1.

Applications

The major role of antibodies to pituitary hormones is that they serve as the primary basis of adenoma classification. A study of surgical series showed 80% of pituitary adenomas to be functional, while a combined surgical/autopsy series found only 50% to be hormonally functional. In adults, adenomas may present with hyperfunction (amenorrhea–galactorrhea, Cushing's disease, Nelson's syndrome, and acromegaly or gigantism), hypofunction (insufficiency of gonadal, thyroidal, or adrenal function), or compressive signs (visual disturbance, headache, or raised intracranial pressure). Aggression of pituitary adenomas is based on the radiological assessment: grade I, microadenomas (<10 mm); grade 2, intrasellar adenoma; grade 3, diffuse adenomas with erosion of sellar floor; grade 4, invasive adenomas with widespread sellar erosion and destruction.

The conventional tinctorial classification of adenomas, based on affinity of tumor cells for acid or basic dyes, correlated crudely with the functional characteristics. Acidophil adenomas were presumed to produce growth hormone, while basophilic adenomas were considered synonymous with ACTH secretion and Cushing's disease. Chromophobe adenomas, in contrast, were considered nonfunctioning, with symptoms being attributed to local destructive or compressive effects. Hence, with the advent of commercially available specific antisera to pituitary hormones, there is a functional classification (Table 2).

Comments

Histopathology laboratories servicing neurosurgical units need to provide a comprehensive functional characterization of pituitary adenomas. The use of the normal pituitary gland will suffice as a positive control for the six hormones.

Selected references

Earle KM, Dillard SH. Pathology of adenomas of the pituitary gland. *Excerpta Medica International Congress Series* 1973; 303: 3–16.

Hardy J, Vezina JL. Transsphenoidal neurosurgery of intracranial neoplasm. *Advances in Neurology* 1976; 15: 261–5.

Robert F. Electron microscopy of human pituitary tumors. In Tindall GT, Collins WF, eds. *Clinical Management of Pituitary Disorders*. New York: Raven Press, 1979, pp. 113–31.

Scheithauer BW. Surgical pathology of the pituitary: the adenomas. Part 1. *Pathology Annual* 1984; 19: 317–69.

NOTES

PLAP (placental alkaline phosphatase)

Sources/clones

Accurate (8B6, polyclonal), American Research (polyclonal), Biogenesis (PLAP001, polyclonal), Biogenex (polyclonal), Dako (8B6, 8A9, polyclonal), Novocastra (polyclonal), Sanbio (MIG-P), Sigma (8B6), Zymed (polyclonal).

Fixation/preparation

The antigen is resistant to fixation, and both polyclonal and monoclonal antibodies are immunoreactive in fixed paraffin-embedded sections. HIER enhances staining.

Background

The alkaline phosphatases (APs) are a heterogeneous group of glycoproteins, which are usually confined to the cell surface. The isoenzymes differ in terms of their biochemical properties, anatomical sites of production, and reactivity with different antibodies. APs probably have a role in cellular transport, regulation of metabolism, gene transcription, and cellular differentiation. At least three genes encode the human AP isoenzymes, one for tissue-nonspecific AP present in the liver, bone, and kidney; one for the synthesis of intestinal AP; and one or more genes for the placental isoenzyme (PLAP). The different isoenzymes differ in molecular weight and amino acid composition and have different properties. The tissue-nonspecific and intestinal variants are heat-sensitive, whereas the PLAP isoenzymes are heat-resistant.

PLAP occurs only in higher primates and displays a high degree of genetic polymorphism. It is a dimer of 65 kDa subunits and is synthesized during the G phase of the cell cycle. The enzyme is produced by trophoblasts and is responsible for the hyperphosphatemia observed during pregnancy. Biochemically, immunologically, and electrophoretically, PLAP can be separated into three distinct subtypes. The phase 1 isoenzyme corresponds to that produced by 6–8-week trophoblasts, the second is a mixture of the early-phase and term-placental isoenzymes, and the phase 3 corresponds to the 13-weeks-to-term gestation AP isoenzymes. PLAP-like reactivity has been reported in the serum of about 5% of patients with tumors that included carcinoma of the lung, ovary, breast, colon, and endometrium, as well as malignant lymphoma and multiple myeloma. Raised levels of serum PLAP were found in 25% of patients with seminoma. Several isoenzymes of AP have been specifically named. The Regan isoenzyme was named after a patient with lung cancer whose serum had the phase 3-type isoenzyme. It was also found in 4–14% of patients with a variety of neoplasms including testicular germ cell tumors and carcinomas of the breast, ovary, lung, stomach, and pancreas, as well as in the serum of patients with ulcerative colitis, familial polyposis, and cirrhosis of the liver. The Nagao isoenzyme was named after a patient with pleural carcinomatosis and bears some similarities to the phase 3 PLAP. The Nagao AP has been found in the serum and tumor cells of patients with adenocarcinoma of the bile ducts and pancreas. The Kashahara variant was detected in tumor extracts of hepatocellular carcinoma and possesses some of the properties of the placental isoenzyme. Other non-Regan isoenzymes have been described in patients with gastrointestinal cancer, benign gynecological disease and female genital cancer, testicular teratomas, and lung tumors.

Applications

Antibodies to PLAP are primarily used as a diagnostic discriminator of germ cell tumors in the context of separation from somatic carcinomas and mediastinal tumors (Appendix 1.5, 1.12). It is also useful for the identification of intraventricular germ cell tumors (Appendix 1.35). Membrane-based PLAP has been documented immunohistochemically in seminoma, embryonal carcinoma, gonadoblastoma, endodermal sinus tumor, and choriocarcinoma, and in metastatic deposits of seminoma, making this marker an important one for the identification of germ cell tumors (Appendix 1.37). Spermatocytic seminoma and immature teratomas were negative. Epithelial neoplasms of the ovary and intratubular neoplastic germ cells also labeled for PLAP. It has been suggested that PLAP immunostaining may help separate partial and complete hydatidiform moles and choriocarcinoma. Partial moles show weak human chorionic gonadotrophin (hCG) and strong PLAP, complete moles show strong expression of hCG and weak PLAP, while choriocarcinomas display strong expression of hCG and weak PLAP and hPL (Appendix 1.34). Intermediate trophoblasts are reported not to express PLAP, an observation that requires confirmation. PLAP has also been observed in cell lines from human bladder cancer and in somatic tumors such as tumors of the female genital tract, intestine, and lung, and less frequently in breast and renal carcinomas (Wick *et al.* 1987). Epithelial membrane antigen (EMA) is said to help in distinguishing these somatic tumors, which express EMA, from germ cell tumors, which do not.

Selected references

Koshida K, Uchibayashi T, Yamamoto H, *et al.* A potential use of a monoclonal antibody to placental alkaline phosphatase (PLAP) to detect lymph node metastases of seminoma. *Journal of Urology* 1996; 155: 337–41.

Losch A, Kainz C. Immunohistochemistry in the diagnosis of the gestational trophoblastic disease. *Acta Obstetrica et Gynecologica Scandinavica* 1996; 75: 753–6.

Manivel JC, Jessurun J, Wick MR, Dehner LP. Placental alkaline phosphatase immunoreactivity in testicular germ cell neoplasms. *American Journal of Surgical Pathology* 1987; 11: 21–9.

Wick MR, Swanson PE, Manivel JC. Placental-like alkaline phosphatase reactivity in human tumors: an immunohistochemical study of 520 cases. *Human Pathology* 1987; 18: 946–54.

PMS2

Sources/clones

Biocare Med (A16–4), Dako (EP51), Diagnostic Biosystems (A16–4), LifeSpan BioSciences (EPR3947), Novocastro (MOR46), Ventana (EPR3947).

Fixation/preparation

The antigen is preserved in formalin-fixed paraffin-embedded sections. HIER enhances immunolabeling.

Background

There are four main mismatch repair genes (*MLH1*, *MSH2*, *MSH6*, and *PMS2*). The products of these genes are necessary to identify and correct errors that occur during DNA replication at microsatellite loci, small repetitive sequences scattered throughout the genome. These areas are prone to DNA slippage, resulting in insertion and deletion loops. The mismatch repair proteins form heterodimers, with the MSH2–MSH6 complex recognizing the impaired bases, while MLH1 and PMS2 excise the mismatched nucleotides. Germline mutations in these genes are associated with Lynch syndrome (hereditary non-polyposis colorectal carcinoma), an autosomal dominant disorder characterized by early-onset colorectal cancer and increased risk of cancer of the endometrium, stomach, ovary, skin, and other sites.

PMS2 (postmeiotic segregation increased 2) comprises 15 exons encoding a protein of 862 amino acids and is located on chromosome 7p22. It was first identified because of its homology with the yeast mismatch repair gene *mutL* homolog (*PMS1*), and it is associated with multiple pseudogenes. Its function as a mismatch repair gene in humans was confirmed when knockout mice lacking both *PMS2* alleles were shown to have microsatellite instability in both germline and tumor DNA. Genetic testing has confirmed the presence of heterozygous truncating mutations in cohorts of hereditary non-polyposis colorectal cancer (HNPCC) families lacking mutations in *MLH1*, *MSH2*, and *MSH6*. Germline mutations in *PMS2* are rare, and patients with these mutations tend to show decreased penetrance in comparison with patients with *MLH1* and *MSH2* mutations.

Applications

In practice, the PMS2 immunohistochemical stain is most commonly used in a panel with MLH1, MSH2, and MSH6, to screen tumors for microsatellite instability and Lynch syndrome. It is important to remember that *PMS2* mutations are usually associated with a truncated protein product and loss of function, and therefore one must assess for the absence of staining in tumor nuclei. As the proliferating epithelium of the gastrointestinal tract should show strong nuclear staining, most slides should have ample tissue as an internal positive control. Although the four-stain panel is most commonly used, studies have shown that a panel consisting of MSH6 and PMS2 is equally sensitive, with the added benefit of reduced cost.

Loss of PMS2 may be seen in three distinct scenarios. The first, and most common, is in the setting of sporadic cancers with hypermethylation of the MLH1 promoter region, causing loss of expression of both MLH1 and PMS2 by immunohistochemistry. Loss of both markers can also be seen in the setting of a germline mutation of *MLH1*, while germline mutations of *PMS2* usually result in loss of expression of PMS2 only. This is most likely related to the biochemical properties of the MLH1 protein, which has the ability to form a heterodimer with PMS1 in the absence of PMS2 (which may also explain the decreased penetrance seen in patients with PMS2 mutations).

Immunohistochemistry to predict microsatellite instability is often used outside of colorectal carcinoma, with increasing frequency. Studies have confirmed its accuracy in detecting microsatellite instability in endometrial carcinomas, and it can also be used to screen for Lynch syndrome in patients with sebaceous neoplasms.

Selected references

Garg K, Leitao MM, Kauff ND, *et al*. Selection of endometrial carcinomas for DNA mismatch repair protein immunohistochemistry using patient age and tumor morphology enhances detection of mismatch repair abnormalites. *American Journal of Surgical Pathology* 2009; 33: 925–33.

Hall G, Clarkson A, Shi A, *et al*. Immunohistochemistry for PMS2 and MSH6 alone can replace a four antibody panel for mismatch repair deficiency screening in colorectal adenocarcinoma. *Pathology* 2010; 42: 409–13.

Hendriks YM, Jagmohan-Changur S, van der Klift HM, *et al*. Heterozygous mutations in PMS2 cause hereditary nonpolyposis colorectal carcinoma (Lynch syndrome). *Gastroenterology* 2006; 130: 312–22.

Modica I, Soslow RA, Black D, *et al*. Utility of immunohistochemistry in predicting microsatellite instability in endometrial carcinoma. *American Journal of Surgical Pathology* 2007; 31: 744–51.

Nicolaides NC, Papadopoulos N, Liu B, *et al*. Mutations of two PMS homologues in hereditary nonpolyposis colon cancer. *Nature* 1994; 371: 75–80.

Shia JR, Tang LH, Vakiani E, *et al*. Immunohistochemistry as first-line screening for detecting colorectal cancer patients at risk for hereditary nonpolyposis colorectal cancer syndrome A 2-antibody panel may be as predictive as a 4-antibody panel. *American Journal of Surgical Pathology* 2009; 33: 1639–45.

Truninger K, Menigatti M, Luz J, *et al*. Immunohistochemical analysis reveals high frequency of PMS2 defects in colorectal cancer. *Gastroenterology* 2005; 128: 1160–71.

Pneumocystis jirovecii

Sources/clones

Accurate (3F6), Axcel/Accurate (3F6), Biodesign (092, 093), Biogenesis (0G1/1), Biogenex (3F6), Chemicon, Dako (3F6).

Fixation/preparation

The Dako antibody reacts with an antigenic epitope of *Pneumocystis jirovecii* (previously known as *P. carinii*), which is resistant to fixation in formalin and picric acid, paraffin embedding, and extraction with ethanol and xylene. This antibody may also be used to detect *P. jirovecii* in smears prepared from bronchoalveolar lavage fluid and sputum samples. However, enzymatic digestion of smears (e.g., trypsin) must be performed before staining.

Background

The Dako antibody (IgMκ) reacts with an 82 kDa parasite-specific component of human *Pneumocystis jirovecii*. No cross-reactivity has been found with a number of parasites and fungi.

Applications

The AIDS epidemic brought about an increased need for specific markers that recognize *Pneumocystis jirovecii*. Antibodies mark cyst and/or trophozoites. While the sensitivity of the immunohistochemical method appears to be greater than that of the Giemsa stain, it is only slightly better than the GMS stain, warranting the use of immunostaining in sputum, where identification of the pathogen is more difficult than in bronchoalveolar lavage. The other advantage of immunostaining is that both cyst wall and trophozoites are stained, whereas the silver stain only labels the cyst wall. However, the former staining pattern may appear amorphous or focally granular, which may be confused with nonspecific staining of mucin or intracellular/free particulate material. The 3F6 monoclonal antibody has been found to be consistently more sensitive at detecting cysts of pneumocystis in both sputum and bronchoalveolar lavage specimens.

Comments

Immunohistochemistry for *Pneumocystis jirovecii* is a useful adjunct to traditional Giemsa and silver stains, particularly in cytopathology laboratories that examine a large number of respiratory specimens from HIV-positive patients.

Selected reference

Amin MB, Mezger E, Zarbo RJ. Detection of Pneumocystis carinii. Comparative study of monoclonal antibody and silver staining. *American Journal of Clinical Pathology* 1992; 98: 13–18.

NOTES

Pregnancy-specific β-1-glycoprotein (SP1)

Sources/clones

Axcel/Accurate, Biodesign (BD4D8), Biogenesis (polyclonal), Biogenex (4E4, polyclonal), Chemicon (polyclonal), Dako (polyclonal), Fitzgerald (M32236), Research Diagnostics (BB4E4), Zymed (polyclonal).

Fixation/preparation

The antigen is fixation-resistant, and immunoreactivity may be improved with proteolytic digestion or HIER.

Background

Pregnancy-specific β-1-glycoprotein (SP1), human chorionic gonadotropin (hCG), and placental alkaline phosphatase (PLAP) are three major proteins produced by the trophoblasts of the human placenta. Immunohistochemical studies suggest that SP1 and hCG are also present in the human amnion. Molecular cloning studies indicate that the human SP1s form a group of closely related placental proteins that, together with the carcinoembryonic antigen family members, comprise a subfamily within the immunoglobulin superfamily. The main source of SP1 is the syncytiotrophoblast, but it has been demonstrated that amniotic as well as chorionic membranes express low levels of SP1 genes, although only certain subpopulations of SP1 transcripts were expressed, with differences in species expression between amnion, chorion, and trophoblasts. The function of the SP1s is largely unknown. The SP1 family induces secretion of anti-inflammatory cytokines in mononuclear phagocytes and the tetraspanin; CD9 has been identified as a receptor of murine SP1.

Applications

The immunohistochemical applications of SP1 have been mainly in the study of placental elements and their corresponding tumors. Differing levels of expression of hCG, human placental lactogen (hPL,) and SP1 were observed in the fetomaternal tissues throughout pregnancy. hCG was strongly localized in the cytoplasm of the syncytiotrophoblast in the 12-day blastocysts, remaining strong until 8–10 weeks before decreasing and becoming almost negative at term. hCG showed variable staining in the implantation site. hPL and SP1 appear later than hCG in the syncytiotrophoblast, increasingly rapidly by week 8 and remaining strong until term. Immunolocalization studies of SP1 in syncytiotrophoblasts suggest a secretory pathway including synthesis in the endoplasmic reticulum, processing by the Golgi and exocytic release into maternal blood in the intervillous space.

The presence of SP1, vimentin, cytokeratin, and PLAP, particularly the first three antigens, has been used to identify intermediate trophoblasts in the placental site nodule (Appendix 1.34).

Comments

SP1 is not specific to placental cells. It is expressed in a variety of non-placental tumors: colonic carcinomas, some high-grade urothelial tumors, and breast carcinoma. SP1 has been employed in the panel for the distinction of mesothelioma from adenocarcinoma, being positive in almost 60% of adenocarcinomas. However, SP1 is also expressed in mesotheliomas, albeit in lower frequency (6%). In lung carcinomas, SP1 was expressed in 85% of non-small-cell carcinomas and in 50% of small-cell carcinomas, with a significant negative correlation of both SP1 and CEA immunoexpression with grade of differentiation in adenocarcinoma.

Selected references

Plouzek CA, Leslie KK, Stephens JK, Chou JY. Differential gene expression in the amnion, chorion, and trophoblast of the human placenta. *Placenta* 1993; 14: 277–85.

Sabet LM, Daya D, Stead R, *et al*. Significance and value of immunohistochemical localization of pregnancy specific proteins in feto-maternal tissue throughout pregnancy. *Modern Pathology* 1989; 2: 227–32.

Waterhouse R, Ha C, Dvcksler GS. Murine CD9 is the receptor for pregnancy-specific glycoprotein 17. *Journal of Experimental Medicine* 2002; 195: 277–82.

Wright C, Angus B, Napier J, *et al*. Prognostic factors in breast cancer: immunohistochemical staining for SP1 and NCRC 11 related to survival, tumour epidermal growth factor receptor and oestrogen receptor status. *Journal of Pathology* 1987; 153: 325–31.

Progesterone receptor (PR)

Sources/clones

Abbott (PgR-ICA), Becton Dickinson (PR33, PR4–12), Biogenesis (1A6), Biogenex (PgR-lA), Dako (1A6, polyclonal), Immunotech (PR10A9), Novocastra (1A6), Zymed (1A6).

Fixation/preparation

Most antibody clones currently available are immunoractive in routinely fixed paraffin-embedded tissues and enhanced after HIER. Enzymatic predigestion is not required.

Background

In selected target tissues, estrogens have been found to stimulate not only mitogenesis but also the synthesis of specific proteins. One of these estrogen-induced proteins is the progesterone receptor (PR). Progesterone and synthetic progestins activate the receptor, provoke its phosphorylation and DNA-binding ability, and induce its regulatory activities. Since the PR is an estrogen-inducible protein, its expression is indicative of an intact estrogen receptor pathway and may identify tumors that are hormonally responsive to estrogen, thereby improving the overall predictive value of steroid receptor assays in selected tumors such as breast carcinoma.

The PR displays the typical three-domain structure of the steroid-thyroid receptor family, with the central domain containing two "zinc finger" structures responsible for the specific recognition of the cognate DNA sequences. The carboxyl-terminal domain contains the hormone and anti-hormone binding sites. The complete organization of the human PR gene has been determined. It spans over 90 kb and contains eight exons. The first exon encodes the N-terminal part of the receptor, the DNA binding domain is encoded by two exons, each corresponding to one zinc finger, and the steroid binding domain is encoded by five exons.

The signal responsible for the nuclear localization of the PR is a complex one. The receptor continuously shuttles between the nucleus and cytoplasm. The receptor diffuses into the cytoplasm and is constantly and actively transported back into the nucleus, similar to the phenomenon for estradiol and glucocorticosteroid receptors. Immunolocalization of PR is confined to the nucleus.

Applications

The value of estrogen and progesterone receptor assays in predicting response to hormonal treatment in advanced breast cancer patients has been well supported both by studies employing cytosol-based ligand binding methods and by immunohistochemical assays, the prognostic utility being strongest in premenopausal women. Approximately 50% of breast cancers are ER+/PR+, 20% ER+/PR−, 5% ER−/PR+, and 25% ER−/PR−.

Those women whose cancers express both ER and PR show the greatest likelihood of responding to endocrine treatment. Using conventional biochemical assays, the response rate is about 77% for ER+/PR+ tumors, 46% for ER−/PR+, 27% for ER+/PR−, and 11% for ER−/PR− tumors. However, it is clinically recognized that a small proportion of women with tumors that are receptor-negative will show a positive response to hormonal therapy, and as many as one-third of those with receptor-positive tumors may fail to respond to such treatment. The significance of breast carcinomas biochemically negative for estrogen receptor (ER), but positive for PR, is poorly understood. It has been proposed that these tumors, more common in younger women, contain ER whose presence is masked in a biochemical binding assay by endogenous estrogen. Such tumors should be positive for ER by immunocytochemical assay, but this was not proven in one study, which found that ER−/PR+ tended to have larger tumor size and higher histologic grade and S-phase fractions compared to ER+/PR+ tumors. It was concluded that biochemically ER−PR+ breast carcinomas are biologically different from ER+/PR+ tumors.

There has been some suggestion that PR may be a more important predictor, as there are more responders among patients with ER−/PR+ compared to ER+/PR− tumors. In some series, the prognostic advantage of steroid receptor positivity was lost after 4–5 years of follow-up. As with the estrogen receptor, there is increasing evidence that immunohistological assays provide more accurate prognostication than cytosol-based methods.

Comments

We employ PgR-ICA, which is enhanced following HIER. Immunostaining is further enhanced following HIER in Target Retrieval Solution (Dako) as compared to citrate buffer. Consistent immunostaining is obtained in cytological preparations that have been fixed in 10% formalin following complete air-drying. HIER should be used.

Selected references

Keshgegian AA. Biochemically estrogen receptor-negative, progesterone receptor-positive breast carcinoma. Immunocytochemical hormone receptors and prognostic factors. *Archives of Pathology and Laboratory Medicine* 1994; 118: 240–4.

Leong AS-Y, Milios J. Comparison of antibodies to estrogen and progesterone receptors and the influence of microwave antigen retrieval. *Applied Immunohistochemistry* 1993; 1: 282–8.

MacGrogan G, Soubeyran I, De Mascarei I, *et al.* Immunohistochemical detection of progesterone receptors in breast invasive ductal carcinomas: a correlative study of 942 cases. *Applied Immunohistochemistry* 1996; 4: 219–27.

Protein gene product 9.5 (PGP 9.5)

Sources/clones

Accurate (31A3, 13C4), Biogenesis (31A3, 13C4).

Fixation/preparation

HIER enhances immunostaining in paraffin-embedded sections in citrate buffer at pH 6.0.

Background

Protein gene product 9.5 (PGP 9.5) is a ubiquitin carboxyl-terminal hydrolase whose gene is mapped to chromosome 4p14, spans 10 kb, and contains nine exons. It displays 5′ features, some common to many genes and others common with neurofilament neuron-specific enolase and Thy-1-antigen gene 5′ regions. PGP 9.5 is a 27 kDa soluble protein which has been shown by immunostaining in all levels of the central and peripheral nervous system and in many neuroendocrine cells, part of the renal tubule, spermatogonia, and non-pregnant corpus luteum. Benign and neoplastic follicular center lymphoid cells also stain for the antigen.

There is some evidence from studies in glioma cell lines that the protein is maximally expressed during the growth phase and that it may play a role in glial cells during brain development, in reactive gliosis, or in tumorigenesis of the glial lineage. PGP 9.5 has been demonstrated in pituitary adenoma, medullary carcinoma of thyroid, pancreatic islet cell tumor, paraganglioma, neuroblastoma, carcinoid tumors from a variety of sites, and Merkel cell carcinoma.

PGP 9.5 is now thought to be a neurospecific peptide that functions to remove ubiquitin from ubiquitinated proteins and prevents them from targeted degradation by proteasomes. Thus, in neoplasms, the increased deubiquitination of cyclins by PGP 9.5 could contribute to the uncontrolled growth of somatic cells that is the hallmark of cancer. PGP 9.5 overexpression has been negatively correlated with outcome in pancreatic and colorectal carcinoma. Interestingly, the examination of gene expression with the SAGE method has demonstrated the presence of PGP 9.5 transcripts in normal lung epithelium, lung tumor cell lines, and resected primary non-small-cell lung carcinoma, suggesting that increased expression of PGP 9.5 may have a role in carcinogenesis.

Applications

PGP 9.5 is distinct from neuron-specific enolase (NSE) and is largely employed as a marker of nervous and neuroendocrine differentiation. However, it is of low specificity, as shown in a study of bronchial carcinomas where, like NSE, PGP 9.5 actually labeled more cases of non-small-cell tumors than small-cell lesions. PGP 9.5 has the advantage of producing a more intense stain with less background than NSE, but if used as a marker of neural and neuroendocrine differentiation, it must be employed in conjunction with chromogranin and synaptophysin, which are more specific markers for this purpose. Other applications of PGP 9.5 include the study of unmyelinated nerve fibers in the skin and colonic mucosa, atrial myxomas, and inclusion bodies in the central nervous system.

PGP 9.5 may also be a useful marker for the identification of malignant peripheral nerve sheath tumors, which often display a lack of S100 protein, especially in the epithelioid variant. However, PGP 9.5 also has low specificity, as it has been found in synovial sarcomas and leiomyosarcomas.

Comments

Before the advent of HIER, it was recommended that fresh tissues be fixed in a solution of 95% alcohol–5% acetic acid for 2–3 hours to obtain optimal results. This is no longer necessary, as HIER produces marked enhancement of immunoreactivity compared to other methods of antigen unmasking, with both increased numbers of positive-staining cells and increased intensity of reaction within individual cells and their processes.

Selected references

Edwards YH, Fox MF, Povey S, Hinks LJ. The gene for human neuron specific ubiquitin C-terminal hydrolase (UCHL1, PGP9.5) maps to chromosome 4p14. *Annals of Human Genetics* 1991; 55: 273–8.

Giambanco I, Bianchi R, Ceccarelli P, *et al.* "Neuron-specific" protein gene product 9.5 (PGP 9.5) is also expressed in glioma cell lines and its expression depends on the cellular growth state. *FEBS Letters* 1991; 290: 131–4.

Gosney JR, Gosney MA, Lye M, Butt SA. Reliability of commercially available immunocytochemical markers for identification of neuroendocrine differentiation in bronchoscopic biopsies of bronchial carcinoma. *Thorax* 1995; 50: 116–20.

Hibi K, Westra WH, Borges M, *et al.* PGP9.5 as a candidate tumor marker for non-small-cell lung cancer. *American Journal of Pathology* 1999; 155: 711–15.

Rode J, Dhillon AP, Doran JF, *et al.* PGP 9.5, a new marker for human neuroendocrine tumors. *Histopathology* 1985; 9; 147–58.

Proto-oncogene tyrosine-protein kinase 1 (ROS1)

Sources/clones
Cell Signaling (D4D6).

Fixation/preparation
- Formalin-fixed paraffin-embedded tissues are suitable.
- Deparaffinize slides using xylene or xylene alternative and graded alcohols.
- Suitable for automated slide staining system.

Background
Proto-oncogene tyrosine-protein kinase 1 (ROS1) is a receptor tyrosine kinase (RTK) of the insulin receptor family. The *ROS1* gene is located on chromosome 6q22. The protein encoded by this gene is a type I integral membrane protein with tyrosine kinase activity. The protein may function as a growth or differentiation factor receptor. Mutations of the *ROS1* gene were originally described in glioblastoma, but more recently they have also been associated with non-small-cell lung carcinoma and cholangiocarcinoma. A small percentage of lung adenocarcinoma (2%) are associated with ROS1 fusions. These patients are usually younger-age light smokers or never-smokers. Tyrosine kinase inhibitor drugs, such as crizotinib, have been shown to cause reduction in tumor burden in those cases of lung adenocarcinoma harboring ROS1 fusion shrinkage.

Applications
Antibodies against ROS1 can be used in the selection of lung adenocarcinomas that are more likely to respond to tyrosine kinase inhibitor drugs (crizotinib). Another possible application is the identification of ALK– inflammatory myofibroblastic tumors (IMTs) with ROS1 rearrangement. These IMTs with ROS1 rearrangement can be potential candidates for targeted therapy directed against ROS1.

Staining pattern

IHC expression in selected neoplasm	IHC staining pattern
Inflammatory myofibroblastic tumor	Cytoplasmic and/or nuclear[a]
ROS1 rearranged lung adenocarcinoma	Granular to diffuse cytoplasmic

[a] Based on one report (Hornick et al. 2014).

Selected references

Bergethon K, Shaw AT, Ou SH, et al. ROS1 rearrangements define a unique molecular class of lung cancers. *Journal of Clinical Oncology* 2012; 30: 863–70.

Charest A, Lane K, McMahon K, et al. Fusion of FIG to the receptor tyrosine kinase ROS in a glioblastoma with an interstitial del(6)(q21q21). *Genes, Chromosomes, and Cancer* 2003; 37: 58–71.

Gu TL, Deng X, Huang F, et al. Survey of tyrosine kinase signaling reveals ROS kinase fusions in human cholangiocarcinoma. *PloS ONE* 2011; 6: e15640.

Hornick JL, Sholl LM, Lovly CM. Expression of ROS1 predicts ROS1 gene rearrangement in inflammatory myofibroblastic tumors. *Modern Pathology* 2014; 27: 18A.

Lindeman NI, Cagle PT, Beasley MB, et al. Molecular testing guideline for selection of lung cancer patients for EGFR and ALK tyrosine kinase inhibitors: guideline from the College of American Pathologists, International Association for the Study of Lung Cancer, and Association for Molecular Pathology. *Archives of Pathology and Laboratory Medicine* 2013; 137: 828–60.

Sholl LM, Sun H, Butaney M, et al. ROS1 immunohistochemistry for detection of ROS1-rearranged lung adenocarcinomas. *American Journal of Surgical Pathology* 2013; 37: 1441–9.

Yoshida A, Tsuta K, Wakai S, *et al.* Immunohistochemical detection of ROS1 is useful for identifying ROS1 rearrangements in lung cancers. *Modern Pathology* 2014; 27: 711–20.

pS2

Sources/clones

Biogenex (PS2.1), Dako (BC04), Labvision Corp. (PS2.1, R47-94).

Fixation/preparation

The antigen survives formalin fixation and is enhanced by HIER.

Background

pS2 is a 6.66 kDa 60 amino acid secretory polypeptide protein that was isolated from the breast carcinoma cell line MCF-7. It belongs to a family of trefoil-shaped growth factors which includes human intestinal trefoil factor (hITF) and human spasmolytic polypeptide (hSP). Although its exact function is unknown, it is believed to be part of a steroid-dependent stimulatory pathway. An estrogen-regulated protein, it has been studied as a marker of an intact estrogen pathway, and hence marker hormone sensitivity and favorable prognosis in breast carcinoma. There is growing evidence that members of the trefoil peptide family are involved in active maintenance of the integrity of gastrointestinal mucosa and facilitating its repair.

Applications

pS2 positivity is preferentially expressed in hormone-dependent cells in breast cancer. Low concentrations of the protein have been associated with a poor prognosis, while strong expression predicts responsiveness to endocrine treatment. The five-year recurrence-free survival and overall survival were 85% and 95% respectively for estrogen receptor (ER)+/progesterone receptor (PR)+/pS2+ tumors, but only 50% and 54% for patients with ER+/PR+/pS2− tumors.

In advanced breast cancer cases, 75% of pS2+ cases had stable disease, complete remission, or partial remission, compared with 37% of the pS2− cases. It is proposed that pS2 may help differentiate the 35–50% of ER+ breast cancer patients who do not clinically respond to hormone therapy, and the rare ER− patients who do. While pS2 immunostaining correlates with age, estrogen receptor and progesterone receptor status, it is not an independent prognostic factor and is not an indicator of increased survival in breast cancer. pS2 is thus best viewed as an estrogen receptor-associated protein and not an independent prognostic marker. It has been suggested that pS2 expression in breast cancers with BRCA1 mutation was significantly lower than in sporadic breast cancer.

pS2 is widely distributed throughout the gastrointestinal tract, particularly adjacent to damaged mucosa. It is consistently expressed in superficial and foveolar epithelium of non-neoplastic gastric mucosa and in 65% of gastric carcinomas, but has little value as a prognostic indicator. Colorectal carcinoma stains with pS2 to a lesser extent, but this too lacks statistical significance.

Expression in normal pancreas is usually absent, but it can be seen focally within occasional ducts in chronic pancreatitis and it is prominent in pancreatic adenocarcinoma and ampullary tumors.

Selected references

May FE, Westley BR. Trefoil proteins: their role in normal and malignant cells. *Journal of Pathology* 1997; 183: 4–7.

Poulsom R. Trefoil peptides. *Baillières Clinical Gastroenterology* 1996; 10: 113–34.

Wysocki SJ, Iacopetta BJ, Ingram DM. Prognostic significance of pS2 mRNA in breast cancer. *European Journal of Cancer* 1994; 30A: 1882–4.

NOTES

PSA (prostate-specific antigen)

Sources/clones

Accurate (ER-PR8), Biodesign (8), Biogenesis (PSA-001, 07), Biogenex (8), Dako (ER-PR8, polyclonal), Enzo, Hybritech, Immunotech, Oncogene (OS94.3), Oxoid (PSB535), Sanbio (8), Serotec (SC.5), Zymed (2009).

Fixation/preparation

The antigen is resistant to formalin fixation and immunostaining is enhanced by HIER.

Background

Prostate-specific antigen (PSA) is a chymotrypsin-like, 33 kDa single chain glycoprotein with selective serine protease activity for cleaving specific peptides. The PSA gene is a member of the human kallikrein gene family and is located on the 13q region of chromosome 19. PSA is selectively produced by the epithelial cells of the acini and ducts of the prostate gland and is secreted into the semen, where it is directly involved in the liquefaction of the seminal coagulum that is formed at ejaculation. The sequence of PSA shows extensive homology with γ-nerve growth factor (56%), epidermal growth factor-binding protein (53%), and OC-nerve growth factor (51%). This feature, together with its ability to digest insulin growth factor-binding protein-III (IGFBP-3) to release biologically active IGF-I, makes PSA a candidate growth factor or a cytokine or modulator of cell growth. PSA has also been suggested to be capable of being produced by cells bearing steroid hormone receptors under conditions of steroid hormone stimulation.

Applications

PSA is a useful biochemical marker, as any disruption of the normal architecture of the prostate allows diffusion of PSA into the stoma where it gains access to the peripheral blood through the microvasculature. Elevated serum PSA levels are thus seen with prostatitis, infarcts, benign hyperplasia, and transiently after manipulation and biopsy. Most importantly, significant elevations are seen with prostatic adenocarcinoma, making it an important tool for diagnosis as well as monitoring response to treatment. Although cancer produces less PSA per cell than normal prostatic epithelium, the greater number of malignant cells and the disruption of stroma in the malignant gland accounts for the elevated serum PSA levels.

Immunostaining for PSA has proven to be an effective method of identifying cells of prostatic origin; however, the presence of PSA cannot be used to differentiate between benign and malignant. Antibodies to PSA show high sensitivity, although very occasionally carcinomas have been reported to be negative for PSA. Correlations of PSA tissue reactivity with Gleason's grade of prostatic cancer have shown that high-grade tumors may be entirely negative by immunolabeling. There was an initial suggestion that the presence of PSA-negative cells in a prostatic carcinoma correlates with a more aggressive clinical course, but this has not been confirmed and most tumors display very heterogeneous staining.

Comments

As the occasional case of prostatic carcinoma and metastatic deposit may show only weak or no staining for PSA, it is best to use this marker in conjunction with other markers of prostatic tissue such as prostate-specific acid phosphatase (PSAP) and CD57 (Leu-7). A combination of these three markers gives the highest diagnostic yield (Appendix 1.15). Furthermore, immunoreactivity to PSA has been shown in a variety of extraprostatic tissues including the epithelium of the urethra, periurethral glands of both males and females, urachal remnants, endometrium transitional epithelium of the bladder, and in cystitis cystica and glandularis, anal mucosa and anal glands, ductal cells of the normal pancreas and normal salivary glands. PSA immunoreactivity is also seen in urethral and periurethral gland adenocarcinoma, extramammary Paget's disease of the penis, and pleomorphic adenoma and carcinoma of the salivary gland. PSA has been found in breast carcinoma cells and was initially suggested to confer a positive prognosis, but more recent controlled studies have not confirmed this earlier finding. Neutrophils and some neuroendocrine tumors also stain for PSA.

Small, closely apposed Cowper's glands can mimic neoplastic prostatic glands especially in core biopsies, and can be distinguished by the absence of prostatic markers such as PSA, PSAP, and carcinoembryonic antigen. While Cowper's glands, like malignant prostatic glands, do not stain for high-molecular-weight cytokeratin, they show a peripheral layer of attenuated myoepithelial cells which can be highlighted by staining for smooth muscle actin.

Specificity is improved by using the monoclonal antibodies. We have had consistent results with clone ER-PR8 from Dako when used with microwave-induced retrieval.

Selected reference

Bostwick DG. Prostate-specific antigen: current role in diagnostic pathology of prostatic cancer. *American Journal of Clinical Pathology* 1994; 102 (Suppl 1): S31–7.

PSAP (prostate-specific acid phosphatase)

Sources/clones

Accurate (P-29, 4LJ, SB19), Biodesign, Biogenesis (501, 503, 504), Biogenex (045), Camon, Chemicon, Dako (PASE/4LJ, polyclonal), Diagnostic, Immunotech (PAP29), Milab/Med, Novocastra, Oxoid (PAY376), Sanbio (4LJ), Saxon, Sera Lab (8), Serotec, Sigma (PAP12, PAP29), Zymed (ZMPAP4).

Fixation/preparation

Both polyclonal and monoclonal antibodies are immunoreactive in fixed paraffin-embedded tissues, and staining is enhanced by HIER.

Background

Acid phosphatases hydrolyze phosphoric acid esters at acid pH. They are found in a variety of tissues, and differences in electrophoretic patterns or sensitivity to isoenzyme inhibitors allowed the distinction of isoforms of the enzyme to specific tissues. Normal prostatic tissue contains several isoforms, but only two are secreted in the seminal fluid. Acid phosphatase activity is mainly localized to the lysosomes of prostatic epithelial cells and ultrastructurally is identified within microvilli of the apical cell membranes and in the secretory granules at the supranuclear or apical regions of benign cells. Although synthesized in rough endoplasmic reticulum, PSAP is not demonstrable in this site, and because it is only recognized in lysosomes it is assumed that antibodies recognize PSAP only when packaged into granules. Basal cells are negative for PSAP. Serum levels of the enzyme reflect the amount of enzyme released into the circulation and are dependent on the tumor mass and also the rate of synthesis and access to the intravascular space. Low levels of the enzyme have been suggested to represent low rates of synthesis by poorly differentiated tumors.

Applications

PSAP immunostaining is a useful discriminator for prostatic tissue, and its diagnostic specificity and sensitivity is increased when used in a panel in conjunction with prostate-specific antigen (PSA) and CD57 (Leu-7). As with PSA, immunoreactivity for PSAP is more intense and homogeneous in benign prostatic tissue than in prostatic carcinoma. PSAP is localized within prostatic acini and ducts, although the latter tend to show weaker and more heterogeneous staining.

Rare cases of squamous metaplasia of the prostatic epithelium show staining for PSAP. There is weak positivity in seminal vesicle epithelium and, like PSA, periurethral glands in both men and women are positive for the enzyme. Other non-prostatic tissues that may show PSAP immunostaining are anal glands in men, neuroendocrine cells of the rectum, transitional epithelium and von Brun's nests of the bladder, renal tubular epithelium, pancreatic islet cells, hepatocytes, gastric parietal cells, and mammary ductal epithelium. Neutrophils show the strongest concentration of PSAP among non-prostatic tissues. Neoplasms that show cross-reactivity are mainly those derived from the cloaca, such as urinary bladder, periurethral glands, and colon, and neuroendocrine tumors.

Comments

In general, PSAP is relatively specific for prostatic neoplasms. However, because of the cross-reactivity of both PSAP and PSA with the tissues listed above, it is still best to use PSAP in conjunction with PSA, particularly in the context of a tumor in the perineum whose differential diagnosis includes prostatic carcinoma, transitional carcinoma and adenocarcinoma of the bladder, and rectal carcinoma. Besides PSAP and PSA, the panel should include an antibody to high-molecular-weight cytokeratin, CK20 and CK7 (Appendix 1.15). Cowper's glands may mimic prostatic adenocarcinoma because they are small closely packed acini lined by a single cell layer and do not stain for high-molecular-weight cytokeratin. However, these glands do not stain for prostatic markers such as PSAP, PSA, and carcinoembryonic antigen and show an attenuated myoepithelial cell layer in the periphery, staining with smooth muscle actin.

Acid phosphatase consists of several isoenzymes, and polyclonal antibodies to PSAP cross-react with isoenzyme 4, which is present in small amounts in most human tissues.

Furthermore, polyclonal antibodies recognize several antigenic sites and may produce weak background staining, but this is not seen with monoclonal antibodies that recognize only one antigenic site. Clone PASE/4LJ from Dako produces satisfactory results.

Selected reference

Epstein JI. PSA and PAP as immunohistochemical markers in prostatic cancer. *Urologic Clinics of North America* 1993; 20: 757–70.

PTEN (phosphatase and tensin homolog deleted on chromosome 10)

Sources/clones

Dako (6H2.1), Life Technologies (PN37), Millipore (A2b1), SpringBio (SP170).

Fixation/preparation

- Formalin-fixed paraffin-embedded tissues are suitable.
- Deparaffinize slides using xylene or xylene alternative and graded alcohols.
- Suitable for automated slide staining system.

Background

Phosphatase and tensin homolog deleted on chromosome 10 (PTEN) is a human protein encoded by the *PTEN* gene. PTEN is a dual protein/lipid phosphatase and its main substrate, phosphatidylinositol-3,4,5-trisphosphate (PIP3), is the product of PI3K. Increase in PIP3 recruits Akt to the membrane where it is activated by other kinases. PTEN contains a tensin-like domain as well as a catalytic domain similar to that of the dual-specificity protein tyrosine phosphatases. *PTEN* is a tumor suppressor gene that is mutated in a large number of cancers and some syndromes (notably Cowden syndrome and Bannayan–Riley–Ruvalcaba syndrome). Unlike most of the protein tyrosine phosphatases, this protein preferentially dephosphorylates phosphoinositide substrates. It negatively regulates intracellular levels of PIP3 in cells and functions as a tumor suppressor by negatively regulating the Akt/PKB signaling pathway. *PTEN* gene mutations have been reported in many types of cancer, and studies suggest that *PTEN* may be the most frequently mutated gene in prostate cancer and endometrial cancer.

Applications

Reduced expression of PTEN has been reported in a variety of malignancies, including breast, prostate, and endometrial cancer. In some cancers, loss of PTEN expression has been shown to correlate with poor prognosis.

Staining pattern

IHC expression in selected neoplasm	IHC staining pattern
Breast carcinoma	Cytoplasmic and/or nuclear
Endometrial carcinoma	Cytoplasmic and/or nuclear
Pancreatic endocrine carcinoma	Cytoplasmic and/or nuclear
Colorectal carcinoma	Cytoplasmic and/or nuclear

Selected references

Djordjevic B, Hennessy BT, Li J, *et al*. Clinical assessment of PTEN loss in endometrial carcinoma: immunohistochemistry outperforms gene sequencing. *Modern Pathology* 2012; 25: 699–708.

Foo WC, Rashid A, Wang H, *et al*. Loss of phosphatase and tensin homolog expression is associated with recurrence and poor prognosis in patients with pancreatic ductal adenocarcinoma, *Human Pathology* 2013; 44: 1024–30.

Govender D, Chetty R. Gene of the month: PTEN. *Journal of Clinical Pathology* 2012; 65: 601–3.

McMenamin ME, Soung P, Perera S, *et al*. Loss of PTEN expression in paraffin-embedded primary prostate cancer correlates with high Gleason score and advanced stage. *Cancer Research* 1999; 59: 4291–6.

Perren A, Weng LP, Boag AH, *et al*. Immunohistochemical evidence of loss of PTEN expression in primary ductal adenocarcinomas of the breast. *American Journal of Pathology* 1999; 155: 1253–60.

NOTES

Rabies

Sources/clones

Accurate (HYB-3R7), Biodesign, Biogenesis (RAB50), Chemicon International (C4-62-15-2), Research Diagnostics (RV7C5).

Fixation/preparation

Anti-rabies monoclonal antibody may be applied to acetone-fixed samples. It is also potentially applicable to formalin-fixed paraffin-embedded tissue sections, although optimization will be necessary with some form of antigen retrieval.

Background

Rabies is a rod- or bullet-shaped virus with a single-stranded RNA genome, and belongs to the family Rhabdoviridae. It is a highly fatal disease of humans and warm-blooded vertebrates, usually transmitted via infected saliva following the bite of a diseased animal, most commonly dogs. Virus introduced into the bite wound enters the peripheral nerves and, following an incubation of weeks to months, spreads to the spinal cord and brain. It produces a neurological derangement, lasting a few days to weeks and resulting in death.

Antibody C4-62-15-2 to rabies virus is specific to the N-nucleoprotein. It enjoys a wide range of species reactivity, including mouse, raccoon, skunk, dog/coyote, and bats.

Applications

During prolonged incubation periods, the sensory neurons of the dorsal root ganglia may be the site of viral sequestration. Efferent spread of virus in the nervous system may extend terminally to the eye and nerve fibers surrounding hair follicles. Hence, demonstration of antigen in corneal impression smears or skin biopsies may be used for confirmation of diagnosis in a live patient. Unless the diagnosis is confirmed during life, an autopsy must be performed with 10–20 mm^3 blocks of cerebrum, cerebellum, hippocampus, medulla, thalamus, and brainstem being taken in duplicate: 50% glycerol-saline for virological examination and 10% buffered formalin for immunohistological examination.

Comments

Antibody to rabies is useful in locating the Negri bodies in sections of brain. In one study of naturally infected domestic and wild animals, rabies antigen was detected in 62% of the brain areas in which inclusion bodies were not found. The antigen is not limited to the Negri bodies but also traceable in the cytoplasm. Most of the work with rabies antibodies has been performed on fresh tissue with direct immunofluorescence techniques, although application to formalin-fixed tissue has met with good success.

Selected references

Feiden W, Feiden U, Gerhard L, et al. Rabies encephalitis: immunohistochemical investigations. *Clinical Neuropathology* 1985; 4: 156–64.

Jogai S, Radotra BD, Banerjee AK. Immunohistochemical study of human rabies. *Neuropathology* 2000; 20: 197–203.

NOTES

Retinoblastoma gene protein (P110^{RB}, Rb protein)

Sources/clones

Accurate (84B311), Biodesign (RB1, 1F8), Biogenesis (RB), Dako (Rb1), Lab Vision (1F8), Novocastra (Rb1), Oncogene Research (AF11, LM95.1), Pharmingen (245), Santa Cruz Lab (C-15).

Fixation/preparation

The antibodies are mostly immunoreactive only in fresh frozen sections. Some antibodies stain fixed paraffin-embedded sections, but only after HIER.

Background

The *RB* gene is located on chromosome 13q14 and spans a region of more than 200 kb, including 27 exons. The Rb protein (p110^{RB}) is the only tumor suppressor that has been shown to directly suppress tumor formation. It is a cell cycle regulator preventing cells from entering the S-phase. The Rb protein has a molecular weight of 105 kDa, and a number of antibodies which recognize specific parts of this protein have been developed. Besides loss of function due to chromosomal abnormalities including chromosomal deletion, translocation, and point mutation, as with p53, phosphorylation may inactivate the Rb protein. In addition, a variety of viral oncoproteins including simian virus 40T antigen, E1A from adenovirus, and E6 from human papillomavirus may bind and inactivate the Rb protein.

Immunostaining may be a valid way to assess the presence of normal Rb protein, but several factors affecting staining should be considered before accepting the relevance of the technique. Firstly, it has been observed that the level of expression of Rb protein is not the same in all cells in any individual tissue, e.g., in the epithelium of the cervix there are low or undetectable levels of staining in the basal layers and staining increases with cell maturation. In contrast, low or absent anti-Rb protein staining has been observed in the well-differentiated epithelial cells of the gastric mucosa such as the foveolar and mucus cells, compared to the cells in the crypts and neck of the glands. Astrocytes and microglia do not show detectable Rb protein by immunostaining, and other subsets of normal cells such as some stromal cells do not display demonstrable Rb protein. The reasons for failure to demonstrate the protein at an equivalent level in all cells may relate to variations in expression as a function of cell cycling activity, cell differentiation, and protein phosphorylation. More importantly, there is a large subset of cells which include endothelial cells, lymphocytes, and stromal cells, in which the ability to demonstrate Rb (p110^{RB}) expression is critically dependent on the method of staining used.

Applications

The p53 and retinoblastoma gene products must be the two most-studied tumor suppressor genes. While alterations in the p53 tumor suppressor gene have been recognized as the most frequent genetic alterations in human neoplasia, the extent of Rb gene alterations is less well known. p53 alterations are mostly detected as overexpression of the protein in immunostaining, whereas most normal cells do not contain stainable wild-type p53 protein. In contrast, the Rb protein is detectable immunohistochemically in normal non-transformed cells, although whether this is so for all normal cells and tissues is currently unknown. As abnormality is based on the absence of stainable Rb protein, it is critical that techniques of maximal sensitivity must be employed, and internal positive controls must be present in the sections.

Alterations in the *RB* gene have been described in a number of human tumors including retinoblastoma, osteosarcoma, other sarcomas, leukemias, lymphomas, and certain carcinomas including those from the breast, prostate,

Retinoblastoma gene protein

lung, bladder, kidney, and testis. *RB* gene alterations have been associated with increasing tumor grade and stage in a variety of tumors, and there is increasing evidence that alterations of this gene are associated with increased risk for metastasis. In breast carcinoma there is some evidence of association with other signs of progression and loss of hormonal receptor expression. A downregulation of the *RB* gene has been shown in the progression of melanocytic tumors, and loss of expression correlated with increase in Clark level and shorter survival rates. All nevi with and without dysplasia showed high expression, and a large percentage of primary melanomas showed Rb-positive cells. There was loss of immunostaining for Rb protein in ovarian carcinomas compared to benign and borderline tumors, and this loss correlated with a higher proliferative index and loss of heterozygosity at the Rb-1 locus. In clear cell renal carcinoma, increased Rb protein and decreased p27 immunoexpression are claimed to be powerful and independent poor prognostic factors.

Rb protein immunohistochemistry is negative in cellular angiofibromas, extramammary myofibroblastomas, and spindle cell lipoma.

Comments

It has been demonstrated that HIER in citrate buffer at pH 6.0 with overnight antibody incubation produced maximal sensitivity when staining fixed paraffin-embedded sections. Fixation in methacarn also requires HIER treatment, and the use of DNAse has produced variable results. The use of low pH buffers can produce false-positive results. Thus, in the assessment of Rb protein, as with other fixation-sensitive antigens, it is clear that the findings of individual laboratories cannot be generalized, owing to differences in fixation and immunolabeling techniques. However, these factors do not preclude the assessment of the Rb protein in laboratories where fixation and other variables are strictly controlled.

Selected reference

Cordon-Cardo C, Richon VM. Expression of the retinoblastoma protein is regulated in normal human tissues. *American Journal of Pathology* 1994; 144: 500–10.

S100

Sources/clones

Accurate (polyclonal), Biodesign (polyclonal), Biogenesis (15E2E2, polyclonal), Biogenex (15E2E2, polyclonal), Chemicon (monoclonal, polyclonal), Cymbus Bioscience (MIG5), Dako (polyclonal), ICN (polyclonal), Immunotech (polyclonal), Medac (S1/61/69), Novocastra (polyclonal), Oncogene (OS94.5), RDI (MIG-5), Sera Lab (polyclonal), Serotec (polyclonal), Sigma (polyclonal), Zymed (polyclonal).

Fixation/preparation

Formalin-fixed tissues are ideally suited for S100 immunostaining, and the antigen is resistant to long durations of fixation in formalin. Its reactivity can still be enhanced by heat-induced antigen retrieval but not by proteolytic digestion.

Background

S100 protein, so named because of its solubility in a saturated ammonium sulfate solution, occurs as three biochemically distinct forms. Each is a protein dimer of two subunits, designated α and β. The three dimers are $S100A_0$ ($\alpha-\alpha$), S100A ($\alpha-\beta$), and S100B ($\beta-\beta$). The α- and β-subunits each have a molecular weight of approximately 10.5 kDa, with extensive amino acid sequence homology between the two subunits. They both have amino acid sequences known to code for the calcium binding sites of the calmodulin family of proteins. S100 is highly acidic and water-soluble, with varying affinities for calcium, zinc, and manganese. These properties are related to many basic cell functions such as cation diffusion across lipid membranes, microtubule assembly and stability, calcium and cyclic nucleotide regulation and increased activity of RNA polymerase, drug–protein interactions, the plasma membrane function of neurons and interaction with chromosomes and synaptosomes. S100 protein is conserved in nature and is present within the cells of all three germ layers in humans, a reflection of its important role in basic cell function.

Applications

S100 has been demonstrated in a wide variety of normal and abnormal tissues. Formalin fixation and paraffin embedding may alter antigenic sites, and aldehyde fixation may prevent diffusion of the highly soluble antigen that can produce artifactual immunolocalization patterns. Indeed, one study has reported granular staining of virtually every cell type when fresh frozen tissue was stained with a monoclonal S100 antibody.

Normal and neoplastic cartilaginous tissue including benign and malignant chondroid tumors express S100 protein, and thus it is useful for the distinction of non-cartilaginous bone tumors, which are mostly negative for the antigen. Cartilaginous tumors can be distinguished from chordomas by the presence of cytokeratin and epithelial membrane antigen (EMA) in the latter and their absence in the former. S100 is also useful for the labeling of myoepithelial cells in mammary ducts, particularly when distinguishing sclerosing adenosis from tubular carcinomas, the former displaying a distinct layer of myoepithelial cells. Sustentacular or satellite cells of the adrenal medulla and paraganglia and their corresponding tumors are labeled by S100 antibodies, as are the folliculostellate cells of the anterior pituitary.

The S100 antigen is a useful marker of peripheral nerve cells. The protein is present in the nuclei and cytoplasm of Schwann cells and satellite cells in parasympathetic and sympathetic ganglia. The β-subunit has been reported in these cells but not in neurons, the latter contain the α-subunit that is not expressed in Schwann cells or satellite cells. Pacinian corpuscles also contain S100 protein. While S100 protein is expressed diffusely in the majority of benign nerve sheath tumors, as many as 40–50% of malignant

Schwann cells do not stain and/or show patchy, focal S100 staining. A population of S100+ Schwann cells can be demonstrated in neurofibromas, but variable numbers of perineural and intermediate cells within these tumors do not stain for S100 protein. Correspondingly, neurogenic sarcomas arising in patients with neurofibromatosis show a spectrum of expression of S100 protein. Both benign and malignant granular cell tumors contain S100 protein expressed as the β-subunit, a feature used to support an origin from Schwann cells.

The other group of cells which are labeled by S100 antibodies are the histiocytes. The interdigitating reticulum cells of the paracortical areas in the lymph node are stained by S100 protein antibodies, as are dendritic reticulum cells of the lymphoid follicles. Langerhans cells of the skin, mucous membranes, and other sites are also positive for S100, expressing S100B (β–β) activity. S100 protein is therefore a useful marker for the identification of Langerhans cell histiocytosis.

One of the most useful applications of the S100 protein is its use as a marker of nevus cells and melanomas. Virtually all benign melanocytic lesions contain S100 protein, which is also observed in over 95% of malignant melanomas. When used in conjunction with a panel comprising cytokeratin, vimentin, and LCA, it allows the separation of malignant melanoma from its common mimics, namely, anaplastic carcinoma and large-cell lymphoma. Similarly, the inclusion of anti-CEA forms a useful panel to distinguish Bowen's disease, Paget's disease of the skin, and superficial spreading malignant melanoma. Because a small number of melanomas may fail to express S100 protein, antibodies to HMB-45 and the melanoma-associated antigen NKI/C3 are useful additional markers for melanoma.

S100 protein is expressed by adipocytes, and a proportion of liposarcomas also stains positive. Tumors of the cutaneous adnexae and salivary glands also express S100 protein.

Comments

Although S100 protein is a useful marker for the identification of melanoma, Langerhans cell histiocytosis, and peripheral nerve tumor, the antibodies should be used in the context of the differential diagnosis derived from morphologic and clinical appearances. A wide variety of carcinomas, including those from the lung, pancreas, and female genitourinary tract, as well as *Mycobacteria ulcerans* organisms, have been reported to show positivity, so S100 antibodies should not be used or interpreted in isolation. We have also observed the staining of benign skeletal and smooth muscle cells with some anti-S100 antibodies.

The use of S100 to identify residual melanoma cells in re-excision biopsies is fraught with problems, as S100+ spindle cells are often present in the scar tissue. These spindle cells may stain for neuron-specific enolase but do not label with HMB-45, Melan-A, or CD57. These cells may occur in re-excisions of non-melanoma tumors and stain with the Schwann cell differentiation markers p75NGFR, CD56/N-CAM, and GAP-43, suggesting that they represent reactive proliferating Schwann cells.

Selected references

Daimaru Y, Hashimoto H, Enjoji M. Malignant peripheral nerve sheath tumours (malignant schwannomas). An immunohistochemical study of 29 cases. *American Journal of Surgical Pathology* 1985; 9: 434–44.

Loeffel SC, Gillespie GY, Mirmiran SA, *et al.* Cellular immunolocalisation of S100 protein within fixed tissue sections by monoclonal antibodies. *Archives of Pathology and Laboratory Medicine* 1985; 109: 117–22.

Nakajima T, Watanabe S, Sato Y, *et al.* An immunoperoxidase study of S100 protein distribution in normal and neoplastic tissues. *American Journal of Surgical Pathology* 1982; 6: 715–27.

Takahashi K, Isobe T, Ohtsuki Y, *et al.* Immunohistochemical study on the distribution of alpha and beta subunits of S-100 protein in human neoplasm and normal tissues. *Virchows Archiv B. Cell Pathology Including Molecular Pathology* 1984; 45: 385–96.

SALL4

Sources/clones

Abnova, Taipei, Taiwan (6E3).

Fixation/preparation

Standardized for formalin-fixed paraffin-embedded tissue. Nuclear staining.

Background

SALL4 is a zinc finger transcription factor that shares homology to the *Drosophila* spalt (*sal*) gene. The *SALL4* gene is located on chromosome 20q13.13–13.2 and is essential for embryological development. It forms a regulatory circuit with OCT4, NANOG, and SOX2 to maintain embryonic stem cell pleuripotency and self-renewal. Immunohistochemical staining for SALL4 can be detected in all types of testicular germ cell tumors (GCTs), in contrast to OCT4, which only labels intratubular germ cell neoplasia (ITGCN), classic seminoma, and embryonal carcinoma (EC). The overall findings indicate that SALL4 is a very sensitive marker for most primary GCTs. In addition, the staining is well maintained in all metastatic tumors including seminomas, ECs, and yolk sac tumors (YSTs) with a 100% sensitivity.

GCTs can be divided into three broad genetic groups, namely, teratomas and YSTs in neonates and infants, classic seminoma and non-seminomatous GCTs in postpubertal patients, and spermatocytic seminoma in old patients. Each of these groups is thought to arise from germ cells at different stages of development. It is thought that germ cell tumors in the pediatric age group arise from the malignant transformation of either embryonic stem cells or early migrating primordial germ cells. YSTs and teratomas of the pediatric age group therefore are thought not to arise from ITGCN. In adult GCTs the malignant transformation occurs at a later stage, while in spermatocytic seminoma it is thought to occur at the stage of primary spermatocytes.

The demonstration of SALL4 in all of the above subtypes of GCTs suggests that dysregulation of SALL4 is a common factor in their pathogenesis. There is stronger staining of SALL4 in poorly differentiated GCTs than in the more differentiated teratoma and spermatocytic seminoma. This finding led them to suggest that SALL4 may be essential for maintaining the poorly differentiated status. SALL4 is an immensely helpful stain in the workup of metastatic germ cell tumors, especially when limited biopsy material is available and the differential diagnosis includes non-germ cell tumors. Below is a short discussion of selected scenarios where SALL4 forms an important and helpful component of a panel of stains.

Differentiation of metastatic germ cell tumors (GCTs) from metastatic non-germ cell tumors (NGCTs)

Seminoma, embryonal carcinoma (EC), and yolk sac tumors (YSTs) often have varied morphologic appearance and may enter the differential diagnosis in the workup of metastatic tumors. In needle biopsies only limited material may be available for immunohistochemical characterization, and therefore a concise, definitive workup is necessary. SALL4 is positive in more than 90% of the GCTs and forms an important part of a limited panel along with OCT4 and epithelial membrane antigen (EMA) and/or cytokeratin 7 (CK7). In institutions where SALL4 is not available, an alternative panel consisting of OCT4, glypican-3, and EMA can be used. A positive SALL4 rules out non-GCTs (with some exceptions – see below). A positive OCT4 is suggestive of seminoma or embryonal carcinoma. A positive SALL4 with a negative OCT4 and positive glypican-3 is consistent with YST. Inclusion of EMA is valuable in this context, as it is positive in most carcinomas but mostly negative in GCTs. Only rare seminomas (2%) and yolk sac tumors (2%) have been reported positive. Embryonal carcinomas have been reported to be positive for EMA in 2–12% of cases. If the specific differential diagnosis involves metastatic adenocarcinoma and YST, the addition of CK7 may be helpful because of its positive reactivity in most adenocarcinomas (with the notable exceptions of prostate, kidney, and colon carcinomas) and negativity in YST. Adding CK20, CDX2, PAX-8, and PSA and/or PSAP may help refine the differential diagnosis further where renal, prostate, or colon primaries are in question.

While SALL4 is highly expressed in all GCTs, it is expressed in a variety of poorly differentiated non-GCTs as well. 30% of ovarian serous carcinomas were positive but all endometrioid and clear cell carcinomas were negative. 25% of gastric adenocarcinomas showed SALL4 positivity, with a great majority showing intestinal-like differentiation with at least focal positivity for CDX2. In this context it is also interesting to note that intestinal epithelia of the mature component of teratomas also showed uniform positivity for SALL4, while the squamous epithelium only revealed focal positivity. Other tumors that show a high percentage of expression of SALL4 include high-grade urothelial carcinomas (~22%), hepatic cholangiocarcinoma and pulmonary small-cell carcinomas (~20% of the cases).

Renal rhabdoid tumors, Wilms tumors, rare cases of desmoplastic small round cell tumors, embryonal rhabdomyosarcomas of uterine cervix, and epithelioid sarcomas have been reported positive to variable degrees.

SALL4 should be used, keeping in mind that while it has a high sensitivity for GCTs, it is also positive in a subset of non-GCTS. SALL4 positivity should be interpreted in the context of a carefully selected panel of stains that best characterize the specific differential diagnosis in question. Additional GCT markers such as PLAP may be added when tumors with overlapping staining patterns are in the differential diagnosis.

Differentiation of germ cell tumors from large-cell lymphoma

Lymphoma may enter the differential diagnosis of primary testicular tumors, especially when the growth pattern is diffuse and the tumor reveals plasmacytoid features or a very high-grade histology. An important differential diagnosis is the distinction of a GCT from large-cell lymphoma. While the majority of lymphomas have a distinct quality of discohesive growth pattern, some may reveal a degree of cohesion.

High-grade nuclei are often seen in embryonal carcinoma, but are also a notable feature of anaplastic large-cell lymphoma and natural killer/T-cell type lymphomas.

A limited panel of lymphoid markers including CD45, CD20, and CD3 along with SALL4 is very useful in making the distinction.

When using SALL4 in the context of a differential diagnosis between GCT and lymphoma, one needs to keep in mind that occasional lymphoblastic lymphomas, anaplastic large-cell lymphomas, and myeloid leukemias may also be positive.

Differentiation of germ cell tumors from sex cord–stromal tumors

Sex cord–stromal tumors are histologically very distinct, and a diagnosis can usually be made with only a limited panel of stains. There are however some case of Sertoli cell tumors that may show a predominantly diffuse pattern of growth, with lymphocytic infiltrate bringing seminoma into the differential diagnosis. A growth pattern with predominantly trabecular or reticulated growth may be confused with YST. A limited panel including SALL4, inhibin, and calretinin help in the differential diagnosis. While the sex cord–stromal tumors are negative for SALL4, they stain positive for calretinin and inhibin. Inhibin is a member of the transforming growth factor-β superfamily that inhibits the production and secretion of gonadotropins from the pituitary gland. A variable number of sex cord–stromal tumors of the testis stain positive for antibodies against the α-subunit. While 100% of Leydig cell tumors are reportedly positive for α-inhibin, only 30–90% of Sertoli cell tumors are reportedly positive. The germ cell tumors will be positive for SALL4 and negative for the other two. SALL4+ tumors then can be further worked up with OCT4, glypican-3/ α-fetoprotein to differentiate between YST and seminoma. Syncytiotrophoblastic cells may be positive for inhibin, but other elements of GCTs are negative. Calretinin stains sex cord–stromal tumors similarly to inhibin.

Other uses of SALL4

SALL4 can be used for distinguishing hepatoid gastric carcinoma (which is SALL4+) from hepatocellular carcinoma (SALL4–). In the ovary YST (SALL4+) can be distinguished from clear cell carcinoma (SALL4–). SALL4 can aid in the diagnosis of extragonadal YST, which may be a challenging diagnosis without immunohistochemical markers.

Selected references

Cao D, Guo S, Allan RW, Molberg KH, Peng Y. SALL4 is a novel sensitive and specific marker of ovarian primitive germ cell tumors and is particularly useful in distinguishing yolk sac tumor from clear cell carcinoma. *American Journal of Surgical Pathology* 2009; 33: 894–904.

Cao D, Humphrey PA, Allan RW. SALL4 is a novel sensitive and specific marker for metastatic germ cell tumors, with particular utility in detection of metastatic yolk sac tumors. *Cancer* 2009; 115: 2640–51.

Cao D, Li J, Guo CC, Allan RW, Humphrey PA. SALL4 is a novel diagnostic marker for testicular germ cell tumors. *American Journal of Surgical Pathology* 2009; 33: 1065–77.

Liu A, Cheng L, Du J, *et al.* Diagnostic utility of novel stem cell markers SALL4, OCT4, NANOG, SOX2, UTF1, and TCL1 in primary mediastinal germ cell tumors. *American Journal of Surgical Pathology* 2010; 34: 697–706.

Miettinen M, Wang Z, McCue PA, *et al.* SALL4 expression in germ cell and non-germ cell tumors: a systematic immunohistochemical study of 3215 cases. *American Journal of Surgical Pathology* 2014; 38: 410–20.

Ushiku T, Shinozaki A, Shibahara J, *et al.* SALL4 represents fetal gut differentiation of gastric cancer, and is diagnostically useful in distinguishing hepatoid gastric carcinoma from hepatocellular carcinoma. *American Journal of Surgical Pathology* 2010; 34: 533–40.

Wang F, Liu A, Peng Y, *et al.* Diagnostic utility of SALL4 in extragonadal yolk sac tumors: an immunohistochemical study of 59 cases with comparison to placental-like alkaline phosphatase, alpha-fetoprotein, and glypican-3. *American Journal of Surgical Pathology* 2009; 33: 1529–39.

NOTES

SDHB (succinate dehydrogenase complex, subunit B)

Sources/clones

Abcam, rabbit monoclonal (EPR10880)
ABnova Corporation, rabbit polyclonal
Acris antibodies GmbH, rabbit polyclonal (C-terminus)
Antibodies online, rabbit polyclonal (C-terminus), rabbit polyclonal
Atlas antibodies, mouse monoclonal (CL0346, CL0347, CL0349), rabbit polyclonal
Aviva Systems Biology, rabbit polyclonal
Biorbyt, rabbit polyclonal
Bioss, rabbit polyclonal
Boster Immunoleader, rabbit polyclonal
Creative Biomart, rabbit polyclonal
Genetex, rabbit polyclonal
LifeSpan Biosciences, rabbit polyclonal
Neobiolab, polyclonal
Novus biologicals, rabbit polyclonal
OriGene, goat polyclonal (C-terminus)
Proteintech Group, rabbit polyclonal
Raybiotech, goat polyclonal (C-terminus)
Santa Cruz Technology, rabbit polyclonal
St.John's Laboratory, rabbit polyclonal
Thermo Scientific, rabbit polyclonal (N-terminus), rabbit polyclonal

Fixation/preparation

Most of these antibodies react in formalin-fixed paraffin-embedded tissue. Please refer to vendor instructions for specific antigen retrieval requirements.

Background

SDHB (succinate dehydrogenase [ubiquinone] iron-sulfur subunit, mitochondrial) is an iron-sulfur protein subunit of succinate dehydrogenase (SDH) that participates in the oxidation of succinate in the mitochondrial electron transport chain's complex II. This complex is composed of four subunits encoded by nuclear DNA named SDHA (a flavoprotein), SDHB, SDHC, and SDHD (two integral membrane proteins), and it facilitates electron transfer from succinate to ubiquinone/coenzyme Q. Complex II behaves as a tumor suppressor, since sporadic and familial mutations in the genes encoding for the different subunits (except for SDHA) have been identified in tumors such as paragangliomas, pheochromocytomas, and gastrointestinal stromal tumors, supporting evidence for a link between mitochondrial/metabolic dysfunction and tumorigenesis.

As a mitochondrial membrane protein, SDHB is expressed in practically all human tissue types, with the highest level of expression in cells containing numerous mitochondria, such as heart muscle, skeletal muscle, hepatocytes, epithelial and endocrine cells, and others, all of which can be used as positive controls.

Applications

Pheochromocytomas are predominantly sporadic neuroendocrine tumors of the adrenal medulla, and paragangliomas likely represent their extra-adrenal counterpart, arising in neural crest-derived peripheral autonomic paraganglia. However, both tumor types can occur in several hereditary tumor syndromes, including neurofibromatosis type 1, von-Hippel–Lindau syndrome, and multiple endocrine neoplasia type 2. In addition, germline mutations in genes encoding for SDH subunits (*SDHB*, *SDHC*, and *SDHD*) are associated with the pheochromocytoma–paraganglioma syndrome, and they are present in 10–30% of apparently sporadic cases. In the majority of tumors associated with these mutations, there is loss of expression of the corresponding subunit as well as destabilization of the respiratory chain complex II, giving rise to partial or total loss of staining with anti-SDHB antibodies in the tumor cells. Thus, SDHB immunohistochemistry can be used in clinical practice as a screening test in sporadic paragangliomas and pheochromocytomas, serving as a surrogate marker of potential *SDH* germline mutations. In addition to susceptibility to pheochromocytomas and paragangliomas, *SDH* germline mutations have been found in patients with hereditary paraganglioma and gastric stromal sarcoma (also called Carney–Stratakis syndrome), apparently sporadic gastrointestinal stromal tumor, and Cowden-like syndrome. Of note, gastrointestinal stromal tumors associated with loss of SDHB expression and germline *SDH* mutations do not show mutations in *KIT* or *PDGFRA*.

Comments

Although there is a strong correlation between loss of SDHB expression and mutations in *SDH* genes, the sensitivity and specificity are not 100%. Genetic testing should be performed for confirmation in cases of loss of SDHB as well as in cases with retained SDHB expression when there is a strong clinical suspicion for germline mutations.

Selected references

Gill AJ, Benn DE, Chou A, *et al.* Immunohistochemistry for SDHB triages genetic testing of SDHB, SDHC, and SDHD in paraganglioma–pheochromocytoma syndromes. *Human Pathology* 2010; 41: 805–14.

Gill AJ, Toon CW, Clarkson A, *et al.* Succinate dehydrogenase deficiency is rare in pituitary adenomas. *American Journal of Surgical Pathology* 2014; 38: 560–66.

Miettinen M, Killian JK, Wang ZF, *et al.* Immunohistochemical loss of succinate dehydrogenase subunit A (SDHA) in gastrointestinal stromal tumors (GISTs) signals SDHA germline mutation. *American Journal of Surgical Pathology* 2013; 37: 234–40.

Serotonin

Sources/clones

Accurate (5HTH209, YC5/45, polyclonal), American Qualex (polyclonal), Axcel/Accurate (5HT-H209), Biodesign (polyclonal), Biogenesis (polyclonal), Biogenex (polyclonal), Caltag Laboratories (polyclonal), Chemicon (polyclonal), Dako (5HT-H209), Fitzgerald (M09203), Immunotech (polyclonal), Pharmingen (YC5-45), Sanbio/Monosan (polyclonal), Sera Lab (polyclonal), Serotec (polyclonal), Zymed (polyclonal).

Fixation/preparation

The antibodies to serotonin are immunoreactive in formalin-fixed paraffin-embedded tissue sections. HIER enhances immunoreactivity.

Background

Serotonin (5-hydroxytryptamine) is a neurotransmitter substance that is found in a broad range of normal, hyperplastic, and neoplastic tissues, including the gastrointestinal tract, central nervous system, adrenergic nerve fibers, platelets, and basophils. The major use of this marker has been to identify serotonin-secreting carcinoid tumors, which mostly arise from the midgut.

Applications

Immunostaining for serotonin has been employed as a marker of neuroendocrine differentiation. However, like other specific neuropeptides such as bombesin, ACTH, calcitonin, and VIP, it is of low sensitivity and specificity and should only be employed in a panel of several antibodies with more specific markers such as chromogranin and synaptophysin. The major application of serotonin lies in the detection of carcinoid tumors, particularly as such tumors may respond to specific therapy with the somatostatin analog octreotide and α-interferons. Serotonin may also be detected in scattered cells within other neuroendocrine tumors from a variety of sites. Whereas all tumors of the lung with dense core granules contained neuron-specific enolase, fewer contained serotonin.

Interestingly, using serotonin staining as a marker of neuroendocrine differentiation, it was shown that androgen ablation promotes neuroendocrine cell differentiation in human and dog prostates. Replacement androgens and estrogens after castration restored this cell population to normal values and induced luminal differentiation and basal metaplasia respectively.

Comments

Serotonin has limited application as a marker of neuroendocrine differentiation. If used for this purpose it should be employed with a panel of more specific and sensitive antibodies such as chromogranin and synaptophysin. Its main application today would be in a secondary panel to identify the specific neuropeptides produced in an established neuroendocrine tumor.

Selected reference

Burke AP, Thomas RM, Elsayed AM, Sobin LH. Carcinoids of the jejunum and ileum: an immunohistochemical and clinicopathologic study of 167 cases. *Cancer* 1997; 79: 1086–93.

NOTES

Simian virus 40 (SV40 T antigen)

Sources/clones

Biogenesis (0H9, 0G5), Chemicon, Oncogene (PAb416, PAb419, PAb280), Pharmingen (Pab101, Pab122), Santa Cruz (PAb101, Pab108).

Fixation/preparation

The use of this antibody was confined to the staining of fixed tissue culture cells until the application of antigen retrieval.

Background

SV40 T antigen (Ab-3) is a mouse monoclonal antibody with specificity for antigenic determinants unique to the SV40 small T antigen and non-reactive with SV40 large T antigen. Both antigens are encoded by the early region of the SV40 genome.

Simian virus 40 (SV40) large T antigen is an 81 kDa multifunctional viral phosphoprotein. Some of its functions are essential to the viral replication in monkey cells. Others contribute to its neoplastic transforming activity.

The large T antigen binds DNA and complexes with p53 protein. It also forms a specific complex with the p105 product of the retinoblastoma susceptibility gene.

Applications

The use of this antibody has been confined to the research laboratory to define the cellular location of small T antigen in subcellular extracts of SV40 infected cells. Pab280 reacted strongly with a cytoplasmic form of small T antigen that appears to be associated with the cytoskeleton. Small T was found to accumulate late in the SV40 lytic cycle and was localized in both the cytoplasm and the nucleus of cells infected with wild-type SV40. Research applications have centered around the use of SV40 as an effective gene transfer vector in vitro, the immortalization of cell lines and the stimulation of developmental abnormalities and tumorigenesis in transgenic mice.

Comments

The demonstration that 60% of human mesotheliomas contain and express SV40 sequences stimulated a great deal of interest. It has also been shown that SV40 large T antigen interferes with the normal expression of the tumor suppressor gene p53 in human mesotheliomas, raising the possibility that SV40 may contribute to the development of human mesotheliomas. The cell cycle inhibitor p21^{WAF1}, a downstream target of p53, shows a significant positive correlation with survival, further supporting the role of SV40 in the pathogenesis of mesothelioma. SV40 has been demonstrated in fixed tissue with the novel application of a DNA thermal cycler for antigen retrieval.

The antigen is nuclear in location.

Selected references

Baldi A, Groeger AM, Esposito V, *et al.* Expression of p21 in SV40 large T antigen positive human pleural mesothelioma: relationship with survival. *Thorax* 2002; 57: 353–6.

Carbone M, Rizzo P, Grimley PM, *et al.* Simian virus-40 large-T antigen binds p53 in human mesotheliomas. *Nature Medicine* 1997; 3: 908–12.

NOTES

SMARCB1

Sources/clones

Abbiotec (polyclonal), Abcam (polyclonal), Abnova (polyclonal), Acris Antibodies (25), Atlas (polyclonal), Aviva (polyclonal), BD Transduction Laboratories (BAF47, 25), Bethyl Laboratories (polyclonal), Biorbyt (polyclonal), Boster Immunoleader (polyclonal), Creative Biomart (MAAG3623), Epitomics (EPR6966), Fitzgerald (polyclonal), Gene Tex (EPR6966), GenWay Biotech (polyclonal), LifeSpan BioSciences (3E10), Millipore (polyclonal), Novus (polyclonal), Ray Biotech (3E10), Sanbio (3E10), Santa Cruz Biotechnology (polyclonal), Serotec (3E10), Sigma-Aldrich (polyclonal), Thermo (polyclonal).

Fixation/preparation

Several of the antibody clones/polyclonal antibodies to SMARCB1/SNF5/INI1/BAF47 are immunoreactive in fixed paraffin-embedded sections. HIER at 120 °C enhances labeling.

Background

SWI/SNF-related, matrix-associated, actin-dependent regular of chromatin, subfamily B, member 1 (SMARCB1) is the protein product of the gene *SMARCB1* (also known as *BAF47*, *INI1*, and *SNF5*) located on chromosome 22q11.2. SMARCB1 has functional roles in ATP-dependent chromatin remodeling, cell cycle control, and regulation of the cytoskeleton. SMARCB1 is widely expressed in cell lines and tissues. The *SMARCB1* gene is mutated in various types of tumors, consistent with a tumor suppressor role for SMARCB1. Loss of SMARCB1 expression correlates with point mutations in the *SMARCB1* gene in malignant rhabdoid tumors and with larger chromosomal deletions in epithelioid sarcoma. Of note, germline mutations in the *SMARCB1* gene have been identified in a subset of the patients with these tumors. In addition, homozygous deficiency for SMARCB1 is lethal in mice with early embryonic death, while SMARCB1 heterozygous mice display a variety of tumors in the soft tissues of the head and neck. SMARCB1 also binds the HIV-1 integrase and stimulates integrase-mediated DNA joining activity. Thus, SMARCB1 is a component of SWI/SNF complexes that may be critical for normal development and tumor suppression, but may also have a role in viral DNA integration into host DNA.

Applications

The loss of SMARCB1 protein expression in tumor cell nuclei correlates with biallelic deletion or mutations in the *SMARCB1* gene. The absence of nuclear SMARCB1 reactivity is useful diagnostically in a few contexts. Loss of SMARCB1 expression is seen in 98% of malignant rhabdoid tumors and 90% of epithelioid sarcomas, whether conventional or proximal type, and in 50% of epithelioid malignant peripheral nerve sheath tumors. Smaller proportions of other tumors demonstrate loss of SMARCB1 expression, including 40% of pediatric and 10% of adult myoepithelial carcinomas, 17% of extraskeletal myxoid chondrosarcomas, poorly differentiated chordoma, undifferentiated hepatoblastoma, and renal medullary carcinoma. Attenuation of SMARCB1 reactivity has been demonstrated in poorly differentiated synovial sarcomas. Germline mutations in *SMARCB1* occur in approximately 60% of patients with the rare hereditary syndrome of familial schwannomatosis, associated with a "mosaic" pattern of protein loss by immunohistochemistry.

The absence of SMARCB1 expression is best used to support the diagnosis of malignant rhabdoid tumor and epithelioid sarcoma.

Comments

Clone BAF47 produces the best results in our hands. Immunoreactivity appears not to be enhanced by boiling or proteolytic digestion and is best demonstrated following retrieval at 120 °C in EDTA buffer at pH 9.0.

Selected references

Biegel JA. Molecular genetics of atypical teratoid/rhabdoid tumor. *Neurosurgical Focus* 2006; 20: E11.

Bourdeaut F, Lequin D, Brugières L, *et al.* Frequent hSNF5/INI1 germline mutations in patients with rhabdoid tumor. *Clinical Cancer Research* 2011; 17: 31–8.

Calderaro J, Moroch J, Pierron G, *et al.* SMARCB1/INI1 inactivation in renal medullary carcinoma. *Histopathology* 2012; 61: 428–35.

Hollmann TJ, Hornick JL. INI1-deficient tumors: diagnostic features and molecular genetics. *American Journal of Surgical Pathology* 2011; 35: e47–63.

Hornick JL, Dal Cin P, Fletcher CD. Loss of INI1 expression is characteristic of both conventional and proximal-type epithelioid sarcoma. *American Journal of Surgical Pathology* 2009; 33: 542–50.

Sullivan LM, Folpe AL, Pawel BR, Judkins AR, Biegel JA. Epithelioid sarcoma is associated with a high percentage of SMARCB1 deletions. *Modern Pathology* 2013; 26: 385–92.

Smooth muscle myosin heavy chain

Sources/clones

Dako (clone SMMS-1).

Fixation/preparation

SMMS-1 may be used on formalin-fixed paraffin-embedded tissue sections, cryostat sections, or cell smears. For optimal results, deparaffinized tissue sections should be treated with a proteolytic enzyme followed by HIER.

Background

Smooth muscle myosin heavy chain (SMM-HC) is a cytoplasmic structural protein/component of smooth muscle cells. SMM-HC expression is developmentally regulated and appears early in smooth muscle development. Although specific for smooth muscle development, it is not a contractile regulatory protein. SMM-HC exists in two isoforms, MHC-1 (205 kDa) and MHC-2 (200 kDa), and is composed of dimerized heavy chains which then bind with two pairs of myosin light chains to form myosin polypeptide. SMM-HC is encoded by a single gene through alternative splicing of mRNA. Both isoforms are specific for smooth muscle cells and are considered markers of "terminal" smooth muscle differentiation.

Positive immunostaining in cryostat sections with SMM-HC antibody has been demonstrated in adult human visceral and vascular smooth muscle cells but not in epithelial cells, endothelial cells, or connective tissue fibroblasts. In normal breast tissue, SMM-HC highlights vascular smooth muscle and myoepithelial cells in lobules, ducts, and lactiferous sinuses in cryostat and routinely processed sections. Similarly, periacinar and periductal myoepithelial cells of salivary gland are also immunopositive with SMM-HC, whereas all of the acinar/ductal epithelial cells are negative.

Anti-SMM-HC also labels intact myoepithelial cells in benign and in-situ malignant breast lesions. Furthermore, while muscle actin-positive myofibroblasts are noted within the stroma of invasive carcinomas, SMM-HC is expressed only on rare myofibroblasts. This predominantly negative immunostaining of myofibroblasts is helpful to avoid confusion between myoepithelial cells and the condensation of myofibroblasts around ducts. SMM-HC immunostaining has also proved to be useful for the demonstration of myoepithelial cells in salivary gland tumors and lymphangioleiomyomatosis.

Applications

Anti-SMM-HC may be of use for the demonstration of myoepithelial cells in the following more common histologic difficulties:

- radial scar vs. infiltrating tubular carcinoma
- cancerization of adenosis by DCIS mimicking microinvasive carcinoma
- invasive cribriform carcinoma mimicking noninvasive lesions
- papillary carcinoma vs. papilloma
- nipple adenoma and syringomatous nipple adenoma vs. infiltrating duct carcinoma

Comments

Anti-SMM-HC has proved to be superior to muscle actin for the demonstration of myoepithelial cells in breast tissue, as the latter also stains the vast number of myofibroblasts in the stroma.

Selected references

Borrione AC, Zanellato AM, Scannapieco G, et al. Myosin heavy-chain isoforms in adult and developing rabbit vascular smooth muscle. *European Journal of Biochemistry* 1989; 183: 413–17.

Eddinger TJ, Murphy RA. Developmental changes in actin and myosin heavy chain isoform expression in smooth muscle. *Archives of Biochemistry and Biophysics* 1991; 284: 232-7.

Savera AT, Gown AM, Zarbo RJ. Immunolocalization of three novel smooth muscle-specific proteins in salivary gland pleomorphic adenoma: assessment of the morphogenetic role of myoepithelium. *Modern Pathology* 1997; 10: 1093-100.

Wang NP, Wan BC, Skelly M, *et al.* Antibodies to novel myoepithelium-associated proteins distinguish benign lesions and carcinoma in situ from invasive carcinoma of the breast. *Applied Immunohistochemistry* 1997; 5: 141-51.

White S. Martin AG, Periasamy M. Identification of a novel smooth muscle myosin heavy chain cDNA: isoform diversity in the SI head region. *American Journal of Physiology* 1993; 264: 1252-8.

Yaziji H, Gown AM, Sneige N. Detection of stromal invasion in breast cancer: The myoepithelial markers. *Advances in Anatomic Pathology* 2000; 7: 100-9.

SOX9

Sources/clones

Abcam (polyclonal, SOX9), Santa Cruz (polyclonal, H-90), Sigma Aldrich (polyclonal, SOX9), Thermo Fisher Scientific (monoclonal, 1B-11).

Fixation/preparation

Formalin-fixed paraffin-embedded tissues are suitable. Blocking buffer is needed for the Abcam clone.

Background

SOX9 (sex determining region Y, box 9) is a transcription factor associated with the testis-determining factor sex-determining region Y (SRY). It is expressed predominantly in adult tissues as well as in fetal testis and skeletal tissue. There are two functional domains: a high-mobility group (HMG) DNA-binding domain and a C-terminal transactivation domain. SOX9 plays a major role in cartilage differentiation (chondrogenesis) and early testis development. Mutation of the *SOX9* gene in humans causes campomelic dysplasia, a severe dwarfism syndrome, and autosomal XY sex reversal. SOX9 is thought to be a master regulator of the differentiation of mesenchymal cells into chondrocytes.

Applications

It is a nuclear marker for cartilaginous tumors, and has been used to separate mesenchymal chondrosarcoma from other small round blue cell tumors.

Selected reference

Wehrli BM, Huang W, De Crombrugghe B, *et al.* Sox9, a master regulator of chondrogenesis, distinguishes mesenchymal chondrosarcoma from other small blue round cell tumors. *Human Pathology* 2003; 34: 3263–9.

NOTES

SOX10

Sources/clones

Abcam (monoclonal, BC34, 1E6), Biocare Medical (monoclonal, BC34), R&D systems (monoclonal, 20B7), Thermo Fisher Scientific (polyclonal, catalog number PA5-40697).

Fixation/preparation

Formalin-fixed paraffin-embedded tissues are suitable. Peroxide block and HIER required.

Background

The *SOX10* gene encodes a member of the SOX (SRY-related HMG-box) family of transcription factors involved in the regulation of embryonic development and in the determination of cell fate. Mutations are associated with Waardenburg–Shah syndrome and Hirschsprung disease. The encoded protein acts as a transcriptional activator after forming a protein complex with other proteins. The SOX10 protein serves as a nucleocytoplasmic shuttle protein, and it is important for neural crest and peripheral nervous system development. SOX10 is therefore a neural crest transcription factor crucial for maturation and maintenance of Schwann cells and melanocytes. Antibodies against SOX10 have been applied to a variety of neural crest-derived tumors, mesenchymal and epithelial neoplasms.

Applications

SOX10 immunostaining is seen in melanoma, breast carcinoma, gliomas, and benign tumors such as schwannomas, and it was also seen to be expressed in 100% of melanocytic nevi. SOX10 is positive in 97–100% of desmoplastic and spindle cell melanomas, the majority of oligodendrogliomas, as well as in a large percentage of astrocytomas, poorly differentiated glioblastomas, and clear cell sarcoma-like tumors. Sustentacular cells are also SOX10-positive. SOX10 is a more sensitive and specific marker of melanocytic and schwannian tumors than S100 protein.

Malignant serous, mucinous, and endometrioid tumors are significantly more likely to express SOX10 than benign and borderline tumors. Expression patterns in adenocarcinomas are different for histologic subtypes: nuclear SOX10 staining is common in clear cell adenocarcinomas and serous adenocarcinomas, whereas mucinous and endometrioid tumors are negative for nuclear staining.

Selected references

Kwon AY, Heo I, Lee HJ, *et al.* Sox10 expression in ovarian epithelial tumors is associated with poor overall survival. *Virchows Archiv* 2016: 468: 597–60.

Nonaka D, Chiriboga L, Rubin BP. Sox10: a pan-schwannian and melanocytic marker. *American Journal of Surgical Pathology* 2008; 32: 1291–8.

NOTES

Spectrin/fodrin

Sources/clones

Accurate (SB-SP1, SB-SP2), American Qualex (polyclonal), Biodesign (polyclonal), Biogenesis (B12G3, D4D7, 2C5, polyclonal), Calbiochem (polyclonal), Chemicon (polyclonal), Finland Novocastra (RBC1.5B1, RPC2.3D5), Helsinki (101AA6), ICN Immunologicals (AA6), Locus Genex, Serotec (D7A3, D4D7), Sigma Chemical (polyclonal), Zymed (Z068).

Fixation/preparation

The antibody is immunoreactive in fresh frozen tissue sections and in fixed paraffin-embedded sections following HIER.

Background

Spectrin is a flexible rod-shaped molecule of 200 nm length found in mammalian and avian erythrocytes. It is composed of two non-identical subunits, α and β, and is linked to the plasma membrane by the protein ankyrin. Along with actin, ankyrin, and band 4.1, spectrin forms a network or membrane skeleton that lies immediately beneath the plasma membrane. The main function of the spectrin cytoskeleton is that of structural support for the bilipid layer of the cell membrane, and the spectrin-based membrane skeleton also controls lateral mobility of the erythrocyte membrane proteins. Thermal denaturation of spectrin leads to disintegration of the erythrocytes into vesicles, and deficiencies or structural abnormalities of the membrane skeleton proteins lead to loss of shape or tensile strength of the erythrocytes resulting in fragmentation and destruction as they pass through the spleen. Defects of spectrin are associated with fragile erythrocytes in hemolytic anemias such as hereditary elliptocytosis, pyropoikilocytosis, and spherocytosis.

Non-erythroid cells also show a membrane skeleton which contains spectrin, although the molecular organization in such cells is less known. Non-erythroid spectrin is known as fodrin,molecular weight of 240 kDa; it exhibits many similarities to spectrin, including immunochemical cross-reactivity, and is found in virtually all non-erythroid cells. Besides the function of maintaining some specialized membrane domains, fodrin appears to be redistributed in a variety of cell surface events, suggesting that it acts as a dynamic mediator between the cell membrane, membrane skeleton, and cytoskeleton. For example, there is significant reorganization of the spectrin network in cells treated with growth factors. In chromaffin cells, stimulation with a calcium ionophore results in secretion and a relocation of spectrin as cytoplasmic aggregates, antibody-induced capping of B-lymphocyte surface immunoglobulin leads to redistribution of spectrin similar to the surface proteins, and in A-431, an epidermoid carcinoma cell line, epidermal growth factor (EGF) induces cell surface remodeling and the accumulation of spectrin in membrane ruffles coincident with its phosphorylation. It is thought that calcium ions influence membrane skeleton assembly and maintenance by binding to spectrin, by calcium-regulated, calmodulin-mediated influence of the interactions between spectrin and other proteins, or by calcium-dependent protease cleavage of spectrin. In skeletal muscle cells it has been shown that fodrin has a significant cytoskeletal role, lining the sarcolemma and remaining relatively uniform even when the cell changes in shape and shrinks.

Applications

The antibody to spectrin/fodrin was initially employed only on fresh frozen tissue sections; however, with the use of microwave antigen retrieval, we were able to demonstrate immunoreactivity in fixed paraffin-embedded sections. The interest in fodrin lies in its role in cell adhesion during embryogenesis and in neoplasms. In comparison to their non-neoplastic counterparts, neoplastic epithelial cells show elevated levels of fodrin immunostaining regardless of tumor type. There was strong and fragmented and circumferential staining for fodrin, which often became accentuated with increasing grades of anaplasia, and loss of membrane staining corresponded with loss of tumor cell cohesiveness. Fodrin is linked to E-cadherin and β-catenin, together having a role in cell-to-cell adhesion. The breakage of this complex is heralded by detachment of β-catenin and associated with change in cell shape and cell adhesion in breast carcinoma. Earlier work with frozen tissue suggested that a number of cutaneous tumors show a diminished amount, or a total lack, of membrane-bound fodrin with increasing depolarization and proliferation of cells in solar keratosis and malignant melanoma. There was also accumulation of cytoplasmic fodrin in the invasive cells of squamous cell carcinoma and melanoma.

Selected reference

Bennett V. The spectrinactin junction of erythrocyte membrane skeletons. *Biochemica et Biophysica Acta* 1989; 988: 107–22.

Surfactant apoprotein A

Sources/clones

Chemicon (polyclonal), Dako (PE10).

Fixation/preparation

The antibodies are immunoreactive in fixed paraffin-embedded tissues, and immunoreactivity is enhanced by HIER.

Background

Pulmonary surfactant apoproteins, together with phospholipids, play an essential role in maintaining the surface tension of intra-alveolar fluid and preventing the alveoli from collapsing at the end of expiration. Surfactant has been localized in two functionally distinct structures within alveolar type II pneumocytes, the lamellar bodies and lysosomes, the former probably involved in surfactant secretion and the latter in degradation. Surfactant has also been demonstrated within tracheobronchial epithelial cells by immunostaining.

Applications

Except for type II pneumocytes and pulmonary macrophages, and the walls and perivascular connective tissues of small to medium-sized blood vessels of the lung, normal cells or tissues are generally not labeled by the PE10 antibody. In particular, it does not react with type I pneumocytes and mesothelial cells and has been shown to be negative in mesotheliomas, so it is a useful marker to distinguish pulmonary adenocarcinomas from mesotheliomas. Immunolabeling for surfactant apoprotein A in human normal and neoplastic breast epithelium is a finding confirmed by the demonstration of surfactant messenger RNA in both benign and neoplastic breast samples.

Surfactant immunoexpression does not appear to distinguish between type II pneumocyte and Clara cell type adenocarcinomas, perhaps because of a common precursor. The protein, together with carcinoembryonic antigen and Clara cell antigen has been demonstrated in the so-called sclerosing hemangioma of the lung.

Immunostaining for surfactant has found application in forensic autopsies in relation to the assessment of the severity and duration of respiratory distress from non-central nervous system or peripheral/alveolar damage. Those cases with hyaline membrane syndrome from a variety of traumas, protracted death from drowning, mechanical asphyxia, and fire death displayed intense granular staining of intra-alveolar surfactant apoprotein. In contrast, there was weak staining following death from alcohol intoxication, poisoning by hypnotics, and carbon monoxide poisoning. Surfactant immunoexpression has been shown to be significantly reduced in lungs from infants with pulmonary hypoplasia, suggesting that there is also suppression or defect in functional maturity in such lungs. Immunoexpression of the protein A has been used as a marker to link rhabdoid tumor of the lung to origin from adenocarcinoma.

Comments

PE10 is a specific marker of type II pneumocyte and Clara cells with a reasonable level of sensitivity. PE10 alone was not found to be useful in discriminating between primary pulmonary tumors and metastatic adenocarcinomas in fine needle aspiration biopsies because of low specificity and sensitivity and had to be employed in a panel with TTF-1, CK7, and CK20 to produce significant results. The demonstration of surfactant apoprotein A and messenger RNA in both normal and neoplastic breast epithelium by immunolabeling and reverse transcriptase-polymerase chain reaction respectively, and the demonstration of the surfactant apoprotein A gene expression in a subgroup of epithelial cells in human large and small intestine, raise the possibility of a wider role of this protein in the regulation of inflammatory processes and tissue specificity.

Selected references

Braidotti P, Cigala C, Graziani D, *et al.* Surfactant protein A expression in human normal and neoplastic breast epithelium. *American Journal of Clinical Pathology* 2001; 116: 721–8.

Yousem SA, Wick MR, singh G, *et al.* So-called sclerosing hemangioma of lung. An immunohistochemical study supporting a respiratory epithelial origin. *American Journal of Surgical Pathology* 1988; 12: 582–90.

Synaptophysin

Sources/clones

Accurate (SVP-38, S5768), Biodesign (SY-38), Biogenesis (SY-38), Biogenex (SY-38), Boehringer Mannheim (SY-38), Calbiochem, Cymbus Bioscience (SY-38), Dako (SY38, polyclonal), Sanbio/Monosan (SY-38), Sera Lab (SY-38), Sigma Chemical (SVP-38).

Fixation/preparation

Applicable to formalin-fixed paraffin-embedded sections. Microwave antigen retrieval in citrate buffer improves the immunostaining of this antibody. Enzyme pretreatment is not recommended for the monoclonal antibody, which is applicable to frozen sections and cell smears. The polyclonal antibody requires enzyme pretreatment before immunostaining.

Background

Synaptophysin is an integral-membrane glycoprotein (38 kDa) of presynaptic vesicles. The protein is a component of the classic, locally recycled small synaptic vesicle present in almost all neurons.

Synaptophysin is localized to "empty" vesicles and is both chemically and topographically different from chromogranin (68 kDa), a membrane protein of the dense-core neuroendocrine granules.

Antibody (SY38) to synaptophysin has been raised against presynaptic vesicles from bovine brain. Hence, the antibody shows reactivity with neuronal presynaptic vesicles of brain, spinal cord, retina, neuromuscular junctions, small vesicles of adrenal medulla, and pancreatic islets of human, bovine, rat, and mouse origin. In normal tissues, neuroendocrine cells of the human adrenal medulla, carotid body, skin, pituitary, thyroid, lung, pancreas, and gastrointestinal mucosa are labeled with this antibody.

The polyclonal antibody (Dako) was raised against the synthetic human synaptophysin peptide coupled to keyhole limpet hemocyanin.

Applications

Antibody to synaptophysin allows specific staining of neuronal, adrenal, and neuroepithelial tumors: these include pheochromocytoma, paraganglioma, pancreatic islet cell tumors, medullary thyroid carcinoma, pulmonary/gastrointestinal/mediastinal carcinoid tumors, and pituitary/parathyroid adenomas. Other neural tumors such as neuroblastomas, ganglioneuroblastomas, ganglioneuromas, central neurocytoma, and ganglioglioma also demonstrate immunoreactions with this antibody. The Dako rabbit anti-human synaptophysin is also useful for the identification of normal and neoplastic neuroendocrine cells.

The so-called pigmented "black" tumor in the pancreas has been shown to be of neuroendocrine origin with definite staining for synaptophysin and chromogranin but not HMB-45, S100, glucagon, or insulin.

Comments

Synaptophysin is a specific and fairly sensitive marker for neural/neuroendocrine tumors of low and high grades of malignancy. While earlier antibodies were sensitive to formalin fixation and worked best in alcohol-fixed material, many of the currently available antibodies are immunoreactive in formalin-fixed paraffin-embedded sections after heat-induced antigen retrieval. Synaptophysin is an excellent marker of neuroendocrine cells and should be used together with chromogranin in the detection of neuroendocrine differentiation. The recommended positive control tissue is pancreas (islets).

Selected references

Chejfec G, Falkmer S, Grimelius L, *et al.* Synaptophysin: a new marker for pancreatic neuroendocrine tumors. *American Journal of Surgical Pathology* 1987; 11: 241–7.

Gould VE, Lee I, Wiedenmann B, *et al.* Synaptophysin: a novel marker for neurons, certain neuroendocrine cells, and their neoplasms. *Human Pathology* 1986; 17: 979–83.

Tau

Sources/clones

Accurate (TAU2, polyclonal), Accurate/Sigma, Biodesign (TAU2), Biosource (AT8, BT2, HT7), Calbiochem, Chemicon, Dako (polyclonal), Labvision Corp. (TAU5), Pharmingen (TAU2.1), Sigma (TAU2, polyclonal), Zymed (T14, T46).

Fixation/preparation

Most of the antibodies are immunoreactive in fixed paraffin-embedded sections.

Background

The major components of the neuronal cytoskeleton are α- and β-tubulin, the microtubule-associated proteins (MAPs), neurofilaments, and actin. Tau is a neuronal microtubule-associated protein, which is the major antigenic component of neurofibrillary tangles and senile plaques in Alzheimer's disease. Comparison of tau-immunoreactive lesions in three relatively uncommon neurodegenerative diseases, namely, supranuclear palsy, Pick's disease, and corticobasal degeneration, demonstrated unexpected pathological similarities, but also fundamental differences between these disorders.

Tau2 was produced using bovine MAP as immunogen. It reacts exclusively with the chemically heterogeneous tau in both the phosphorylated and non-phosphorylated form. Tau2 does not react with other MAPs or with tubulin and localizes along microtubules in axons, dendrites, somata, and astrocytes, and on ribosomes. Tau2 cross-reacts with bovine, monkey, and chicken tissue. A variety of antibodies to phosphorylated neurofilament proteins have been shown to cross-react with phosphorylated epitopes of tau.

Applications

Applications of tau are mainly in the field of neuropathological research in neurodegenerative disorders. In the diagnostic setting, conventional silver impregnation stains such as Bielchowsky or Bodian are used for the demonstration of neurofibrillary tangles. These can also be detected with antibodies to phosphorylated tau epitopes and ubiquitin. Tau is not only a basic component of neurofibrillary degeneration but is also an etiologic factor, as demonstrated by mutations on the tau gene responsible for frontotemporal dementias, with parkinsonism linked to chromosome 17. The abnormal accumulation of tau protein in glial cells in many neurodegenerative diseases suggests that in some instances the disease process may also target the glial tau, with neuronal degeneration as a secondary consequence of this process. Prominent filamentous tau pathology and brain degeneration in the absence of extracellular amyloid deposition thus characterize a number of neurodegenerative disorders other than Alzheimer's disease, including progressive supranuclear palsy, corticobasal degeneration, and Pick's disease, collectively referred to as the tauopathies. Tau protein has also been demonstrated in gastrointestinal stromal tumors in an intense diffuse staining pattern in both epithelioid and spindle cell tumors in as many as 76% of both gastric and small bowel tumors. Tau also immunostains other intra-abdominal tumors including neuroendocrine carcinomas, paragangliomas, and desmoplastic round cell tumors.

Selected references

Cork LC, Sternberger NH, Sternberger LA, *et al.* Phosphorylated neurofilament antigens in neurofibrillary tangles in Alzheimer's disease. *Journal of Neuropathology and Experimental Neurology* 1986; 45: 56–64.

Feany MB, Dickson DW. Neurodegenerative disorders with extensive tau pathology: a comparative study and review. *Annals of Neurology* 1996; 40: 139–48.

Joachim CL, Morris JH, Kosik KS, Selkoe DJ. Tau antisera recognize neurofibrillary tangles in a range of neurodegenerative disorders. *Annals of Neurology* 1987; 22: 514–20.

NOTES

T-cell receptor

Sources/clones

TCR-βF1 (detects α/β-expressing T cells): Abcam (mouse monoclonal; clone = 8A3); Thermo Scientific (mouse monoclonal; clone = 8A3)

TCR-γ (detects γ/δ-expressing T cells): Novus (mouse monoclonal; clone = 7A5); Thermo Scientific (mouse monoclonal; clone = gamma 3.20)

Fixation/preparation

The antigen is preserved in formalin-fixed paraffin-embedded tissue.

Background

T lymphocytes recognize antigens via the T-cell receptor (TCR), a disulfide-linked heterodimer that is associated with the CD3 molecule on the cell surface. There are two types of TCR heterodimers, alpha–beta (αβ) and gamma–delta (γδ), which can be detected via immunohistochemical techniques. Each of these polypeptide chains is composed of variable (V), joining (J), constant (C), and diversity (D) segments, which undergo VDJ rearrangements during T-cell development. TCR rearrangement occurs in the thymus and is a fairly early event in T-cell maturation, with the TCR-γ and TCR-δ genes rearranging before TCR-α and TCR-β genes. Rearrangement of the TCR-α gene results in deletion of the TCR-δ gene, and the expression of either αβ or γδ heterodimers is exclusive on a given normal T cell. The majority of circulating T cells express the αβ T-cell receptor. TCR-γδ-expressing T cells constitute only a small proportion of the circulating T cells (<5%); however, they can be found in higher abundance in some mucosal and epithelial sites, such as skin, intestine, and reproductive tract, and within the sinusoidal areas of the splenic red pulp.

Applications

According to the 2008 WHO Classification of Haematopoietic and Lymphoid Tissues, peripheral T-cell lymphomas are classified based in part upon the expression of TCR-αβ or TCR-γδ. Therefore, immunohistochemical determination of TCR type can be very important in the diagnostic workup of T-cell lymphomas in formalin-fixed paraffin-embedded tissues, as antibodies are available that detect the β-chain of the TCR-αβ complex (TCR-βF1 antibody) and the γ-chain of the TCR-γδ complex (TCR-γ antibody), thereby identifying TCR-αβ-expressing and TCR-γδ-expressing T cells, respectively.

The majority of peripheral T-cell lymphomas derive from αβ T cells; however, two distinct γδ T-cell lymphoma categories are recognized by the 2008 WHO classification: hepatosplenic γδ T-cell lymphoma (HSTL) and primary cutaneous γδ T-cell lymphoma (PCGD-TCL). HSTL has a male predominance and characteristically occurs in young adults with chronic immune suppression or prolonged antigen stimulation. The neoplastic cells typically lack expression of CD4, CD8, and CD5 and characteristically express TCR-γδ; however, the diagnosis of HSTL can be made in the appropriate clinical and morphologic context in rare instances of TCR-αβ expression. PCGD-TCL often affects the extremities, can exhibit a variety of clinical appearances, and often involves the deep dermal/subcutaneous tissues. The neoplastic cells exhibit strong expression of cytotoxic markers and derive from γδ-T cells. While TCR-γδ expression is a characteristic feature of PCGD-TCL, TCR-γδ expression has been described in a small percentage of other cutaneous T-cell lymphoproliferative disorders, including mycosis fungoides and lymphomatoid papulosis. In the author's experience, biopsies of inflammatory dermatoses contain predominantly αβ T cells, with only rare γδ T cells identified by immunohistochemistry. γδ-T cells usually comprise 10% or less of the lymphocytic infiltrate in erythema multiforme, graft-versus-host disease, lichen planus, lupus panniculities, spongiotic dermatitis, and mycosis fungoides.

The spectrum of γδ-derived T-cell lymphomas is expanding beyond the 2008 WHO defined diagnoses of HSTL and PCGD-TCL, as γδ-T cell lymphomas have been reported involving mucosal, extranodal (other than liver/spleen), and rarely nodal sites. For example, extranodal NK/T-cell lymphomas, lymphomas that typically exhibit aggressive/destructive behavior and are associated with EBV infection, have been shown to include cases of γδ origin. Enteropathy-associated T-cell lymphoma (EATL) is an intestinal T-cell lymphoma characterized by intraepithelial T cells, villous atrophy, and crypt hyperplasia, and it is often classified into two distinct but overlapping subtypes of EATL. Type I cases are associated with celiac disease, frequently show gains in chromosomes 1q and 5q, and usually lack expression of CD8 and CD56; type II EATLs exhibit a more monomorphoic cytologic appearance, frequently express CD56 and CD8, show frequent gains in 8q24, and only rarely show gains of 1q or 5q. TCR-γδ expression is frequently seen in type II EATL; however, TCR expression cannot be used to definitively distinguish type I from type II. Of note, there are reports of T-cell lymphomas without demonstrable TCR-αβ or TCR-γδ expression (i.e., a TCR "silent" immunophenotype); therefore, the lack of TCR-β expression by immunohistochemistry cannot be used to definitively predict γδ T-cell origin. In addition, rare cases of T-cell lymphomas expressing both TCR β- and γ-chains by immunohistochemistry have been reported.

Selected references

Ozsan N, Feldman AF, Caron BL, *et al*. A new immunohistochemistry method to detect T-cell receptor gamma-chain expression in paraffin-embedded biopsies identifies a unique set of peripheral T-cell lymphomas co-expressing T-cell receptor beta and gamma chains. *Modern Pathology* 2011; 24: 313a.

Rodriguez-Pinilla SA, Ortiz-Romero PL, Monsalvez V, *et al*. TCR-γ expression in primary cutaneous T cell lymphomas. *American Journal of Surgical Pathology* 2013; 37: 375–384.

Tenascin

Sources/clones

Biogenex (DB7, monoclonal), Dako (M636, rabbit anti-human), Dako (TN2, monoclonal).

Fixation/preparation

These antibodies react positively with tenascin in formalin-fixed paraffin-embedded tissue sections. Enzyme pretreatment with pepsin is recommended with the use of the monoclonal antibodies prior to the immunohistochemical procedure.

Background

Tenascin is a large glycoprotein of the extracellular matrix with a unique six-armed multidomain macromolecular structure. It is expressed in fibroblasts and the extracellular matrix during embryogenesis and growth. Tenascin is synthesized by fibroblasts and is believed to have active functions in epithelial–mesenchymal interactions.

Tenascin expression is also induced during wound healing and inflammatory processes. The amino acid sequence of tenascin comprises epidermal growth factor (EGF)-like repetitions, which bind to EGF receptors of tumor cells, implying that tenascin may play a role in tumor invasion and metastasis. Tenascin has also been demonstrated in the extracellular matrix of mature tissue and benign and malignant neoplasms.

Hence, tenascin has been demonstrated to be a stromal marker of malignancy in breast carcinoma, with a positive correlation between tenascin expression, five-year disease-free survival, and distant metastases in breast carcinomas. Increased tenascin immunoexpression has also been demonstrated in the stroma of gastric, endometrial, and colon carcinomas. In comparison to normal tissue and benign tumors, increased tenascin expression has therefore been regarded as a stromal marker of tumor progression.

Tenascin immunoexpression has also been demonstrated in mesenchymal tumors, including schwannomas, leiomyosarcomas, fibromas, liposarcomas, and other fibrohistiocytic tumors. The corona-like expression of tenascin around lymphofollicular infiltrates appears to be a distinctive feature of lymphocytic thyroiditis. A similar pattern of tenascin staining has been described in lymphoid hyperplasia of the thymus associated with myasthenia gravis, another autoimmune disorder. This has been interpreted as the lymphoid follicles stimulating/activating the surrounding mesenchyme to produce tenascin as part of the extracellular matrix, during the course of the autoimmune disease process.

Tenascin is an extracellular matrix glycoprotein that plays a role in endometrial proliferation and possibly endometrial carcinogenesis.

Applications

Tenascin immunopositivity at the dermal–epidermal junction overlying dermatofibroma but not dermatofibrosarcoma protuberans has been shown to be useful in distinguishing these skin tumors. However, there was no difference in staining patterns between the two tumors. Malignant pheochromocytomas (defined by the presence of metastases) demonstrated strong stromal tenascin positivity, while pheochromocytomas that had not metastasized were negative; the adrenal medulla was negative. In contrast, paragangliomas showed a heterogeneous pattern with no difference between "benign" and malignant paragangliomas.

Selected references

Erickson HP, Bourdon MA. Tenascin: an extracellular matrix protein prominent in specialized embryonic tissues and tumors. *Annual Review of Cell Biology* 1989; 5: 71–92.

Koukoulis GK, Gould VE, Bhattacharyya A, *et al*. Tenascin in normal, reactive, hyperplastic and neoplastic tissues:

biologic and pathologic implications. *Human Pathology* 1991; 22: 636–43.

Sedele M, Karaveli S, Pestereli HE, *et al.* Tenascin expression in normal, hyperplastic and neoplastic endometrium. *International Journal of Gynecological Pathology* 2002; 12: 161–6.

Terminal deoxynucleotidyl transferase (TdT)

Sources/clones

Accurate (polyclonal), Biodesign (monoclonal), Biogenex (6A6.09), Chemicon, Dako (HT1, HT3, HT4, polyclonal), Gentrak, Immunotech (HTdT, polyclonal), Sera Lab (HTdT-1, polyclonal), Sigma (8-1 E4).

Fixation/preparation

While both immunofluorescent and immunoenzyme techniques were initially applied to cryostat sections and cell suspensions, immunohistochemical staining of formalin-fixed paraffin-embedded sections is now possible. Paraffin section immunostaining is greatly enhanced by heat-induced antigen retrieval so that terminal deoxynucleotidyl transferase (TdT) can be demonstrated on routine and archival specimens without the need for DNAse digestion and prolonged incubation previously necessary. Both 4 M urea and citrate buffer pH 6.0 are suitable retrieval solutions. Polyclonal antibodies are preferable to monoclonal antibodies for formalin-fixed paraffin-embedded sections.

Background

Terminal deoxynucleotidyl transferase (TdT) is a 58 kDa protein encoded by a 35 kb gene on chromosome 10q23–25. It is a nuclear enzyme that catalyzes the random addition of deoxynucleotidyl residues on the 3′OH termini of single-stranded DNA and of oligo-deoxynucleotide primers, and it differs from other DNA polymerases by not requiring template instruction for polymerization.

TdT is recognized to exert its DNA polymerase function during the early variation of genes coding for T and B cells, perhaps by addition of non-germline-encoded nucleotides (N-regions), although its function is still debated.

TdT is normally present only in hematopoietic tissues such as thymus and bone marrow, where it is restricted to a proportion of multipotent cell precursors and immature T and B lymphocytes. TdT positivity is never observed in normal peripheral blood cells.

Approximately 1–2% (more in young individuals) of bone marrow cells show TdT positivity, and these mostly express B-cell precursor phenotype in cell suspension studies. In trephine biopsies, TdT+ cells do not display preferential localization and are sparsely dispersed in interstitial spaces.

In the thymus, T lymphocytes can be defined into three maturation stages corresponding to their microenvironment. Stage I thymocytes, accounting for 0.5–5% of thymocytes, reside in the subcapsular zone of the thymus and comprise large TdT blast cells which express CD7, CD2, CD5, and cCD3 (cytoplasmic). Stage II thymocytes, accounting for 60–80% of thymocytes, are TdT-positive and express CD7, CD5, cCD3, CD2, CD1, CD4, and CD8. Stage III thymocytes, accounting for 15–20% of thymocytes, reside in the medulla, do not express TdT or CD1, and show differentiation into either CD4+ or CD8+ cells.

Applications

TdT as a marker is mostly used in the diagnosis of lymphomas and leukemias. TdT activity is seen in acute lymphoblastic leukemias (ALL) of both B- and T-cell lineages, so TdT is a useful diagnostic marker for lymphoblastic leukemias. In addition, as many as 30% of patients with chronic granulocytic leukemia develop a lymphoid blast crisis that is characterized by a lymphoblastic phenotype with nuclear TdT expression. These TdT lymphoblastic crises have a better prognosis than TdT-non-lymphoid blast crises, and respond to ALL-like therapy.

There are about 20% of cases of acute non-lymphoid leukemias that also express TdT and in which the proportion of TdT blasts co-expressing various myeloid markers is variable. It has been suggested that the expression of TdT in such cases is a marker of poor prognosis, but this is controversial. Such cases often show the phenomenon of phenotypic and genotypic "lineage infidelity" in which there is expression of lymphoid antigens such as CD7 and there is rearrangement of Ig and T-cell receptor genes.

The L3 ALL in the FAB classification, which represents Burkitt-type leukemia, is an exception as the blast cells of this type of leukemia represents a "mature" B-cell phenotype with surface immunoglobulin expression.

TdT is a reliable marker to distinguish lymphoblastic lymphoma (LL) from other lymphomas, which are always TdT-negative. LLs are related to T-ALL, and their distinction from the latter can be difficult; nevertheless, clinical and phenotypic differences have been observed, with the latter tending to show a more immature immunophenotype. While LL is frequent in children, forming about one-third of all non-Hodgkin lymphoma, it also makes up about 5% of cases in adults, and cases of non-T, non-B, or pre-B-cell LL have been reported in extranodal sites in both children and adults. TdT is particularly useful for the separation of LL from the other small-cell tumors of childhood (Appendix 1.3).

TdT is thus a useful marker for diagnosis as well as for staging, as it helps identify tumor cells from reactive lymphocytes. TdT staining can be used for the detection of early involvement and in staging, especially in extranodal sites such as the testes, CNS (through cerebrospinal fluid examination), skin, liver, kidney, and other sites of extramedullary involvement, and for monitoring minimal residual disease following chemotherapy. In the assessment of residual LL, it should be noted that a small population of TdT+ lymphoblasts resides in benign lymph nodes and tonsils. In benign lymph nodes from pediatric patients, TdT+ cells were found adjacent to medullary and cortical sinuses in a frequency of 1–180 cells per high-power field, as single cells or small clusters. These cells had a B-precursor phenotype, staining for CD79a, CD34, and CD10. In the tonsil, TdT+ cells were demonstrated in adults and children studied by immunostaining, indicating that tonsils, like bone marrow and thymus, are sites of lymphopoiesis.

In the identification of thymomas, particularly when sited in unusual sites such as the pleura, the presence of a TdT+/CD1a+/CD2+/CD99+ phenotype in the associated lymphoid population is supporting evidence of thymoma, as is the aberrant expression of CD20 in the cytokeratin-positive neoplastic cells.

Up to 70% of Merkel cells are TdT-positive.

Comments

TdT represents a powerful tool in leukemia and lymphoma diagnosis but it should be used in the context of a complete panel of markers and relevant histochemical enzyme stains. The ability to stain for this DNA polymerase in paraffin-embedded tissues, especially with polyclonal antibodies, following heat-induced antigen retrieval has greatly enhanced its diagnostic utility. When immunostaining cryostat sections it is necessary to employ brief fixation in buffered formalin or Zamboni's fixative, and to reduce diffusion of the enzyme the sections must be immersed in fixative immediately after cryosectioning. We employ the rabbit anti-TdT from Dako.

Selected references

Chilosi M, Pizzolo G. Review of terminal deoxynucleotidy transferase. Biological aspects, methods of detection, and selected diagnostic applications. *Applied Immunohistochemistry* 1995; 3: 209–21.

Onciu M, Lorsbach RB, Henry EC, Behm FG. Terminal deoxynucleotidyl transferase-positive lymphoid cells in reactive lymph nodes from children with malignant tumor: incidence, distribution pattern, and immunophenotype in 26 patients. *American Journal of Clinical Pathology* 2002; 118: 248–54.

Orazi A, Cattoretti G, Joh K, Neiman RS. Terminal deoxynucleotidyl transferase staining of malignant lymphomas in paraffin sections. *Modern Pathology* 1994; 7: 582–6.

TFE3

Sources/clones

Abbexa (polyclonal), Abcam (EPR11591), Acris Antibodies (polyclonal), Antibodies-online.com (polyclonal), Atlas Antibodies (polyclonal), Aviva Systems Biology (polyclonal), Biorbyt (polyclonal), Gene Tex (polyclonal), LifeSpan BioSciences (polyclonal), Cell Marque/Ventana Medical Systems (MRQ-37), Novus Biologicals (polyclonal), Santa Cruz Biotechnology (sc 5958, polyclonal), Thermo Fisher Scientific (polyclonal).

Fixation/preparation

Several of the antibody clones/polyclonal antibodies to TFE3 are immunoreactive in fixed paraffin-embedded sections. HIER at 120 °C enhances labeling.

Background

The transcription factor for immunoglobulin heavy chain enhancer region 3 (TFE3) is a member of the microphthalmia transcription factor (MiTF) family that is ubiquitously expressed in humans and is presumed to regulate many genes. Genetic translocations involving the TFE3 gene on the X chromosome (Xp11.2) include the ASPL:TFE3 translocation characteristic of alveolar soft part sarcoma, and several different translocation partners present in Xp11 translocation renal cell carcinomas. TFE3 gene translocation results in the activation of the MET oncogene, with activation of the rapamycin intracellular signaling pathway.

Applications

Antibodies to TFE3 are used in several diagnostic situations. Moderate to strong nuclear TFE3 reactivity is detected in almost all tumors featuring TFE3 gene fusions (alveolar soft part sarcoma 98%). Differential recognition of two different ASPL:TFE3 gene translocations have been demonstrated. TFE3 gene arrangements have been identified in a subset of PEComas, and Xp11.2 translocation renal cell carcinomas often display TFE3 reactivity.

Nuclear TFE3 immunoreactivity is present in some types of tumors that lack the TFE3 gene translocation. Owing to their scarcity, these tumors have been studied in small numbers. Almost all granular cell tumors are TFE3-positive, with most showing weak to moderate TFE3 reactivity. TFE3 expression can be detected in tumors with melanocytic or myomelanocytic differentiation, including angiomyolipoma (80%), melanoma (55%), and clear cell sarcoma (70%). Scattered weak to focally moderate staining intensity of native TFE3 protein has been reported in non-tumor cells.

Comments

Monoclonal (MRQ-37) produces consistent results. Immunoreactivity appears not to be enhanced by boiling or proteolytic digestion and is best demonstrated following retrieval at 120 °C EDTA buffer at pH 9.0.

Selected references

Argani P, Aulmann S, Illei PB, et al. A distinctive subset of PEComas harbors TFE3 gene fusions. *American Journal of Surgical Pathology* 2010; 34: 1395–406.

Argani P, Lal P, Hutchinson B, et al. Aberrant nuclear immunoreactivity for TFE3 in neoplasms with TFE3 gene fusions: a sensitive and specific immunohistochemical assay. *American Journal of Surgical Pathology* 2003; 27: 750–61.

Argani P, Olgac S, Tickoo SK, et al. Xp11 translocation renal cell carcinoma in adults: expanded clinical, pathologic, and genetic spectrum. *American Journal of Surgical Pathology* 2007; 31: 1149–60.

Dickson BC, Brooks JS, Pasha TL, Zhang PJ. TFE3 expression in tumors of the microphthalmia-associated transcription factor (MiTF) family. *International Journal of Surgical Pathology* 2011; 19: 26–30.

Inamura K, Fujiwara M, Togashi Y, *et al.* Diverse fusion patterns and heterogeneous clinicopathologic features of renal cell carcinoma with t(6; 11) translocation. *American Journal of Surgical Pathology* 2012; 36: 35–42.

Lazar AJ, Lahat G, Myers SE, *et al.* Validation of potential therapeutic targets in alveolar soft part sarcoma: an immunohistochemical study utilizing tissue microarray. *Histopathology* 2009 55: 750–5.

Reis H, Hager T, Wohlschlaeger J, *et al.* Mammalian target of rapamycin pathway activity in alveolar soft part sarcoma. *Human Pathology* 2013; 44: 2266–74.

Thrombomodulin

Sources/clones

Advanced Immunochemical (polyclonal), American Diagnostic (polyclonal), Axcel (24FN, 3E2), Dako (1009).

Fixation/preparation

Antibodies to thrombomodulin are applicable to formalin-fixed paraffin-embedded tissue.

Background

Thrombomodulin (TM) is a transmembrane glycoprotein composed of 575 amino acids (molecular weight 75 kDa) with natural anticoagulant properties. It is normally expressed by a restricted number of cells, such as endothelial and mesothelial cells. In addition, synovial lining and syncytiotrophoblasts of human placenta also express TM. Although TM contains six domains that are structurally similar to epidermal growth factor (EGF), there is no cross-reaction of anti-TM with EGF. The anticoagulant activity of TM results from the activation of protein C and the subsequent action on factors Va and VIIIa, and from the binding of thrombin.

Applications

Several immunohistochemical endothelial markers are available, and thrombomodulin serves as another marker, staining blood and lymphatic channels and their corresponding channels consistently. In one study, TM antibody stained 95% of benign lymphatic lesions (including lymphangioma and lymphangiectasia). In addition, TM demonstrated positivity in 100% of benign vascular tumors (pyogenic granuloma and hemangioma) and 95% of malignant vascular tumors (Kaposi's sarcoma, angiosarcoma, and epithelioid hemangioendothelioma). Hence, TM serves as a sensitive marker for lymphatic endothelial cells and their tumors. There has also been interest in the use of TM as an immunohistochemical marker for mesothelial cells and malignant mesotheliomas. The results have been rather variable, with some studies claiming high specificity while others have found that it is less specific in distinguishing mesothelioma from adenocarcinoma. The positivity rates for TM in mesothelioma range from 50% to 100%, and in pulmonary adenocarcinoma from 8% to 75%.

Based on these data, it appears that TM cannot be totally depended upon for the purpose of distinction between mesothelioma and pulmonary adenocarcinoma. TM may have a higher sensitivity for the small-cell variant of mesothelioma.

TM has been immunohistochemically demonstrated in the endothelial cells of sinusoidal vessels in 95% of subdural hematomas, and in surface cells and endothelium of neoplastic vessels in cardiac myxoma.

Thrombomodulin is immunoexpressed in a variety of tumors including squamous cell carcinomas of the lung, synovial sarcoma, angiosarcoma, transitional cell carcinoma, renal cell carcinomas, and thymomas.

Comments

Clearly, the major role of TM remains in the confirmation of lymphatic and vascular tumors, although some advocate the use of TM as a mesothelioma-binding antibody in the standard panel of antibodies used for the evaluation of malignant mesothelioma.

Selected references

Appleton MAC, Attanoos RL, Jasani B. Thrombomodulin as a marker of vascular and lymphatic tumors. *Histopathology* 1996; 29: 153–7.

Attanoos RL, Goddard H, Gibbs AR. Mesothelioma-binding antibodies: thrombomodulin, OV632 and HBME-1 and their use in the diagnosis of malignant mesothelioma. *Histopathology* 1996; 29: 209–15.

Collins CL, Ordonez NG, Schaefer R, *et al.* Thrombomodulin expression in malignant pleural mesothelioma and pulmonary adenocarcinoma. *American Journal of Pathology* 1992; 141: 827–33.

Ordonez NG. Value of thrombomodulin immunostaining in the diagnosis of mesothelioma. *Histopathology* 1997; 31: 25–30.

Thyroglobulin

Sources/clones

Axcel/Accurate (polyclonal, DAK-Tg6), Biodesign (polyclonal, 101, 102, 103, 104), Biogenesis (polyclonal), Biogenex (polyclonal), Caltag Laboratories (14/14), Chemicon (polyclonal), Dako (polyclonal, DAK-Tg6), Fitzgerald (M370108, M310136, M310137, M310138, M310139), Immunotech SA (J7B49, J7C9-3, J7C76-20), Labvision Corp. (2H11, 6E1), Novocastra (polyclonal, ID4), Sanbio/Monosan (14/14), Zymed (polyclonal).

Fixation/preparation

The antibodies to thyroglobulin are applicable to formalin-fixed paraffin sections, acetone-fixed cryostat sections and fixed cell smears.

Background

DAK-Tg6 (isotype: IgG1κ) and 1D4 (IgG2a) were raised against purified human thyroglobulin. These antibodies react with thyroglobulin (300 kDa) in normal, hyperplastic, and neoplastic thyroid glands. Circulating iodide, derived from dietary sources and deiodination of thyroid hormones, is selectively trapped by the thyroid gland. Oxidation of iodine to the organic form is then effected by a thyroid peroxidase enzyme, which is sited at the apical border of the follicular cell. This is recognized as the antigen to thyroid antimicrosomal antibody in autoimmune disease. Organic iodide is incorporated into mono- and di-iodotyrosine by binding to tyrosine residues on thyroglobulin stored in colloid. Thyroglobulin contains 140 tyrosine residues, but not all of these are iodinated, and T4 and T3 synthesis occurs only at specific sites. Hormone release is brought about by endocytosis of thyroglobulin at the apical pole of the follicular stem cell, fusion of endocytotic vesicles with lysosomes, and release of T3 and T4 by the proteolytic cleavage of thyroglobulin. These hormones are then secreted into the peripheral blood via the basal pole.

Applications

Apart from being immunoexpressed in all papillary and follicular carcinomas, thyroglobulin may also be useful in poorly differentiated and anaplastic carcinomas. Although both latter entities have been shown biochemically to synthesize 19S thyroglobulin, immunohistochemistry often fails to detect thyroglobulin in these tumors. Hürthle cell tumors also demonstrate immunopositivity with thyroglobulin. The other major role of antibodies to thyroglobulin is in the identification of metastatic thyroid carcinomas. A note of caution is necessary, since thyroglobulin may be demonstrated in medullary carcinoma of the thyroid gland. In such instances, attention to morphology as well as application of calcitonin antibodies would be crucial in avoiding an erroneous diagnosis. Antibodies to thyroglobulin do not react with epithelial cells from the gastrointestinal tract, pancreas, kidney, lung, and breast, nor the malignancies that arise in these organs.

Comments

The main role of thyroglobulin antibody lies in the identification of poorly differentiated/anaplastic thyroid carcinomas and metastatic thyroid carcinoma. The development of antibodies to thyroid transcription factor (TTF-1) provides another relatively specific marker of comparable sensitivity to thyroglobulin for thyroid carcinoma. The use of thyroglobulin in an appropriate panel allows the distinction of thyroid follicular, papillary, and medullary carcinoma and metastatic carcinoma (Appendix 1.30). Normal thyroid tissues may be used as positive controls. Because most antibodies are polyclonal, care should be taken to titrate optimal dilutions to avoid background staining.

Selected references

De Micco C, Ruf J, Carayon P, *et al.* Immunohistochemical study of thyroglobulin in thyroid carcinomas with monoclonal antibodies. *Cancer* 1987; 59: 471–6.

Wilson NW, Pambakian H, Richardson TC, *et al.* Epithelial markers in thyroid carcinoma: an immunoperoxidase study. *Histopathology* 1986; 10: 815–29.

TLE1

Sources/clones

Abcam (1F5, EPR9386(2)), BioSBvlone (1F5), Gene Tex (polyclonal), LifeSpan BioSciences (1D6), NovaTeinBio (polyclonal), Novus (polyclonal), Origene (3H3), Proteintech Group (polyclonal), Santa Cruz (M-101, polyclonal), Thermo Fisher Scientific (polyclonal).

Fixation/preparation

Several of the polyclonal antibodies to TLE1 are immunoreactive in fixed paraffin-embedded sections. HIER at 120 °C enhances labeling.

Background

Transducin-like enhancer of split 1 (TLE1) is one of the human homologs for the *Drosophila* Groucho protein. TLE1 has been previously discussed in the literature as ESG and GRG1. It acts as a transcriptional co-repressor implicated in the regulation of hematopoietic, neuronal, and epithelial differentiation. Analysis of the differential expression of TLE1 mRNA demonstrates wide expression in fetal and adult tissues. TLE proteins act through the Wnt/β-catenin signaling pathway, which has been associated with synovial sarcoma. Gene expression profiling studies show significant overexpression of TLE1 in synovial sarcoma. The synovial sarcoma fusion protein SS18-SSX appears to perform a bridging function between activating transcription factor 2 (ATF2) and TLE1, resulting in repression of ATF2 target genes. Blocking this pathway results in growth suppression and apoptosis, which supports a pathogenetic role for TLE1 and ATF2 in synovial sarcoma.

Applications

The majority of synovial sarcomas exhibit moderate to strong nuclear TLE1 reactivity, with a sensitivity for synovial sarcoma of 73–100%. High-grade sarcomas with *SYT* gene disruptions, demonstrated by fluorescent in-situ hybridization, also expressed TLE1, thus demonstrating high sensitivity of TLE1 in poorly differentiated synovial sarcoma.

TLE1 immunoreactivity has been identified in other types of neoplasms and tissues. A subset of malignant peripheral nerve sheath tumors are positive for TLE1 (up to 20%) with weak to moderate nuclear TLE1 reactivity reported. Combined analysis of tissue microarrays and whole tissue sections reveals rarer positive TLE1 reactivity in leiomyosarcomas and solitary fibrous tumors. In addition, TLE1 has been reported to be positive in acral myxoinflammatory fibroblastic sarcoma, endometrial stromal sarcoma, schwannoma, occasional cases of epithelioid sarcoma, liposarcoma, rhabdomyosarcoma, neurofibroma, lipoma, fibroxanthoma, carcinosarcoma, clear cell sarcoma, high-grade chondrosarcoma, undifferentiated pleomorphic sarcoma, and rare cases of Ewing's sarcoma and gastrointestinal stromal tumor. Nuclear TLE1 reactivity is present in basal keratinocytes, adipocytes, perineurial cells, endothelial cells, and mesothelial cells. One study has demonstrated immunohistochemical detection of TLE1 overexpression in lung carcinoma cases of varying types. TLE1 is expressed by diverse types of epithelial neoplasms.

The limitations in specificity notwithstanding, TLE1 has utility in a panel for the diagnosis of synovial sarcoma.

Comments

Polyclonal antiserum produces the best results in our hands. Immunoreactivity appears not to be enhanced by boiling or proteolytic digestion and is best demonstrated following retrieval at 120 °C in EDTA buffer at pH 9.0.

Selected references

Chen G, Courey AJ. Groucho/TLE family proteins and transcriptional repression. *Gene* 2000; 249: 1–16.

Foo WC, Cruise MW, Wick MR, Hornick JL. Immunohistochemical staining for TLE1 distinguishes synovial sarcoma from histologic mimics. *American Journal of Clinical Pathology* 2011; 135: 839–44.

Jagdis A, Rubin BP, Tubbs RR, Pacheco M, Nielsen TO. Prospective evaluation of TLE1 as a diagnostic immunohistochemical marker in synovial sarcoma. *American Journal of Surgical Pathology* 2009; 33: 1743–51.

Kosemehmetoglu K, Vrana JA, Folpe AL. TLE1 expression is not specific for synovial sarcoma: a whole section study of 163 soft tissue and bone neoplasms. *Modern Pathology* 2009; 22: 872–8.

Terry J, Saito T, Subramanian S, *et al*. TLE1 as a diagnostic immunohistochemical marker for synovial sarcoma emerging from gene expression profiling studies. *American Journal of Surgical Pathology* 2007; 31: 240–6.

Topoisomerase IIα

Sources/clones

Kamiya (monoclonal JH2.7), Novocastra (polyclonal, monoclonal 3F6).

Fixation/preparation

Applicable to fixed paraffin-embedded sections following high-temperature heat-induced antigen retrieval in EDTA at pH 8.0.

Background

The phylogenetic antiquity of DNA topoisomerases indicates their vital function in the cell. The structure and maintenance of genomic DNA depend on the activity of these enzymes, without which replication and cell division are impossible. DNA topoisomerase type II activity is required to change DNA topology and it is important in the relaxation of DNA supercoils generated by cellular processes such as transcription and replication. It is also essential for the condensation of chromosomes and their segregation during mitosis. In mammals this activity is derived from at least two isoforms, namely, topoisomerase IIα (Topo IIα) and β. Because of its essential role in cell replication, Topo IIα is the target for many drugs used for cancer therapy. Reduced expression of this enzyme is the predominant mechanism of resistance to several chemotherapeutic agents, and a wide variation in the range of expression of this protein is noted in many different tumors. The immunostaining pattern of Topo IIα is similar to that of the cell cycling marker Ki-67, so immunostaining of this protein has also been employed as a cell proliferation marker.

Applications

From the preceding discussion, it is not unexpected that the applications of this marker lie in its value as a predictor of chemotherapeutic response to enzyme inhibitors and in the determination of tumor cell proliferation. Increased Topo IIα immunostaining has been shown to correlate with recurrent colon cancers and with chemosensitivity in ovarian and endometrial carcinomas, and with anthracycline-based adjuvant therapy in node-positive breast cancer. Topo IIα cell counts have been shown to correlate well with Ki-67 counts in meningiomas, multiple myeloma, adrenocortical tumors, and pituitary adenomas, and they are a predictor of survival in patients with astrocytoma and ovarian cancer.

Comments

Use of Topo IIα immunostaining for predicton of chemosensitivity to enzyme inhibitors is limited in many tumors; however, detection of this protein has been shown to be a reliable substitute for Ki-67 as a cell proliferation marker. Tonsils serve as suitable controls.

Selected references

Di Leo A, Larsimont D, Gancberg D, et al. HER-2 and topo-isomerase IIα as predictive markers in a population of node-positive breast cancer patients randomly treated with adjuvant CMF or epirubicin plus cyclophosphamide. *Annals of Oncology* 2001; 12: 1081–9.

Gotleib WH, Goldberg I, Weisz B, et al. Topoisomerase II immunostaining as a prognostic marker for survival in ovarian cancer. *Gynecologic Oncology* 2001; 82: 99–104.

NOTES

Transthyretin (prealbumin, TTR)

Sources/clones

Abbiotec: rabbit polyclonal
Abcam: mouse monoclonal (CL0290, 10E1), rabbit monoclonal (C-terminus-EP2929Y, EPR3219, EPR2928(2)), sheep polyclonal, chicken polyclonal, rabbit polyclonal, goat polyclonal
Abgent: rabbit polyclonal (C-terminus)
Abnova Corporation: rabbit polyclonal
Acris Antibodies GmbH: mouse monoclonal (9G6, 10E1), goat polyclonal, rabbit polyclonal
Antibodies-online: rabbit monoclonal (C-terminus), rabbit polyclonal, chicken polyclonal, goat polyclonal, guinea pig polyclonal
Atlas antibodies: mouse monoclonal (CL0290), rabbit polyclonal
Aviva Systems Biology: chicken polyclonal, rabbit polyclonal (C-terminus)
Biorbyt: chicken polyclonal, rabbit polyclonal, goat polyclonal
Bioss Inc.: rabbit polyclonal
Biotrend Chemicals: chicken polyclonal
Bioworld Technology: rabbit polyclonal
Creative Biomart: sheep polyclonal
GeneTex: rabbit monoclonal (C-terminus-EP2929Y, EPR3219, EPR2928(2)), chicken polyclonal
LifeSpan BioSciences: mouse monoclonal (9G6, 10E1), rabbit monoclonal (EPR3219, EPR2928(2)), chicken polyclonal, goat polyclonal
MyBioSource.com: rabbit polyclonal
NeoBioLab: rabbit polyclonal
Novus Biologicals: mouse monoclonal (9G6, 10E1), rabbit monoclonal (EP2929Y), rabbit polyclonal
OriGene Technologies: mouse monoclonal (10E1), rabbit monoclonal (C-terminus-EP2929Y, EPR3219, EPR2928(2)), chicken polyclonal, goat polyclonal, rabbit polyclonal
ProSci: mouse monoclonal (9G6, 10E1), rabbit polyclonal
Proteintech Group: mouse monoclonal, rabbit polyclonal
RayBiotech: mouse monoclonal (9G6, 10E1), chicken polyclonal, goat polyclonal, rabbit polyclonal
Santa Cruz Biotechnology: mouse monoclonal (E1), goat polyclonal (C-15, C-20, K-15), rabbit polyclonal
St. John's Laboratory: rabbit polyclonal
Thermo Scientific: chicken polyclonal, rabbit polyclonal

Fixation/preparation

Most of these antibodies are validated in formalin-fixed paraffin-embedded tissue. Please refer to vendor instructions for specific antigen retrieval requirements.

Background

Transthyretin (TTR), previously known as prealbumin, is a plasma and cerebrospinal fluid carrier protein that transports thyroid hormones and retinol (vitamin A). It is a homotetramer synthetized in the liver, pancreas, choroid plexus, and pigmented epithelium of the retina.

Germline mutations in this gene are mostly associated with amyloid deposition, involving peripheral nerve and cardiac muscle.

More than 80 different mutations in this gene have been reported; most are related to amyloid deposition, affecting predominantly peripheral nerve and/or the heart, and a small portion of the gene mutations is non-amyloidogenic. The diseases caused by mutations include amyloidotic polyneuropathy, euthyroid hyperthyroxinemia, amyloidotic vitreous opacities, cardiomyopathy, oculoleptomeningeal amyloidosis, meningocerebrovascular amyloidosis, and carpal tunnel syndrome.

Mutant and wild-type *TTR* give rise to various forms of amyloid deposition (amyloidosis). Defects in TTR are the cause of amyloidosis transthyretin-related (AMYL-TTR), hyperthyroxinemia dystransthyretinemic euthyroidal (HTDE), and carpal tunnel syndrome type 1 (CTS1).

Applications

Immunohistochemistry classification of amyloidosis has been attempted using antibodies against transthyretin amongst other proteins such as AA amyloid, amyloid P-component, fibrinogen, λ-light chain, κ-light chain, and others.

Within the CNS, TTR is the only known protein synthesized solely by the choroid plexus. Positive immunostaining for TTR has been reported as a sensitive diagnostic marker of choroid plexus tumors.

Selected references

Hasselblatt M, Böhm C, Tatenhorst L, *et al.* Identification of novel diagnostic markers for choroid plexus tumors: a microarray-based approach. *American Journal of Surgical Pathology* 2006; 30: 66–74.

Megerian CA, Pilch BZ, Bhan AK, McKenna MJ. Differential expression of transthyretin in papillary tumors of the endolymphatic sac and choroid plexus. *Laryngoscope* 1997; 107: 216–21.

Tyrosinase

Sources/clones

Novacastra (T311).

Fixation/preparation

A heat-induced epitope retrieval (HIER) system is essential for antigen unmasking.

Background

Tyrosinase is an enzyme involved in the initial stages of melanin biosynthesis. T311 is a murine monoclonal antibody generated to the tyrosinase recombinant protein. On paraffin-embedded material, T311 revealed intense immunoreactivity confined to cells showing melanocytic differentiation. No immunostaining was present in unrelated normal tissues and tumors. 85–95% of metastatic malignant melanomas were immunoreactive with T311. Nevi showed intense staining at the junctional zone, while the dermal component revealed decreasing reactivity towards deeper areas. Immunopositivity correlated inversely with clinical stage, with an exclusively homogeneous pattern in early stages of melanoma to a more heterogeneous pattern in later stages.

Tyrosinase immunoreactivity has been demonstrated in approximately 85% of amelanotic metastatic melanomas, which is comparable to HMB-45 and Melan-A, and in 90% of conventional metastatic melanomas. Tyrosinase is strongly expressed in virtually all epithelioid melanomas, but rarely expressed in the spindled variants. However, tyrosinase has been shown to be less useful in desmoplastic melanomas.

Tyrosinase is the most sensitive marker for sinonasal melanomas and closely approaches the sensitivity of S100 protein for oral mucosal melanomas. Tyrosinase has also been demonstrated to be a sensitive and specific marker to distinguish epithelioid melanocytic nevi from epithelioid histiocytic tumors. Tyrosinase is not recommended for routine use in the diagnosis of renal and hepatic angiomyolipomas. Tyrosinase can also stain pigmented neurofibromas.

Applications

Tyrosinase is useful in the diagnosis of both primary and metastatic melanomas. It is less useful in the identification of spindled melanomas, especially desmoplastic melanomas.

Selected references

Hofbauer GF, Kamarashev J, Geertsen R, *et al.* Tyrosinase immunoreactivity in formalin-fixed, paraffin-embedded primary and metastatic melanoma: frequency and distribution. *Journal of Cutaneous Pathology* 1998; 25: 204–9.

Jungbluth AA, Iversen K, Copian K, *et al.* T311: an anti-tyrosinase monoclonal antibody for the detection of melanocytic lesions in paraffin embedded tissues. *Pathology, Research and Practice* 2000; 196: 235–42.

Kaufmann O, Koch S, Burghardt J, *et al.* Tyrosinase, Melan-A, and KBA62 as markers for the immunohistochemical identification of metastatic amelanotic melanomas on paraffin sections. *Modern Pathology* 1998; 11: 740–6.

NOTES

Tyrosine hydroxylase

Sources/clones

Abcam (ab112), Cell Signaling Technology (#2792), EMD Millipore (Ab152), Novus Biologicals (NB300-109), R&D Systems (#779427), Sigma (T2928).

Fixation/preparation

Fresh frozen tissue and cytologic preparations, and formalin-fixed paraffin-embedded tissue.

Background

Tyrosine hydroxylase (TH) plays an important role in the physiology of adrenergic neurons. It belongs to the biopterin-dependent aromatic amino acid hydroxylase family and is the rate-limiting enzyme of catecholamine biosynthesis; it uses tetrahydrobiopterin and molecular oxygen to convert tyrosine to DOPA. Its amino-terminal 150 amino acids comprise a domain whose structure is involved in regulating enzyme activity. The gene is located in the short arm of chromosome 11 at position 15.5 (11p15.5). The protein consists of 528 amino acids and has a molecular weight of 62 kDa. There are four potential splice variants.

Applications

TH is strongly localized in adrenal medulla, pheochromocytomas, and paragangliomas, and patchily expressed in neuroblastoma. TH activity is high in pheochromocytomas and paragangliomas as compared to the normal adrenal gland, whereas it is low in a neuroblastoma and is undetectable in other tumors. Immunostaining of TH and the measurement of its activity in adrenomedullary and related tumors may provide some information about the process of cell differentiation in these tumors.

Immunostaining for TH in paragangliomas is present in the majority of tumor cells in their cytoplasm with variable intensity regardless of their cytological features such as cellular and nuclear pleomorphism; loss of immunostaining for TH may be observed in metastatic tumors.

TH is also positive in esthesioneuroblastomas, nasal catecholamine-producing tumors of neural crest origin that might be derived from certain sympathetic neuronal cell nests in the superior nasal cavity.

TH is mostly localized on the cytoplasm of the differentiating neuroblasts of neuroblastic tumors of infancy, while immature elements are rarely positive. Although no correlation is found between the immunoreactive pattern and the site of origin or the staging of the neuroblastic tumors, there is a positive relationship between the urinary catecholamine output and the density of tyrosine hydroxylase-immunoreactive cells. TH is positive in 43% of midgut carcinoid tumors.

Comments

TH a useful marker for dopaminergic and noradrenergic neurons, and is mainly expressed in the brain and adrenal glands.

Selected references

Ceccamea A, Carlei F, Dominici C, et al. Correlation between tyrosine hydroxylase immunoreactive cells in tumors and urinary catecholamine output in neuroblastoma patients. *Tumori* 1986; 72: 451–7.

Iwase K, Nagasaka A, Nagatsu I, et al. Tyrosine hydroxylase indicates cell differentiation of catecholamine biosynthesis in neuroendocrine tumors. *Journal of Endocrinological Investigation* 1994; 17: 235–9.

Meijer WG, Copray SC, Hollema H, et al. Catecholamine-synthesizing enzymes in carcinoid tumors and pheochromocytomas. *Clinical Chemistry* 2003; 49: 586–93.

Takahashi H, Wakabayashi K, Ikuta F, Tanimura K. Esthesioneuroblastoma: a nasal catecholamine-producing tumor of neural crest origin. Demonstration of tyrosine hydroxylase-immunoreactive tumor cells. *Acta Neuropathologica* 1988; 76: 522–7.

Ubiquitin

Sources/clones

Accurate/Novocastra (FPM1), Biodesign (polyclonal), Biogenesis (242.9, polyclonal), Dako (polyclonal), Fitzgerald (polyclonal), Serotec (polyclonal), Zymed (UBI1).

Fixation/preparation

This antibody is applicable to formalin-fixed paraffin-embedded tissue sections.

Background

Ubiquitin is an 8.5 kDa polypeptide found almost universally in plants and animals. The best-documented function for ubiquitin involves its conjugation to proteins as a signal to initiate degradation via the ubiquitin-mediated proteolytic pathway. Ubiquitin-mediated proteolysis is involved in the turnover of many short-lived regulatory proteins. This pathway leads to the covalent attachment of one or more multi-ubiquitin chains to target substrates that are then degraded by the 26S multicatalytic chains proteasome complex. Ubiquitin modification of a variety of protein targets within the cells also plays an important role in many cellular processes: regulation of gene expression, regulation of cell cycle and division, involvement in the cellular stress response, modification of cell surface receptors, DNA repair, import of proteins into mitochondria, uptake of precursors into neurons, and biogenesis of mitochondria, ribosomes, and peroxisomes.

Applications

Ubiquitin immunostaining has been shown to be a highly sensitive and specific method for the detection of Mallory bodies, thereby making it a valuable tool in the study of alcoholic liver disease, adding objectivity to the diagnosis of alcoholic hepatitis. In the human spongiform encephalopathies, ubiquitin immunoreactivity has been demonstrated in a punctate distribution at the periphery of prion protein amyloid plaques and in a finely granular pattern in the neuropil around and within areas of spongiform change. Analysis of the relationship of ubiquitin-positive dots and granular structures with pretangle neurons and neurofibrillary tangles suggested that the ubiquitin-positive structures are the result of degeneration and might be related to the initiation of neurofibrillary degeneration. Ubiquitin-positive neuronal and tau2-positive glial inclusions are a marker of frontotemporal dementia of motor neuron type. Ubiquitin is present with GFAP in the cytoplasm and cell processes of tumor cells of astrocytomas. The demonstration of ubiquitin immunolabeling in both ductus efferentes and ductus epididymidis epithelia has concluded that ubiquitinated proteins are secreted into the epididymal lumen. Ubiquitin expression has been demonstrated in the lung and adrenal gland in autopsy cases after death by fire accident, suggesting that the adrenal gland reacts strongly to heat shock. Evidence of ubiquitin-positive myocytic intranuclear or cytoplasmic inclusions or positive-staining rimmed vacuoles in the setting of an inflammatory myopathy may be suggestive of a diagnosis of inclusion body myositis. On the therapeutic front, prevention of p53 ubiquitination (and subsequent degradation) in human papillomavirus (HPV)+ cervical tumors should lead to programmed cell death.

Selected reference

Ciechanover A, Schwartz AL. The ubiquitin-mediated proteolytic pathway: mechanisms of recognition of the proteolytic substrate and involvement in the degradation of native cellular proteins. *FASEB Journal* 1994; 8: 182–91.

NOTES

Ulex europaeus agglutinin 1 lectin (UEA-1)

Sources/clones

Dako (UEA-1).

Fixation/preparation

Carbohydrates reactive with UEA-1 are generally active in formalin-fixed paraffin-embedded tissue sections. Background staining may be reduced by the addition of 5% human serum to the anti-UEA-1 dilution buffer.

Background

UEA-1 is a plant lectin isolated from *Ulex europaeus* (gorse) seeds by affinity chromatography. The lectin is homogeneous, containing 4.2% neutral sugar and 1.4% glucosamine. Its molecular weight is approximately 110 kDa, comprising two covalently bound basic subunits. UEA-1 is specific to certain terminal α-L-fucosyl residues of glycoconjugates and also detects blood group H antigen.

Applications

UEA-1 has been used successfully as a marker for endothelial cells. It has been shown to be more sensitive for benign vascular tumors than thrombomodulin or factor VIII-related antigen. In fact, it has been shown to be a more sensitive marker for endothelial cells of vascular tumors than factor VIII-related antigen. UEA-1 does not distinguish between the endothelial cells of blood vessels and lymphatics. In some tissues *Ulex* lectin has demonstrated additional binding to epithelial structures. This latter immunoreaction has been exploited, with UEA-1 demonstrating specific binding to collecting duct carcinoma of the kidney, enabling distinction from other types of renal cell carcinoma.

Comments

A study evaluating endothelial markers in well- and poorly differentiated areas of angiosarcomas found that CD31 and *Ulex europaeus* were the most sensitive markers, staining both well-differentiated and poorly differentiated ares of the tumors. Anti-FVIII-RA and CD34 did not stain undifferentiated malignant endothelial cells. *Ulex europaeus* and CD34 showed very low specificity. It would appear that the use of UEA-1 is confined to identifying collecting duct carcinoma of the kidney. Benign vascular tissue makes appropriate positive controls for UEA-1.

Selected references

Holthofer H, Virtanen I, Kariniemi AL, et al. *Ulex europaeus* I lectin as a marker for vascular endothelium in human tissues. *Laboratory Investigation* 1982; 47: 60–6.

Meittinen M, Holthofer H, Lehto VP, Miettinen A, Virtanen I. *Ulex europaeus* I lectin as a marker for tumors derived from endothelial cells. *American Journal of Clinical Pathology* 1983; 79: 32–6.

Ordonez NG, Batsakis JG. Comparison of *Ulex europaeus* I lectin and factor VII-related antigen in vascular lesions. *Archives of Pathology and Laboratory Medicine* 1984; 108: 129–32.

NOTES

VEGF (vascular endothelial growth factor)

Sources/clones

Oncogene Research Products (VEGF antibody-3, monoclonal), R&D Research, Minneapolis (MAB293, clone 26503.11), Santa Cruz Biotechnology (VPF/VEGF, used for immunofluoresence staining with fresh frozen tissue), Santa Cruz Biotechnology (polyclonal VEGF, reacts with the 165, 189, and 121 amino acid splice variants of VEGF).

Fixation/preparation

These antibodies are applicable to paraffin sections. A heat-induced epitope/antigen retrieval system for proteinase digestion is recommended prior to the immunohistochemical procedure.

Background

Vascular endothelial growth factor (VEGF) is a dimeric 46 kDa, endothelial-cell-specific, glycosylated, heparin-binding cytokine. It has both angiogenic and vascular permeability factor functions. VEGF exerts paracrine effects by binding to specific tyrosine kinase-receptors on vascular endothelial cells. It may also exert autocrine effects by stimulating tumor growth. Hence, VEGF is one of the most potent, highly specific angiogenic factors.

VEGF is synthesized by both tumor and normal cells and acts specifically on endothelial cells. VEGF stimulates and induces migration and proliferation of endothelial cells. Hence, VEGF is a useful marker of tumor angiogenesis.

Cytoplasmic immunoreactivity for VEGF has been demonstrated in 40% of melanomas, but not in atypical compound melanocytic nevi, cellular blue nevi, or Spitz nevi. Further immunoreactivity for VEGF was related to tumor thickness and to the absence of regression. Hence, although VEGF is not a useful prognostic indicator for malignant melanoma, it may be useful in discriminating between melanoma and benign melanocytic lesions.

VEGF immunoexpression has not been found to be a prognostic marker for head and neck squamous cell carcinomas. However, tumor-associated inflammatory cells show high levels of VEGF expression in all carcinomas, suggesting a possible role in tumor angiogenesis.

VEGF expression has been seen in 60% of squamous lung carcinomas and 50% of breast carcinomas.

The immunohistochemical localization of VEGF (comparable to the localization of VEGF mRNA) was expressed in all thyroid tumors, including all types of thyroid carcinomas (including papillary, follicular, medullary, and anaplastic) and follicular adenomas. In contrast, in the normal thyroid, VEGF was identified in epithelium of isolated follicles. It was concluded that the histological type of thyroid tumor may determine the vascular pattern through a paracrine mechanism involving VEGF.

The characteristic vasculature and edema of sclerosing stromal tumors of the ovary has been demonstrated to be associated with the expression of VEGF.

In the prostate gland, VEGF expression was confined to the basal cell layer in benign glands. In high-grade prostatic intra-epithelial neoplasia, immunolabeling was no longer confined to the basal cell layer, but was seen in all neoplastic secretory cells. All carcinomas were immunopositive for VEGF. Hence, there was a trend for increasing immunolabeling intensity with increasing cellular dedifferentiation. Kollerman concluded that VEGF may have an important role in the process of malignant transformation and tumor progression.

Strong VEGF immunoexpression in malignant chondrocytes was confined exclusively to high-grade chondrosarcomas, interestingly showing a strong correlation with intracartilaginous vessels. Acquisition of these patterns of vasculature may be associated with metastatic potential of cartilage tumors.

Applications

VEGF may be useful in distinguishing between melanomas and melanocytic nevi. VEGF immunoexpression may also be predictive of potential metastasizing cartilaginous tumors. VEGF expression correlates with vascularity, metastasis, and proliferation of tumors and may therefore prove to be a useful prognostic marker.

Selected references

Mattern J, Koomagi R, Volm M. Association of vascular endothelial growth factor expression with intratumoral microvessel density and tumour cell proliferation in human epidermoid lung carcinoma. *British Journal of Cancer* 1996; 72: 931–4.

Salven P, Keikkila P, Anttonen A, *et al*. Vascular endothelial growth factor in squamous cell head and neck carcinoma: expression and prognostic significance. *Modern Pathology* 1997; 10: 1128–33.

Toi M, Inada K, Suzuki H, *et al*. Tumor angiogenesis in breast cancer: its importance as a prognostic indicator and the association with vascular endothelial growth factor expression. *Breast Cancer Research and Treatment* 1995; 36: 193–204.

Zymed Laboratories. Polyclonal rabbit anti-VEGF (data sheet).

Villin

Sources/clones

Accurate, Biodesign (ID2C3), Biogenesis (20/24), Chemicon (15E2), Immunotech (ID2C3), Serotec (ID2C3).

Fixation/preparation

HIER is required for fixed paraffin-embedded sections. Fixation in Carnoy's solution or methacarn preserves immunoreactivity. The antibody is also immunoreactive in fresh cell preparations and frozen sections.

Background

Microvilli increase the absorptive surface of epithelial cells by as much as 20 times. They comprise a highly specialized plasma membrane of a thick extracellular coat of polysaccharide and digestive enzymes and a core comprising a central rigid bundle of 20–30 parallel actin filaments that extend from the tip of the microvillus down to the cell cortex. The actin filaments are all oriented with their plus ends pointing away from the cell body and are held together at regular intervals by actin-bundling proteins. Besides fimbrin, which occurs in microspikes and filopodia, the most important bundling protein is villin, which is found only in microvilli. Like fimbrin, villin cross-links actin filaments into tight parallel bundles, but in a different actin binding sequence, and is capable of stimulating the formation of long microvilli in cultured fibroblasts which do not normally contain villin and have only a few small microvilli.

Villin, a 95 kDa Ca^{2+}-regulated actin-binding protein, is found in absorptive cells that develop a brush border such as those of the small and large intestines, ductal cells of the pancreas and biliary system, and cells of the proximal renal tubules. Villin is also found in undifferentiated normal and tumoral cells of intestinal origin in vivo and in cell culture, so that its expression is seen in cells that do not necessarily display microvilli-lined brush borders.

Applications

Villin has been employed as a marker of gastrointestinal tumors, particularly those from the colon, stomach, and pancreas, all such tumors staining positive in one study. Gall bladder and hepatocellular carcinomas were also demonstrated to express villin. A subset of non-gastrointestinal tumors including some adenocarcinomas of the ovary, endometrium, and kidney were also positive. About 30% of signet ring cell carcinoma of the lung were positive, and rare lung adenocarcinomas were also positive but no staining was observed in breast carcinoma and mesothelioma. The presence of villin in renal carcinomas is variable; it is frequently seen in clear cell and chromophilic tumors but not in chromophobe cell tumors. Villin also appears to be expressed in the tubular and glandular areas of better-differentiated tumors and is not observed in sarcomatoid renal carcinoma, leading to the suggestion that villin may be a potential grading marker. Its expression in renal carcinomas suggests that they display proximal rather than distal tubular differentiation. It is also observed in the glandular areas of Wilms tumor. Villin immunoexpression occurs in 85% of gastrointestinal carcinoids and small-cell carcinomas of the lung and in 40% of lung carcinoids, with a characteristic apical membranous staining pattern. Villin has also been demonstrated in Merkel cells, highlighting their microvilli.

Comments

Villin shows apical localization but may also be seen in the basement membrane area surrounding tumor nests. Clone ID2C3 shows reactivity with human, porcine, and chicken villin.

Selected reference

Bacchi CE, Gown AM. Distribution and pattern of expression of villin, a gastrointestinal-associated cytoskeletal protein, in human carcinomas: a study employing paraffin-embedded tissue. *Laboratory Investigation* 1991; 64: 418–24.

Vimentin

Sources/clones

Accurate (V9, J144, Vim-13.2), Amersham, Biodesign (V9), Biogenesis (Vim-01, LN6), Biogenex (LN6, V9), Boehringer Mannheim (3B4, V9), Chemicon, Dako (VIM3B4, V9), Enzo, Immunotech (V9, V3260), Medac, Milab, Novocastra, Oncogene (V9), Pierce (ZSV5), Serotec (J144), Sigma (LN9), Zymed (ZSV5, ZC64).

Fixation/preparation

Most antibody clones currently available are immunoreactive in fixed paraffin-embedded tissues, and HIER enhances immunostaining.

Background

Vimentin is a 58 kDa protein which has been purified from a variety of sources and has been shown to form homophylic filaments with an average diameter of 10 nm. Its name is derived from the Latin word *vimentum*, which means an array of flexible rods. Similar to the other intermediate filaments, vimentin is a protein monomer of highly elongated fibrous molecules with an amino-terminal head, a carboxyl-terminal tail, and a central rod domain. The latter consists of an extended α-helical region containing long tandem repeats of a distinctive amino acid sequence motif called the hepatad repeat. This central rod domain shows a striking sequence homology between intermediate filaments of different species, and an even more marked homology of as high as 30% between cytokeratin, desmin, glial fibrillary acidic protein, neurofilaments, and vimentin of the same species. Immunohistochemical staining revealed vimentin filaments as part of a wavy network of filaments in the cytoplasm of fibroblasts, associated with both nuclear and plasma membranes. It has been suggested that vimentin, like other intermediate filaments, serves as a modulator between extracellular influences governing calcium flux into the cell and nuclear function at a transcriptional or translational level, and it may thus have a role in gene expression. Vimentin filaments can be precipitated as juxtanuclear whorls following treatment of cells with colcemid or vinblastine.

Applications

Vimentin is the most widely distributed intermediate filament, expressed in virtually all mesenchymal cells and also by most other cell types in culture. With the widespread application of intermediate filament analysis to human neoplasms, it soon became apparent that although individual cell types and their corresponding tumors generally express a single intermediate filament class, several neoplasms may express more than one intermediate filament class. In many instances, this co-expression of one or more intermediate filament class occurs in a predictable manner and may be employed as a diagnostic discriminator. Vimentin expression, traditionally accepted to be class-specific for cells of the mesenchyme, can be co-expressed with cytokeratin in a number of epithelial cell types and their corresponding tumors. These include the endometrium, thyroid, gonadal epithelial cells, renal tubules, adrenal cortex, lung, salivary gland, hepatocytes, and bile duct. A variety of high-grade epithelial tumors may acquire the expression of vimentin intermediate filaments. Vimentin expression has been described in carcinomas of the skin, urinary bladder, breast, prostate, gastric mucosa, and uterine cervix. Several reports have indicated a correlation of vimentin expression with high tumor grades in breast carcinoma and ovarian epithelial malignancy. It has been suggested that vimentin expression is a poor prognostic marker in node-negative breast carcinoma. Expression of vimentin in epithelial tumors also corresponds to change in cell shapes and forms from epithelioid to fibroblastoid or spindle forms so that vimentin is regularly expressed in spindle cell carcinomas. Remodeling of vimentin cytoskeleton correlates with increased motility of promyelocytic leukemia, and a decrease and redistribution of this protein has been observed in aging Kupffer cells.

Many tissues in embryos and fetuses, including surface ectoderm, neural groove and brain, gut mucosa and musculature, and renal tubular epithelium, display co-expression of vimentin with another intermediate filament during their developmental stages before being replaced by the intermediate filament protein specific for the mature tissue type. Vimentin is expressed in epithelial cells in vitro, in culture preparations and cell suspensions, and in exfoliated and metastatic cells in body fluids, suggesting that altered cell-to-cell contact and changes in cell shape may account for this apparent aberrant expression. Studies of cell cultures of mouse parietal endodermal cells led to the hypothesis that the acquisition of vimentin may be related to reduced cell-to-cell contact and the ability of epithelial cells to survive independently.

Immature muscle fibers contain desmin and vimentin, and mature fibers lack vimentin. Regenerating muscle fibers react with anti-vimentin antibodies and more intensely for desmin than mature fibers. The detection of vimentin has therefore been applied to identify muscle regeneration, especially in cases of infantile spinal muscular atrophy, and the high incidence of reactive fibers in some congenital and early-onset disorders may indicate developmental arrest.

Comments

Because of variability in fixation and HIER, vimentin has been used as an internal control or reporter molecule to assess the quality of antigen preservation and the uniformity of tissue fixation in fixed paraffin-embedded tissue sections.

Selected reference

Azumi N, Battifora H. The distribution of vimentin and keratin in epithelial and non-epithelial neoplasms. *American Journal of Clinical Pathology* 1987; 88: 286–97.

VS38

Sources/clones

Dako (VS38c)

Fixation/preparation

The antibody is reactive in paraffin-embedded sections, and staining is enhanced by heat-induced antigen retrieval.

Background

VS38 was shown to detect a protein similar to the p63 protein. The latter is a non-glycated, reversibly palmitoylated type II transmembrane protein, which is found in rough endoplasmic reticulum. VS38 was originally described as a marker of neoplastic and non-neoplastic plasma cells.

Applications

It is known that the protein detected by VS38 is not exclusive to plasma cells but serves to distinguish plasma cells from other lymphoid cells because of their high secretory activity. It is included in a panel of antibodies for the immunostaining of bone marrow trephines fixed in common fixatives including Bouin's solution.

VS38 immunostaining has been reported in neuroendocrine tumors and in melanocytic lesions, and it is frequently positive in primary and metastatic melanomas. Occasionally, clear cell sarcoma of soft tissue can be positive. Caution should therefore be exercised when using this marker to identify plasma cell lineage. VS38 is also immunoexpressed in osteoblasts and stromal cells of bone tumors.

Comments

There is a need for a specific marker of plasma cell differentiation as a variety of neoplastic cells can display plasmacytoid features, and the converse, that is, poorly differentiated plasma cells and plasmacytoid cells can be difficult to recognize morphologically. In endometritis, besides labeling plasma cells, VS38 also stains epithelium and stromal cells of the endometrium. In contrast, CD138 produces strong labeling of plasma cells and not the other endometrial components, suggesting that CD138 may be a more specific marker of plasma cell differentiation.

Selected references

Banham AH, Turley H, Pulford K, *et al*. The plasma cell associated antigen detectable by antibody VS38 is the p63 rough endoplasmic reticulum protein. *Journal of Clinical Pathology* 1997; 50: 485–9.

Turley H, Jones M, Erber W, *et al*. VS38: a new monoclonal antibody for detecting plasma cell differentiation in routine sections. *Journal of Clinical Pathology* 1994; 47: 418–22.

NOTES

WT1

Sources/clones

Dako (polyclonal 6F-H2 directed to the amino terminus of the protein), Santa Cruz (C-19 raised against an 18 amino acid peptide at the carboxyl terminus of the human WT1 protein; F-6 raised against the amino terminal 180 amino acid domain of the WT1 protein).

Fixation/preparation

These antibodies are applicable to formalin-fixed paraffin-embedded tissue and immunoreactivity is enhanced by heat-induced antigen retrieval in citrate buffer followed by 0.4% pepsin digestion.

Background

Wilms tumor gene (*WT1*) is a tumor-suppressor gene located on chromosome 11p13. The Wilms tumor gene encodes a protein (WT1) that is expressed in the developing fetal kidney and urogenital tract, in the developing spleen, and in fetal coelomic lining cells, including mesothelium. WT1 is also expressed in mature benign mesothelial cells and may play a role in the malignant transformation of certain cells. Using non-commercial anti-WT1 antibodies, studies have demonstrated discriminatory expression between mesotheliomas and adenocarcinomas, with strong differential nuclear staining in mesotheliomas and cytoplasmic or no staining in adenocarcinoma. Using a commercially available polyclonal antibody to WT1, strong WT1 nuclear staining is seen in 75% of mesotheliomas. There is no nuclear staining in primary pulmonary adenocarcinomas although cytoplasmic staining can be seen often. Hence, nuclear staining for WT1 is highly specific for mesothelioma, and in the appropriate clinical setting it can be a helpful adjunct in the distinction between adenocarcinomas and mesotheliomas.

Antibody to clone 6F-H2 shows WT1 nuclear expression, with varying degrees of intensity, in the vast majority of ovarian serous carcinomas. Ovarian mucinous neoplasms and pancreaticobiliary adenocarcinomas are negative for WT1. In normal female genital organs, WT1 expression is recognized in ovarian surface epithelium, inclusion cysts, and tubal epithelium, but not in cervical or endometrial epithelium.

The desmoplastic small round cell tumor (DSRCT) is a highly malignant neoplasm usually presenting in the abdomen of adolescent males. This neoplasm has been characterized with a translocation involving the Ewing's sarcoma gene on chromosome 22 and the Wilms tumor gene *WT1* on chromosome 11, producing a fusion gene with expression of the DNA binding area of *WT1*. DSRCT shows strong immunostaining with an anti-WT1 antibody but WT1 is negative in the majority of EWS/PNET.

Applications

In the appropriate setting, WT1 (within a panel of antibodies) may be helpful in the distinction between adenocarcinomas and mesotheliomas. WT1 appears to have a high sensitivity and specificity for DSRCT and is therefore useful for differentiating from EWS/PNET. WT1 has a strong predilection for ovarian serous tumors, which may be helpful in differentiation from other Müllerian neoplasms and their metastases.

Comments

The nuclear antigen is sometimes associated with cytoplasmic staining. However, in the absence of nuclear staining, cytoplasmic staining should be regarded as spurious or may represent cross-reactivity with an epitope unrelated to WT1.

Selected references

Barnoud R, Sabourin JC, Pasquier D, *et al.* Immunohistochemical expression of WT1 by desmoplastic small round cell tumor: a comparative study with other small round cell tumors. *American Journal of Surgical Pathology* 2000; 24: 830–6.

Charles AK, Moore IE, Berry PJ. Immunohistochemical detection of the Wilms' tumour gene WT1 in desmoplastic small round cell tumour. *Histopathology* 1997; 30: 312–14.

Foster MR, Johnson JE, Olson SJ, Allred DC. Immunohistochemical analysis of nuclear versus cytoplasmic staining of WT1 in malignant mesotheliomas and primary pulmonary adenocarcinomas. *Archives of Pathology and Laboratory Medicine* 2001; 125: 1316–20.

SECTION 2
Appendices

Appendices

Appendix 1
Selected antibody panels for specific diagnostic situations

Appendix 1.1 Bone/soft tissue – chondroid-like tumors

	Brachyury	CK	S100	EMA	CEA	GFAP	CD57	SOX9
Chordoma	+	+	+	+	+	–/+	–	–
Myoepithelial tumor	–	+	+	+	–/+	–/+	–	–
Chondroblastoma	–	–	+	+	–	–	–	+
Chondroid chordoma	+	+	+	+	–	–	–	–
Myxoid chondrosarcoma (chordoid sarcoma)	–	–	+	–	–	–	–	–
Mesenchymal chondrosarcoma	–	–	+[a]	–	–	–	+	+
Clear cell sarcoma	–	–	+	–	–	–	–	–

[a] Chondroid cells.

Appendix 1.2 Brain – metastatic carcinoma vs. glioblastoma vs. meningioma

	CK	EMA	VIM	GFAP
Metastatic carcinoma	+	+	–/+	–
Glioblastoma	–[a]	–	+/–	+
Meningioma	–/[b]	+	+	–

[a] May show focal AE1/AE3 positivity.
[b] Secretory meningioma may be focally keratin–positive; CK18 is the most commonly expressed CK; CK8 is expressed by secretory, anaplastic and atypical variants.

Appendix 1.3 Childhood round cell tumors

	LCA	VIM[a]	CK	DES	MSA	CD99	Myogen	MyoD1	NSE	SYN	FLI-1	Chgn	NF
Hematolymphoid tumor[b]	+/–	+	–	–	–	–/+	–	–	–	–	+/–	–	–
Neuroblastoma	–	+	–/+	–	–	–	–	–	+	+/–	–	+/–	+
Ewing's sarcoma	–	+	–/+	–	–	+	–	–	–/+	–	+	–	–/+
PNET	–	+	+	–/+	–/+	+	–	–	+	+	+	–/+	–/+
DSRCT	–	+	+	+	+	–/+	–	–	+	+	+	–/+	–
Rhabdomyosarcoma	–	+	–	+	+	–/+	+	+	–	–	–	–	–

PNET, peripheral/primitive neuroectodermal tumor; DSRCT, desmoplastic small round cell tumor (stains positive for WT1, which is not identified in the other tumors considered in differential diagnosis); NF, neurofilaments.
[a] Vimentin labeling shows up the cytoplasm, which is often not visible on H&E stains.
[b] Lymphoblastic lymphoma is positive for terminal deoxynucleotidyl transferase (TdT).

Appendix 1.4 Gastrointestinal and aerodigestive tract mucosa – basaloid squamous vs. adenoid cystic vs. neuroendocrine carcinoma

	CD117	HMWCK	CEA	S100	p63	Chgn	SYN	CD56
Basaloid squamous carcinoma	–	+	+	–	+	–	–	–
Adenoid cystic carcinoma	+	–/+	+[a]	–/+	–	–	–	–
Neuroendocrine carcinoma	–	–	–	–	–	+	+	+

[a] Confined to luminal aspects of gland–like spaces.

Appendix 1.5 Gonads – germ cell tumors vs. somatic adenocarcinoma

	PLAP	αFP	HCG	CD30	CD117	CK	EMA	Vim	OCT3/4	hPL	SALL4
Seminoma	+	–	–[a]	–	+	–[a]	–	+	+	–	+
Embryonal carcinoma	+	+/–	–	+	–	+	–	–	+	–	+
Yolk sac tumor	+/–	+	–	–	+	+	–	–	–	–	+
Choriocarcinoma	+/–	–	+	–	–	+	+	–/+	–	+	+
Somatic carcinoma	–/+[b]	–	–/+	–	–	+	+	–	–	–	–/+[c]

[a] Occasional trophoblasts may be positive.
[b] Müllerian tract, breast, gut, and pulmonary tumors may occasionally be positive.
[c] May also be positive in tumors of urothelial origin, tumors of lung, tumors of pancreas, serous carcinoma of the ovary, squamous cell carcinoma, ductal carcinoma of the breast.

Appendix 1.6 Granulocytic sarcoma vs. lymphoma vs. carcinoma vs. plasmacytoma

	CD45	CD138	CK	NE	CD15[a]	EMA	CD117
Granulocytic sarcoma	+	–	–	+	+	–	+
Lymphoma	+	–	–	–	–	–	–
Plasmacytoma (poorly differentiated)	+/–	+	–	–	–	+	–
Carcinoma	–	–	+	–	–/+	+	–/+

[a] Other markers of granulocytic sarcoma include neutrophil elastase, myeloperoxidase, lysozyme, CD34, CD68.

Appendix 1.7 Intracranial tumors

	GFAP	VIM	CK	NF	CR	OLIG2
Astrocytoma	+	+	–/+	–	–	+
Oligodendroglioma	+	+	–	–	–	+
Ependymoma	–	–/+	+ (surface)	–	–	+
Neuroma/neurocytoma	–	–	–	+	+	–
Schwannoma	–/+	+	–	–	–/+	–
Metastatic carcinoma	–	–/+	+	–	–	–

CR, calretinin.

Appendix 1.8 Liver – hepatocellular carcinoma vs. metastatic carcinoma vs. cholangiocarcinoma

	CEA	AFP	CK7	CK19	VIM	Hep Par 1	Albumin	Glypican-3	MOC-31	Arginase-1
Hepatocellular carcinoma	+[a]	–/+	–/+	–/+	–/+	+	+/–	+	–	+
Cholangiocarcinoma	+	–	+	+	–/+	–/+	–	–/+[b]	+	–/+
Metastatic carcinoma	+/–	–	+/–	+/–	–/+	–	–	–	+	–/+

[a] Staining of canaliculi in hepatocellular carcinoma by polyclonal CEA.
[b] Positive in other tumors e.g. melanoma, non-seminomatous germ cell tumors.

Appendix 1.9 Lung – clear cell tumors

	CAIX	CK	VIM	Chgn	SYN	HMB-45	S100	PAX-8 stains	Napsin
Non-renal carcinoma with clear cell change	–	+	–	–	–	–	–	–/+	+[b]
Clear cell tumor ("sugar" tumor)	–	–	–[a]	–	–	+	–[a]	–	–
Renal carcinoma, metastatic	+	+	+	–	–	–	–	+	–
Carcinoid	–	+	–	+	+	–	–	–	–

[a] Rare cells may stain positive.
[b] Positive for clear cell carcinoma of ovary.

Appendix 1.10 Lymph node – round cell tumors in adults

	CD45	CK	VIM	S100	HMB-45	Melan-A	MiTF
Melanoma	–	–	+	+	+	+	+
Carcinoma	–	+	–	–/+	–	–	–
Lymphoma	+	–	+	–	–	–	–

Appendix 1.11 Undifferentiated round cell tumors

	CK	S100	CD45	Des	FLI	CD99	HMB-45	Mart-1	Myogenin	TLE1
Small-cell carcinoma	+	–	–	–	–	–/+	–	–	–	–
Melanoma	–	+	–	–	–	–	+	+	–	–
Lymphoma	–	–	+	–	–	–/+	–	–	–	–
PNET	–/+	–	–	–/+	+	+	–	–	–	–
DSRCT	+/–	–	–	+/–	+/–	–/+	–	–	–	–
Rhabdomyosarcoma	–	–/+	–	+	–	–/+	–	–	+	–/+
Synovial sarcoma	+	+/–	–	–/+	–	+	–	–	–	+

DSRCT, desmoplastic small round cell tumor; PNET, peripheral/primitive neuroectodermal tumor.

Appendix 1.12 Mediastinal tumors

	CD45	CK	EMA	PLAP	CD99	SALL4	p63
Thymoma	−	+	+	−	+[a]	−	+
Lymphoma	+	−	−	−	−/+	−	−[b]
Germ cell tumor	−	+	+	+	−	+	−

[a] Staining of associated small lymphocytes that also stain for CD1a.
[b] Anaplastic large-cell lymphoma may be positive.

Appendix 1.13 Nasal tumors

	VIM	CK	S100	HMB-45	NF
Neuroblastoma	+	−	+(SC)	−	+
Melanoma	+	−	+	+	−
Carcinoma	−/+	+	−/+	−	−

SC, supporting stromal cells and areas of ganglineuromatous differentiation stain positive.

Appendix 1.14 Pelvis – metastatic colonic adenocarcinoma vs. ovarian endometrioid carcinoma

	VIM	CEA	CA-19.9	CA125	CK7	CK20	PAX-8	CDX2
Colonic adenocarcinoma	−/+	+	+	−/+	−	+	−	+
Ovarian endometrioid carcinoma	+/−	−	−	+	+	−	+	−

Appendix 1.15 Perineum – prostatic vs. bladder vs. rectal carcinoma

	CK7	CK20	PSA	PSAP	CEA	AR	GATA3
Prostatic carcinoma	−	−/+	+	+	−/+	+	−
Bladder carcinoma	+	+	−	−/+	+	−	+
Rectal carcinoma	−	+	−	−	+	−	−

Appendix 1.16 Peritoneum – myxoid tumors

	SMA	Des	S100	Col IV	CD34	MUC4
Myxoma	−	−	−	−	−	−
Myxoid neurofibroma	−	−	+	+L	+	−
Myxoid liposarcoma	−	−	+	+C	+	−
Myxoid fibrosarcoma	−	−	−	−	−	−
Myxoid leiomyosarcoma	+	−/+	−	+L	−/+	−
Aggressive angiomyxoma	+	−/+	−	+F	−	−
Angiomyofibroblastoma	+	+	−	+F	−/+	−
Low-grade fibromyxoid sarcoma	+/−	−	−	+F/−	−	+

C, circumferential; F, fragmented, thin; L, linear, continuous.

Appendix 1.17 Pleura – mesothelioma vs. carcinoma

	LMWCK	HMWCK	CK5/6	VIM	EMA	αSMA	CEA	CR	CD15[a]	Ber-EP4	WTI	B72.3
Mesothelioma[b]	+	+	+	+	+[c]	+/–	–	+	–	–	+/–	–
Secondary carcinoma	+	–	–	–/+	+	–	+	–/+	+	+	–	+

CR, calretinin.

[a] Can be substituted with other myelomonocytic markers, e.g. LN-1 (CDw75), tN2 (CD74), MAC387.
[b] Mesotheliomas also stain for N-cadherin. In contrast carcinoma stain for E-cadherin and not for N-cadherin.
[c] Circumferential, with long microvilli; EMA may be substituted with HBME-1, which also highlights the characteristic microvilli.

Appendix 1.18 Retroperitoneum – renal cell carcinoma vs. adrenocortical carcinoma vs. pheochromocytoma

	EMA	VIM	CK	Chgn	SYN	S100	MART-1	CR	Inhib	SF1	PAX-8
Renal cell carcinoma	+	+/–	+	–	–	–/+	–	–	–	–	+
Adrenocortical carcinoma	–	+	–/+	–	–/+	–	+	+	+	+	–
Pheochromocytoma	+	–	+	+	+[a]	+[a]	–	–	–	–	–

[a] Sustentacular cells.

Appendix 1.19 Retroperitoneum – vacuolated/clear cell tumor

	Vim	CK	CDX2	S100	GFAP	CEA	PAX-8	Brachyury
Chordoma	+	+	–	+	–/+	–	–	+
Colonic adenocarcinoma	–/+	+	+	–	–	+	–	–
Renal cell carcinoma	+	+/–	–	–/+	–	–	+	–
Myxopapillary ependymoma	+	+/–	–	+/–	+	–	–	–

Appendix 1.20 Skin – adnexal tumors

	CK20	S100	EMA	CEA	GCDFP-15	SA	CD15	Chgn	NF	LYS
Squamous carcinoma	–	–	–	–	–	–	–	–	–	–
Eccrine tumor	–	+	+/–	+/–	–/+	+/–	+/–	–	–	–
Apocrine tumor	–	–	+/–	+/–	+	+/–	+/–	–	–	+
Sebaceous tumor	–	–	+	–	–	–	+	–	–	–
Pilar tumor	–	–	–	–	–	–	–	–	–	–
Merkel cell carcinoma	+	–	+	–	–	–	–	+	+[a]	–

[a] Merkel cell carcinoma often shows juxtanuclear whorls of neurofilaments and/or cytokeratin.

Appendix 1.21 Skin – basal cell carcinoma vs. squamous carcinoma vs. adnexal carcinoma

	EMA	BerEP4
Basal cell carcinoma	–	+
Squamous carcinoma	+	–
Adnexal carcinoma	+	+

Appendix 1.22 Skin – pagetoid tumors

	LMWCK	HMWCK	S100	CEA	VIM
Melanoma	–	–	+	–	+
Paget's disease	+	–	–/+	+	–
Bowen's disease	+	+	–	–	–

Appendix 1.23 Skin – spindle cell tumors

	CK	VIM	CD34	CD31	αSMA	S100	HMB-45	Leu-7	Des	CD99	p63	ERG	SOX10
Spindle SCC	+	+	–	–	–	–	–	–	–	–	+	–	–
Melanoma	–	+	–	–	–	+	+	–/+	–	–	–	–	+
AFX	–	+	–/+	–	–	–	–	–	–	NK	–	–	–
DFSP	–	+	+	–	–	–	–	–	–	NK	–	–	–
(M)PNST	–	+	–/+	–	–	+/–	–	+/–	–	+	–/+	–	+
Smooth muscle tumor	–/+	+	–/+	–	+	–/+	–/+	–	+/–	–/+	–/+	–	–
Kaposi's sarcoma	–	+	+	+	–	–	–	–	–	NK	–	+	–
Angiosarcoma	–/+	+	+	+	–	–/+	–	–	–	NK	–/+	+	–
Glomus tumor	–	+	–	–	+	–	–	–/+	–/+	–	–	–	–

AFX, atypical fibroxanthomas; DFSP, dermatofibrosarcoma protuberans; PNST, peripheral nerve sheath tumor; SCC, squamous cell carcinoma; NK, not known.

Appendix 1.24 Soft tissue – epithelioid tumors

	CK	VIM	EMA	CD34	CD31	Des	αSMA	CD57	S100	CD99	Mart-1	MUC4	TLE1	HMB-45	INI-1	ERG-1	TFE3
Metastatic carcinoma	+	–/+	+	–	–	–	–	–	–/+	–/+	–/+	–/+[b]	–	–	+	–	–
Synovial sarcoma	+	+	+	–	–	–[a]	–	–	–	+/–	–	–/+	+	–	+	–	–
Epithelioid sarcoma	+	+	+	+/–	–	–	–	–	–	–	–	–	–	–	–	–	–
Angiosarcoma	–/+	+	–	+	+	–	–	–	–	–	–	–	–	–	+	+	–
(M)PNST	–[a]	+	–/+	+/–	–	–	+/–	+/–	–/+	–	–	–/+	–	+	–	–	–
Leiomyosarcoma	–/+	+	–	+/–	–	+	+	–	–	–	–	–	–	–	+	–	–
Melanoma	–	+	–	–	–	–	–/+	+/–	+	–	+	–	+	+	+	–	–
Epithelioid fibrosarcoma	–	+	–	–	–	–	–	–	+	–	+	–	–	+	+	–	–
PEComa	–	+	–	–	–	–	+	–	+	–	–	–	+	+	+	–	+

PNST, epithelioid peripheral nerve sheath tumor.
[a] Occasional cells stain positive.
[b] Positive in adenocarcinomas.

Appendix 1.25 Soft tissue – spindle cell, fasciculated

	Myogenin/MyoD1	SMA	MSA	Des	ScA	S100	Col IV	TLE1	β-catenin	SOX10
Fibromatosis	–	+/–	+/–	–/+	–	–	+F	–	+	–
MPNST	–	–	–	–	–	+	+L	–	–	+
Fibrosarcoma	–	–/+	–/+	–	–	–	–/+F	–	–	–
Leiomyosarcoma	–	+	+	+/–	–	–/+	+L	–	–	–
Spindle cell rhabdomyosarcoma	+	–	+	+	+	–	+L	–	–	–
Synovial sarcoma	–	–/+	–/+	–	–	–/+	+C	+	–	–

C, circumferential, around groups and individual cells; F, fragmented; L, linear continuous.

Appendix 1.26 Soft tissue – myxoid tumors

	S100	SMA	MSA	Des	EMA	CK	CD34	CD99	MUC4	Brachyury
Myxoma	–	–	–/+	–	–	–	+	NK	–	–
Aggressive angiomyxoma	–	+	+	+	–	–	–/+	NK	–	–
Angiomyofibroblastoma	–	+	+	–/+	–	–	–/+	NK	–	–
Myxoid neurofibroma	+	–	–	–	+	–	–/+	NK	–	–
Neurothekoma	+	–/+	+/–	–	+	–	–/+	NK	–	–
Chordoma	+	–	–	–	+	+	–	NK	–	+
Myxoid lipoma/liposarcoma	+/–	–	–	–	–	–	+/–	–	–	–
Myxoid chondrosarcoma	+/–	–	–	–	–/+	–/+	–/+	–	–	–
Myxoid MFH	–	–/+	+/–	–	–	–	+	–/+	–	–
Myxoid leiomyosarcoma	–	+	+	–/+	–	–/+	+/–	–/+	–	–
Botryoid embryonal RMS	–	–	–	+	–	–	–	–/+	–	–
Myxofibrosarcoma	–	–/+	–/+	–	–	–	–	–/+	–	–
Low-grade fibromyxoid sarcoma	–	–	–	–	–	–	–	–	+	–
Synovial sarcoma (epithelioid)	–	–	–	–	–	–	–	–	–/+	–

MFH, malignant fibrous histiocytoma; NK, not known; RMS, rhabdomyosarcoma.

Appendix 1.27 Soft tissue – pleomorphic tumors

	VIM	Des	S100	MSA	ScA	HMB-45	CK	MyoD1	Myogen
Rhabdomyosarcoma	+	+	–	+	+	–	–	+	+
Undifferentiated pleomorphic sarcoma	+	–	–/+	–/+	–	–	–	–	–
Melanoma	+	–	+	+	–	+	–	–	–
Carcinoma	–/+	–	–	–	–	–	+	–	–

Appendix 1.28 Extraskeletal myxoid/chondroid tumors

	S100	Cam 5.2	CK7	CK19	EMA	CEA	MSA
Myxoid chondrosarcoma	+	–	–	–	–	–	–
Chordoma	+	+	+/–	+	+	+	–
Myoepithelioma	+	+	–	–	+	–	–
Mixed tumor	+	+	NK	NK	+	–	+/–
Myxoid liposarcoma	+/–	–	–	–	–	–	–

NK, not known.

Appendix 1.29 Stomach – undifferentiated spindle cell tumors

	CD34	SMA	MSA	S100	Chgn	SYN	CK	CD117 (c-kit)	VIM	β-catenin	DOG1
LyMo/LyMSa	–/+ (weak)	+	+	–/+	–	–	–/+	–/+	+	–	–
GIST	+	–	–	–	–	–	–	+/–	+	–	+
PNST	–	–	–	+	–	–	–	–	+	–	–
Plexiform fibromyxoma	–	+	+	–	–	–	–	–	+	–	–
Desmoid tumor	+	–	–	–	–	–	–	–	+	+	–
Solitary fibrous tumor	+	–	–	–	–	–	–	–	+	–	–

GIST, gastrointestinal stromal tumor (this term is used for spindled tumors, which do not show evidence of myogenic or neurogenic differentiation, morphologically and immunophenotypically); LyMo/LyMSa, leiomyoma/leiomyosarcoma; PNST, peripheral nerve sheath tumor.

Appendix 1.30 Thyroid carcinomas

	34βE12	Vim	Thy	Chgn	SYN	CEA	Cal	TTF-1	HBME-1	CK19	Galectin 3	CD56
Papillary carcinoma	+	+	+	−	−	−	−	+	+/−	+/−	+	−
Follicular carcinoma	−	+	+	−	−	−	−	+	+/−	−	+/−	+
Medullary carcinoma	−	−/+[a]	−	+	+	+	+	−	−	+/−	−/+	+
Metastatic carcinoma	−/+	−/+	−	−	−	−	−	−/+	var	var	var	var

var, variable.
[a] Vimentin expressed in spinde cells of medullary carcinoma.

Appendix 1.31 Urinary tract – spindle cell proliferations

	CK	EMA	Des	MSA	SMA	S100	Myog	SOX10
Inflammatory pseudotumor	−	−	−	+	+	−	−	−
Leiomyosarcoma	−/+	−	+/−	+	+	−/+	−	−
Spindle cell carcinoma	+	+	−	−	−	−/+	−	−
Rhabdomyosarcoma	−	−	+	+	−	−	+	−
Undifferentiated pleomorphic sarcoma	−	−	−	−/+[a]	−/+[a]	−/+	−	−
MPNST	−	−	++[b]	−/+[b]	−	+/−	−	+
Malignant melanoma	−	−	−	−	−	+	−	+
Postoperative spindle cell nodule	−/+	−	−	+	+	−	−	−

[a] Reactive myofibroblasts.
[b] Triton tumor.

Appendix 1.32 Uterine cervix – endometrial vs. endocervical carcinoma

	Vim	CK20	CK7	CEA	ER	CDX2	PAX-8
Endometrial carcinoma	+/−	−	+	−/+	+	−	+
Endocervical carcinoma	−/+	−	−	+/−	−	−	+
Colonic carcinoma (metastatic)	−/+	+	−	+	−	+	−

Appendix 1.33 Uterus – trophoblastic cells

Trophoblastic cell	1st Trimester		2nd Trimester		3rd Trimester	
	hCG	hPL	hCG	hPL	hCG	hPL
Cytotrophoblast	−	−	−	−	−	−
Intermediate trophoblast	+	++	−/+	+++	+	+/++
Syncytiotrophoblast	++++	+	++	+++	+	++++

Percentage of cell staining for the respective antigen: + = 1–24%; ++ = 25–49%; +++ = 50–74%; ++++ = >75%.

Appendix 1.34 Uterus – immunophenotyping of syncytiotrophoblasts in trophoblastic proliferations

	hCG	hPL	PLAP	SP1	CK	VIM	P57	GATA3
Partial mole[a]	+ diffuse	+/++ diffuse[b]	+/+++ diffuse[b]	NK	+++ diffuse	−	+	+
Complete mole	+++ diffuse	+/++ focal	+ focal		+++ diffuse	+++ diffuse	−	−	+
Choriocarcinoma	+++ diffuse	+ focal	+ focal	NK	+++ diffuse	−	+/−	+
Implantation site intermediate trophoblast, placental site tumor, trophoblastic tumor[c]	+++ focal	+++ diffuse	+++ diffuse	+++ diffuse	+++ diffuse	+++ diffuse	+	+
Chorionic-type intermediate trophoblast, placental site nodule, and epithelioid trophoblastic tumor[d]	+ focal	+ focal	++++ diffuse	NK	++ diffuse	+++ diffuse	+/−	+

NK = not known; + = weak; ++ = intermediate; +++ = strong staining.

[a] In the 1st trimester, the pattern of expression of hCG in partial and complete moles is very similar. Similarly, the immunophenotypic profile of hydropic abortus and partial moles is very similar to that of normal pregnancy in the 1st trimester.
[b] Expression increases with advancing pregnancy.
[c] Stains strongly for α-inhibin and Mel-CAM (CD146).
[d] Stains for α-inhibin and weakly and focally for Mel-CAM (CD146).

Appendix 1.35 Brain intraventricular tumors

	PLAP	EMA	CK	CEA	Chgn	Syn	S100	GFAP
Ependymoma	−	−/+ [a]	−/+ [a]	−	−	−	+	+
Choroid plexus tumors	−	+	+	+/−	−	−	+	−/+
Subependymoma	−	−	−	−	−	−	+	+
Subependymal giant cell astrocytoma	−	−	+	−	−	−	+	+
Pilocytic astrocytoma	−	−	+/−	−	−	−	+	+
Central neurocytoma	−	−	−	−	−/+	+	+/−	−/+
Pineal tumors	−	−	−	−	−/+	+	+	−/+
Germ cell tumors	+	+	+	+	−	−	−	−
Colloid cyst	−	+	+	−/+	−	−	+	−/+
Meningioma	−	+	+/−	−	−	−	−/+	−

[a] Surface staining only.

Appendix 1.36 CNS small-cell tumors

	EMA	CK	Chgn	Syn	S100	GFAP	CD45	HMB-45
Metastatic carcinoma	+	+	−	−	−	−	−	−
Malignant lymphoma	−	−	−	−	−	−	+	−
Metastatic melanoma	−	−	−	−	+	−	−	+
Medulloblastoma	−	−	−	+	+/−	+/−	−	−
Hemangiopericytoma	−	−	−	−	−	−	−	−
Plasmacytoma/myeloma	+	−	−	−	−	−	+/−	−
Pineocytoma/pineoblastoma	−	−	−/+	+	+	−/+	−	−
Esthesioneuroblastoma	+/−	+/−	+	+	+/−	−	−	−

Appendix 1.37 Tissue-associated antigens in "treatable tumors"

Lymphoma/leukemia	LCA (CD45)
Germ cell tumor	PLAP, SALL4
Breast carcinoma	GCDFP-15, GATA3
Thyroid carcinoma	Thyroglobulin, TTF−1
Prostatic carcinoma	PSA, PSAP, AR
Trophoblastic tumor	hCG, hPL, Mel-CAM, GATA3
Rhabdomyosarcoma	Des, MyoD1, Myogen, Myoglob[a]
Ewing's sarcoma / PNET	CD99
Neuroblastoma	NF
Neuroendocrine tumor	Chgn, SYN, SOX10

[a] Low sensitivity.

Appendix 1.38 Epithelial tumors which may co-express vimentin intermediate filaments

Thyroid carcinoma
Endometrial carcinoma
Adrenocortical carcinoma
Ovarian epithelial tumors
Gonadal tumors
Salivary gland tumors
Renal cell carcinoma
Choroid plexus tumors
Breast carcinoma
Prostatic carcinoma
Ependymal tumors
Lung carcinoma
Hepatocellular carcinoma
Pheochromocytoma
Adamantinoma
Primitive/peripheral neuroepithelial tumor (PNET)

Any carcinoma, when sufficiently dedifferentiated, may co-express vimentin; these tumors show this property with some regularity.

Appendix 1.39 Mesenchymal tumors which may co-express cytokeratin

Angiosarcoma
Leiomyosarcoma
Chordoma
Chondroid chordoma
Chondroblastoma
Synovial sarcoma (monophasic and biphasic)
Epithelioid sarcoma
Mesothelioma
Meningioma
Malignant peripheral nerve sheath tumor[a]
Malignant melanoma[b]
Anaplastic large-cell lymphoma Ki-1
Dendritic cell sarcoma
GIST

[a] Glandular component.
[b] Only in cryostat sections.

Appendix 1.40 Tumors which may co-express three or more intermediate filaments

Astrocytoma	GFAP, Vim, CK
DSRCT	Vim, CK, Des, NF
ES/PNET	Vim, CK, Des
Leiomyosarcoma	Vim, Des, CK
Pheochromocytoma	CK, NF, Vim
Rhabdomyosarcoma	Des, Vim, CK
Pleomorphic adenoma	CK, Vim, GFAP
Endothelial cells	Vim, CK, Des
Teratoma	CK, Des, GFAP, NF, Vim
True mixed tumors (including Müllerian tumors)	CK, Des, Vim
Mesothelioma	CK, Des, Vim

CK, cytokeratin; Des, desmin; DSRCT, desmoplastic small round cell tumor; ES/PNET, Ewing's sarcoma/primitive peripheral neuroepithelial tumor; GFAP, glial fibrillary acidic protein; NF, neurofilaments; Vim, vimentin.

Appendix 2
Antibody panels for lymphoid neoplasms

Appendix 2.1 Useful markers in B-cell neoplasms

Ig light chain restriction (Igκ, Igλ)
CD20 (some pre-B, mostly mature B cells, rare myeloma)
CD79a (immature B cells, mature B cells, plasma cells)
CDw75 (follicle center cells) – no one uses this
CD45RA (neoplastic follicles) – no one uses this for B-cell
Bcl-2 (neoplastic follicles)
CD43 (neoplasms derived from small B cells)
CD5 (neoplastic B cells)
CD10 (CALLA) (follicle center cells, immature B cells)
Bcl-6 (germinal center differentiation)
LMO2 (germinal center differentiation)
PAX-5 (immature B and B cells)
Mum1 (late GC and post-GC cells)
CD138 (plasma cells)
c-myc (usually high-grade B-cell lymphomas)
TdT (immature B cells)
CD25 (hairy cell leukemia)
CD123 (hairy cell leukemia)
Cyclin D1 (mantle cell lymphoma)
CD30
MIB1

Appendix 2.2 Useful markers of T-cell neoplasms

CD2
CD3
CD4
CD5
CD7
CD8
CD10 (some T-cell lymphomas)
CD45RO not used for T-cell lymphoma, only ALPS (not malignant)
CD1a (precursor T cells)
TdT (precursor T cells)
CD25 (some T-cell lymphomas)
PD-1
FOXP1
TIA1
Granzyme B
Perforin
MIB1
CD30
TCL-1 (T-cell prolymphocytic leukemia)
CXCL13 (angioimmunoblastic T-cell lymphoma)
ALK-1 (anaplastic large-cell lymphoma)

Appendix 2.3 Markers of Reed–Sternberg cells[a]

PAX-5
CD15
CD30
MUM1
CD45-negative
CD20−/+
CD79a-negative
CD3-negative
EMA-negative
ALK-negative

[a] Surrounding small lymphocytes are T cells with CD4+, TIA-1+.

Appendix 2.4 Useful markers of monocytes/macrophages

CD45 (variable)
CD4
Myeloperoxidase (subset)
Lysozyme
CD56 (atypical)
HLA-DR
CD15 (variable)
CD68
CD14
α-1-AT
α-1-ACT
S100 –ve not used for monocytes/macrophages (dendritic cells)
CD163
CD123 –ve

Appendix 2.5 Markers of myeloid cells

CD34 (immature, stem cell)
CD45
CD14
CD15
CD10
Lysozyme
Neutrophil elastase
Myeloperoxidase
CD99, CD43, CD68 and CD117 may also mark
TIA-1 (weak, in subset)
CD33

Appendix 2.6 Useful markers of natural killer (NK) cells

CD57
CD56
TIA1
Granzyme B
Perforin
CD16
HLA-DR ±

Appendix 2.7 Markers of follicular dendritic cells

CD35
CD21
CD23
CD68
CD14

Appendix 2.8 Panel for small-cell lymphomas

	CD43	CD5	CD23	Cyclin DI	CD10	CD38
SLL/BCLL	+	+	+	−	−	−
MCL	+	+	−	+	−	−
MZL	+/−	−	−	−	−	−
LPL	+	−	−	−	−	+
FL	−	−	−	−	+	−

FL, follicle center cell lymphoma; LPL, lymphocytic leukemia; MCL, mantle cell lymphoma; MZL, marginal zone lymphoma; SLL/BCLL, small lymphocytic lymphoplasma/ B-cell lymphocytic leukemia.

Appendix 3
Antibody applications

Antibody	Useful diagnostic applications
α-Fetoprotein	Yolk sac tumors, hepatocellular carcinoma
α-Smooth muscle actin (α-SMA)	Smooth muscle, myofibroblasts, myoepithelium, leiomyosarcoma
ALK protein (p80)	Anaplastic large-cell lymphoma with t(2; 5)
Amyloid	Subtypes of amyloid
Androgen receptor	Prostatic cancer
Anti-apoptosis	Apoptotic cells
Antigen (EMA)	Staining in mesothelioma
AR	Prostatic adenocarcinoma
Arginase-1	Hepatocellular carcinoma
Bcl-2	Follicular lymphoma vs. reactive follicles, possible prognostic marker
Ber-EP4	(epithelial glycoprotein) Some adenocarcinomas, negative in mesothelioma
β-Hcg	Trophoblastic cells and tumors including choriocarcinoma
Brachyury	Chordoma
Broad-spectrum cytokeratin (AE1/3, MNF116, polyclonal Antibovine)	Cytokeratins
CA125	Serous cytic tumors of the ovary and various adenocarcinomas
Cadherin	Putative marker of epithelial differentiation, absent in lobular carcinoma of the breast, possible prognostic marker
Calcitonin	Medullary carcinoma of the thyroid
Calretinin	Mesothelioma
Carcinoembryonic antigen (CD66)	Polyclonal antibody, stains hepatocyte canuliculi, various adenocarcinomas, but absent in mesothelioma
Catenins	Associated with E-cadherin
Cathepsin D	Prognostic marker in breast cancer
CD10 (CALLA)	Follicular center cells, follicular center lymphoma, Burkitt lymphoma, myoepithelial cells
CD103 (HML-1)	Memory B lymphocytes and intraepithelial lymphocytes
CD117 (c-*kit*)	Hematopoietic progenitor cells, gastrointestinal stroma tumors, mast cells
CD15	Reed–Sternberg cells, neutrophils, various adenocarcinomas
CD19	(frozen sections only) B-cell lymphomas
CD1a	Langerhans cells, Langerhans cell histiocytosis
CD2	(frozen sections only) Pan-T-cell marker
CD20	B cells and B-cell lymphomas
CD21	B cells and follicular dendritic cells and their corresponding tumors
CD23	Small lymphocytic lymphoma B-cell type
CD3	Mature T cells, T-cell lymphoma

Antibody	Useful diagnostic applications
CD30	Reed–Sternberg cells, Ki-1 lymphoma, embryonal carcinoma
CD31	Endothelial cells and tumors
CD34	Endothelial cells and tumors, leukemias, gastrointestinal stromal tumors
CD35	Follicular dendritic cells and follicular dendritic cell sarcoma
CD38	Plasma cells
CD4	T-cell helper subset
CD40	Reed–Sternberg cells
CD43	T cells, macrophages, and often co-expressing B-cell lymphomas
CD44	Various isoforms, possible prognostic marker in various tumors
CD45 (leukocyte common antigen)	Almost all hematolymphoid cells and progenitors
CD45RA	Mantle zone B cells, T cells, reactive vs. neoplastic follicles
CD45RO	T cells, macrophages, granulocytic precursors
CD5	T cells, mantle zone cells, small lymphocytic lymphoma B-cell type
CD54 (ICAM-1)	Monocytes, endothelial cells, T cells, and B cells
CD56 (NCAM)	Natural killer cells and corresponding tumors, neural tumors
CD57	Nerve sheath tumors, natural killer cells
CD66 (CEA family)	Various adenocarcinomas, bile cannuliculi of hepatocellular carcinoma, negative on mesothelioma
CD68	Macrophages and cells rich in lysozomes
CD7	(frozen sections only) Immature and mature T cells and nature killer cells
CD74 (LN-2)	B-cell lymphoma, some T-cell lymphoma, Reed–Sternberg cells
CD79a	B cells
CD8	T-cell suppressor subset
CD9	Both B and T cells and their corresponding neoplasms
CD99 (p30/32^{MIC2})	Ewing's tumor/PNET
CDw75 (LN-1)	Follicular lymphoma L&H cell
c-erbB-2 (Her2/neu, Herceptest)	Breast cancer prognostic marker, predictor of treatment response
Chlamydia	Chlamydia (all species)
Chromogranin	Dense core granule in neuroendocrine differentiation
c-myc	c-myc
Collagen type IV	Basal lamina
Cyclin D1 (Bcl-1)	Mantle cell lymphoma
Cytokeratin 1/10 (34βE12)	Squamous cell carcinoma, loss of basal cell staining in prostatic carcinoma
Cytokeratin 20	Gastrointestinal tumors, transitional cell carcinoma, Merkel cell carcinoma
Cytokeratin 5/6	Mesothelioma, squamous cell carcinoma
Cytokeratin 7	Carcinoma subset
Cytokeratins	Cytokeratins
Cytomegalovirus (CMV)	Cytomegalovirus
Cytotoxic molecules (TIA-1, granzyme B, perforin)	Cytotoxic cells including NK cells and cytotoxic T cells
DBA.44 (hairy cell leukemia)	Hairy cell leukemia
Desmin	Skeletal and smooth muscle tumors
Desmoplakins	Follicular dendritic cells and tumors, epithelial cells (fixation-sensitive)
Epidermal growth factors (TGF-α, EGFR)	Squamous carcinomas, possible prognostic relevance in various carcinomas
Epithelial membrane antigen	Some carcinomas, meningioma, Ki-1 lymphoma, plasma cell tumors, microvilli
Epstein–Barr virus (EBR1)	(in-situ hybridization) EB virus infection, Hodgkin lymphoma, post-transplant lymphoproliferative disorders
Epstein–Barr virus (LMP)	Latent membrane protein of EB virus

Antibody	Useful diagnostic applications
Estrogen receptor (ER)	Prognostic marker in breast and other carcinomas
Factor VIIIRA (von Willebrand factor)	Endothelial cells, megakaryocytes
Factor XIIIa	Dermal dendrocytes, dermatofibroma, atypical fibroxanthoma
Fas (CD95), Fas-ligand (CD95L)	Apoptotic cells
Ferritin	Bone marrow iron stores, low sensitivity for hepatocytes
Fibrin	Glomerular diseases
Fibrinogen	Glomerular diseases
Fibronectin	Adenoid cystic carcinoma of salivary gland and breast
Galectin 3	Carcinoma of thyroid
Gata3	Urothelial carcinoma, other carcinomas
Glial fibrillary acidic protein (GFAP)	Gliomas
Glypican-3	Hepatocellular carcinoma, melanoma, non-seminomatous germ cell tumor
Gross cystic disease fluid protein-15 (GCDFP-15, Brst-2)	Breast, salivary, sweat gland tumors
HAM 56	Macrophages/monocytes
HBME-1	Membrane staining of mesothelioma cells, carcinoma of thyroid
Heat shock proteins (HSPs)	Possible prognostic marker in various tumors
Helicobacter pylori	*Helicobacter* organisms
Hep Par 1	Hepatocytes, hepatocellular carcinoma, mixed hepatocyte/cholangiocarcinomas
Hepatitis B core antigen (HBcAg)	Hepatitis B infection
Hepatitis B surface antigen (HBsAg)	Hepatitis B infection
Herpes simplex virus I and II (HSV I & II)	Herpes infection
HLA-DR	B-cell lymphomas, activated T cells
HMB-45	PEComa
HMB-45 (gp100)	Melanoma, nevus cells
HMLH-1	(mismatch repair gene product) Hereditary non-polyposis colonic carcinoma (HNPCC) and sporadic colorectal carcinomas with microsatellite instability
HMLH-2	(mismatch repair gene product) Hereditary non-polyposis colonic carcinoma (HNPCC) and sporadic colorectal carcinomas with microsatellite instability
Human immunodeficiency virus (HIV. p24)	HIV infection
Human milk fat globule (HMFG)	Microvilli on mesothelioma
Human papillomavirus (hPV)	Human papillomavirus infection
Human parvovirus B19	Parvovirus infection
Human placental lactogen (hPL)	Intermediate trophoblasts, trophoblastic tumors
Immunoglobulins: Igκ, λ, A, D, E, G, M	Immunoglobulin-producing cells
Inhibin	Granulosa cell tumor, adrenal cortical tumors
Ki-67 (MIB1, Ki-S5)	Cell proliferation marker
Laminin	Basal lamina
Lysozyme (Muramidase)	Macrophage/monocytes, granular cell tumor
MAC387	Macrophage/monocyte
MDM-2 protein	Putative prognostic marker in various tumors
Measles	Measles infection, subacute sclerosing panencephalitis (SSPE) inclusions
Metallothioneins	Possible prognostic marker in various tumors
Microphthalmia transcription factor (MiTF)	Melanoma and melanocytic tumors
MOC-31	Cholangiocarcinoma
MUC4	Low-grade fibromyxoid sarcoma, epithelioid fibrosarcoma
Muscle-specific actin (MSA, HHF-35)	Myoepithelium, smooth, skeletal muscle differentiation and corresponding tumors

Antibody	Useful diagnostic applications
Myelin basic protein (MBP)	Nerve sheath tumors, oligodendrogliomas, ganglioneuroblastomas and ganglioneuromas
Myeloperoxidase	Granulocytes and histiocytes and corresponding leukemias
MyoD1	Rhabdomyosarcoma
Myogenin	Rhabdomyosarcoma
Myoglobin	Rhabdomyosarcoma
Nerve growth factor receptor (NGFR. p75^{NPR})	Nerve sheath differentiation
Neurofilaments	Neurons and neuronal tumors
Neuron-specific enolase (NSE)	Peripheral nerves, melanoma, neuroendocrine cells and tumors with neuroendocrine differentiation, testicular germ cell tumors
Neutrophil elastase	Granulocytic tumors, leukemia
nm23/NME1	Possible prognostic marker, anti-tumor metastases
p21^{waf1}	Tumor suppressor gene, possible prognostic marker
p27^{kip1}	Cyclin-dependent kinase inhibitor, possible prognostic marker in breast and other tumors
p53	Tumor suppressor gene product, marker of poor prognosis
P57	Complete mole
P63	Squamous differentiation, myoepithelial cells
p80 (ALK protein)	Anaplastic large-cell lymphoma with t(2; 5)
Pancreatic hormones (insulin, somatostatin, vasoactive intestinal polypeptide, gastrin, glucagon, pancreatic polypeptide)	Various hormone-secreting tumors
Parathormone	Parathyroid tissue and tumors
Parathyroid hormone-related protein (PTHrP)	Squamous cell carcinomas, cholangiocarcinomas, negative in hepatocellular carcinomas
PAX-8	Renal cell carcinoma, ovarian endometrioid carcinoma, carcinoma of thyroid
p-glycoprotein (p-170, mDR-1)	Chemoresistant marker, bile cannuliculi
Pituitary hormones (ACTH, FSH, hGH, LH, PRL, TSH)	Hormone-secreting pituitary tumors of different subsets
Placental alkaline phosphatase (PLAP)	Seminoma and other germ cell tumors
Pneumocystis jirovecii	*Pneumocystis* infection
Pregnancy-specific β-1-glycoprotein (SP1)	Placental cells and tumors as well as various other carcinomas
Progesterone receptor (PR)	Prognostic marker in breast, endometrial, ovarian, and meningeal tumors
Proliferating cell nuclear antigen (PCNA)	Cell proliferation marker, fixation-sensitive
Prostate-specific acid phosphatase (PSAP)	Prostatic carcinoma
Prostate-specific antigen (PSA)	Prostatic carcinoma
Protein gene product 9.5 (PGP 9.5)	Neuroendocrine differentiation
PS2	Estrogen inducible protein
Rabies	Rabies infection
Retinoblastoma gene protein (Rb, P110^{RB})	Tumor suppressor gene product
S100	Melanoma, Langerhans cell, Shaun cells, neural supporting cells
SALL4	germ cell tumor
Serotonin	Subset of carcinoid tumors
SF1	Adrenocortical carcinoma
Simian virus 40 (SV40T antigen)	Cross-reacts with JC viral inclusions in polymorphonuclear leukoencephalopathy (PML)
SOX9	Chondroid tumors
SOX10	Neuroendocrine tumors, melanoma, clear cell sarcoma-like tumors
Spectrin/fodrin	Linked to E-cadherin and β-catenin
Surfactant (POA, apoA1)	Non-small-cell carcinomas of the lung
Synaptophysin	Neuroendocrine differentiation
TAU	Neurofibrillary tangles

Antibody	Useful diagnostic applications
Terminal deoxynucleotidyl transfer (TdT)	Lymphoblastic lymphoma
Thrombomodulin	Lymphatic and vascular tumors, mesothelial cells and mesothelioma
Thyroglobulin	Thyroid follicular cells
Thyroid transcription factor 1 (TTF-1)	Thyroid and lung carcinomas
TLE1	Synovial sarcoma
Toxoplasma gondii	*Toxoplasma* infection
Ubiquitin	Mallory bodies, astrocytomas
Ulex europaeus agglutinin 1 lectin (UEA-1)	Endothelial cells, various epithelial tumors
Villin	Adenocarcinoma subset, especially gastrointestinal carcinomas
Vimentin	Sarcomas, lymphomas, co-expressed with cytokeratin in some carcinomas
VS38	Plasma cells, neuroendocrine differentiation, some melanocytic tumors
Wilms tumor gene product (WT1)	Desmoplastic small round cell tumor, mesothelioma, Wilms tumor, endometrial carcinoma, ovarian surface epithelial tumors